CHILD DEVELOPMENT

SOCIAL WORK PRACTICE WITH CHILDREN AND FAMILIES

Nancy Boyd Webb, *Series Editor*

Group Work with Adolescents:
Principles and Practice, Second Edition
Andrew Malekoff

Child Development:
A Practitioner's Guide, Second Edition
Douglas Davies

Mass Trauma and Violence:
Helping Families and Children Cope
Nancy Boyd Webb, Editor

Culturally Competent Practice with Immigrant
and Refugee Children and Families
Rowena Fong, Editor

Social Work Practice with Children,
Second Edition
Nancy Boyd Webb

Complex Adoption and Assisted Reproductive Technology:
A Developmental Approach to Clinical Practice
Vivian B. Shapiro, Janet R. Shapiro, and Isabel H. Paret

Child *Development*

A PRACTITIONER'S GUIDE

SECOND EDITION

DOUGLAS DAVIES

Series Editor's Note by Nancy Boyd Webb

THE GUILFORD PRESS
New York   London

Last digit is print number: 9   8   7   6   5   4   3   2   1

Library of Congress Cataloging-in-Publication Data

Davies, Douglas, 1942–
    Child development: a practitioner's guide / Douglas Davies.—2nd ed.
        p.   cm. — (Social work practice with children and families)
    Includes bibliographical references and index.
    ISBN 1-59385-076-X (cloth)
    1. Social work with children.   2. Child development.   I. Title.   II. Series.
    HV713 .D395   2004
    362.7—dc22

                                                        2004012698

For my grandchildren
Hannah, Hayden, and Sage

In memory of Ian

About the Author

Douglas Davies, MSW, PhD, is Clinical/Practice Associate Professor at the School of Social Work, the University of Michigan, Ann Arbor. He is an infant mental health specialist and has published several articles on intervention with young children and their families. In his practice, he works with children and families, supervises clinicians, and offers consultation to mental health agencies and child care centers. He frequently presents professional workshops on practice with infants and toddlers, play therapy, treatment of child witnesses of domestic violence, child care consultation, and developmental approaches to child therapy.

Series Editor's Note

Anyone who works with children or educates practitioners will appreciate this updated second edition of Douglas Davies's comprehensive book, *Child Development: A Practitioner's Guide.* It covers children's growth and development from birth through preadolescence and provides alternating chapters on normal development and detailed cases examples illustrating practice with infants, toddlers, preschoolers, and school-age children. Davies succeeds in presenting complex theoretical information about children's growth and development in lucid prose that makes the concepts vivid. The case examples artfully demonstrate the ever-changing interplay between the child's inherent capabilities and the responses of his or her surrounding caretaking environment. Resting on a firm foundation of developmental knowledge, Davies details the process of individualizing intervention planning, using maturational, transactional, and ecological perspectives.

This completely revised and updated edition is grounded in attachment theory as the foundation for the child's ongoing and future relationships. Davies's examples depict both helpful and dysfunctional interactions that influence the nature of the child's expectations regarding how other people will respond. These reciprocal interactions may originate in either the child or the caretaker. A new chapter on brain development provides a real service to the field in spelling out how the child's brain is shaped by experience. This is particularly relevant in working with children who have been exposed to chronic trauma and emotional neglect. Other new content in this volume includes expanded material on risk and protective factors that influence development, plus new understanding about the development of empathy in childhood and about the influence of peers and friendships in childhood.

As part of the series Social Work Practice with Children and Families, this book is a valuable resource for faculty, students, and practitioners. It can be used in practice courses that focus on work with children and families as well as in social work and psychology courses on human growth and development. Appendices provide an overview of expected milestones at different age periods as well as a summary of the risk and resiliency/protective factors, including the nature of the social environment that either supports or threatens the developing child.

It is a pleasure to have had a role in the production of this valuable contribution to the social work literature on helping children and families. I believe that it provides a needed reference and a guide to understanding the rhythmic transactional dance between the developing child and his caretaking environment.

NANCY BOYD WEBB, DSW
University Distinguished Professor of Social Work
James R. Dumpson Chair in Child Welfare Studies
Fordham University
New York, New York

Preface

This book describes child development and how it can be applied to practice with children. Beginning practitioners often feel intrigued and perplexed by the behavior of children and wonder what is "normal." Developmental knowledge provides a framework for assessing where a child falls within normal expectations and where she or he does not. Any given piece of behavior can be normal, mildly abnormal, or reflective of serious problems, depending on its developmental timing. It is normal and typical, for example, for a 4-year-old to believe in monsters and ghosts, at least at bedtime, while the same beliefs in a 10-year-old are often indicators of generalized or trauma-based anxiety and impairments in reality testing. By demonstrating the value of a developmental framework, I intend to make the book as useful as possible to practitioners working with children.

Knowledge of the abilities and developmental tasks that are typical of children of a given age can inform our clinical work and casework in powerful ways. Knowing what developmental tasks the child is currently struggling with helps us empathize with the child's sense of reality, allowing us to enter the child's world, as opposed to merely seeing him or her as a bundle of symptoms. Knowing where a child is functioning developmentally, especially in the area of the presenting symptoms, helps us define what skills and capacities to target in our treatment plans. Knowing what skills and capacities will soon be appearing as a result of development helps us plan interventions that utilize and support these emerging abilities. Knowing how children at a particular developmental level represent themselves—through behavior, play, or words—informs us about how to communicate with them and helps us plan treatment activities with appropriate materials. Knowing what a child *cannot* do because she or he has not reached a particular developmental level creates realistic expectations about the goals of treatment and allows us to communicate the child's developmental realities to parents. Finally, knowing the next steps in development helps us evaluate the effects of intervention, going beyond the goal of decreasing symptoms, and adding positive developmental progress as a normal measure of change.

Developmental knowledge also provides us with a lens for reviewing a child's history. To understand how earlier experiences have influenced the child's development and contributed to current problems, we need to know the child's strengths and limitations for handling stress and trauma at a given age and how, as a result, the child may have responded internally to past trauma and stress. For example, we interview the mother of a depressed 6-year-old boy and find out that his father abandoned the family when the child was 3. Drawing on our knowledge of development we recall that 3-year-olds are still egocentric and have magical views of cause and effect, which means that they see themselves as the center of the world and believe that their thoughts and behavior can cause things to happen. This leads to a question that can be pursued in the evaluation: To what extent does the child's depression reflect guilt and self-blame based on a belief that his father left because of something he did? A knowledge of development does not automatically provide answers, but it helps the practitioner decide what lines of inquiry will be most fruitful to understand the relationships between a child's past and present realities.

PLAN OF THE BOOK

Part I introduces the idea that the child's development is the outcome of transactions between innate maturational processes and the child's environment. I begin with a brief discussion of the transactional model of development. This is followed by chapters describing attachment and relationships with parents, brain–environment interaction, and risk and protective factors as contexts that influence the course of development. The application of these concepts is illustrated with examples from practice.

Part II presents information about the course of child development. Chapters 5, 7, 9, and 11 cover infancy, toddlerhood, the preschool period, and middle childhood, respectively, and include salient facts, tasks, and processes in development from birth to age 11. In addition to presenting information from the research literature, frequent vignettes of observations of children in their "natural" settings—home, child care center, school, playground, neighborhood—as well as in practice settings, are also provided.

Each of these informational chapters is followed by a practice chapter (Chapters 6, 8, 10, and 12) that presents ways of applying theoretical and factual information about development. These chapters illustrate how each period in development has special issues and characteristics that must shape our practice so that we can respond helpfully to our child clients and their parents. Each period provides opportunities and limitations that must guide our work. For example, we will not get far by trying to *talk* about worries with a 4-year-old. But the 4-year-old's imaginative play often provides us with a dramatized account of what worries her. Since the best way to make developmental concepts real is to observe children at different developmental levels, I suggest observational exercises at the end of each practice chapter. My aim throughout is to demonstrate how to think developmentally in practice with children and their parents.

DOUGLAS DAVIES

Acknowledgments

There are many people to thank for their help on this project and many others who have indirectly contributed to this book through what I have learned from them. I am especially grateful to my child clients and their parents who have taught me about the realities of child development during 25 years of practice. The cases presented in this book are composites based on more than one client. To preserve confidentiality, I have also altered all information that might identify individuals.

The staff at The Guilford Press was uniformly professional and supportive of this project. Jim Nageotte, Senior Editor, and Nancy Boyd Webb, Series Editor, provided astute commentary and welcome support as I worked on this edition. Oliver Sharpe, Production Editor, shepherded the manuscript through the copyediting and production process.

My son Aaron Lane-Davies, MD, a pediatrician, reviewed the chapter on brain development and helped make my discussion of neuroscience information clearer. An anonymous reviewer also provided comments that strengthened this chapter. I also "tried out" this new chapter on two of my classes at the University of Michigan School of Social Work; as usual, my students helped me sort out what was most helpful to them as developing practitioners. My son Justin Davies, an elementary school teacher, invited me to observe and participate in his classrooms and helped me think about how to integrate new material on the interaction between school and development. Marsha Greenberg, MSW, Director, The Child Care Center, University of Michigan Hospitals, provided an insightful review of the material on child care policy. I was fortunate to have the help of two research assistants, David Votruba II, MSW, and Wendy Kern, MSW candidate, who provided excellent summaries of new child development research. I am very grateful to Paula Allen-Meares, Dean of the School of Social Work, for providing a grant to support my research, and to Associate Deans Siri Jayaratne and Richard Tolman for arranging my teaching schedule to allow for maximum time to write. My wife, Tobi Hanna-Davies, served as my in-house editor for the first edition and helped me think through what was important to add to this edition. But more important than her enthusiasm for my work, her love sustains me. I am grateful also for the loving support I have constantly received from my sister, April Jones Van Devender, my daughters-in-law, Elizabeth Lane-Davies and Laurel Wong, and my mother-in-law, Gillian Hanna.

A portion of Chapter 4 is adapted from Blos and Davies (1993) (copyright 1993 by Zero to Three/National Center for Clinical Infant Programs; adapted by permission). I am very grateful to Dr. Peter Blos, Jr. for granting me permission to adapt our collaborative work, and for his helpful comments on the chapter. The play therapy case in Chapter 10 is substantially based on Davies (1992) (copyright 1992 by Plenum Publishing Corporation; adapted by permission). I am grateful for permission to quote in Chapter 6 two passages from Nelson (1989) (copyright 1989 by Harvard University Press; reprinted by permission of Harvard University Press).

Contents

PART I. Contexts of Development: A Transactional Approach

Introduction to Part I: Perspectives on Development   3

The Maturational Perspective   3
The Transactional Model of Development   4
Developmental Pathways and Intervention   5

CHAPTER 1. Attachment as a Context of Development   7

How Attachment Develops   8
Functions of Attachment   8
Patterns of Attachment   11
Attachment Classifications   12
Attachment, Class, and Culture   19
The Universality of Attachment   21
Attachment and Future Development   21
Parental Models of Attachment   24
Attachment Theory and Family Systems Theory   28
The Attachment Perspective in the Assessment of Young Children   29
Kelly and Her Mother: A Case Example   30

CHAPTER 2. Brain Development   39

Sequence of Brain Development   40
Early Brain Growth: Synaptogenesis and Myelination   41
Synaptic Overproduction and Pruning   42
Plasticity and Experience   43
Bonding, Attachment, and Brain Development   43
Can Parents Build Better Brains?   45
Risk and Protective Factors Influencing Brain Development   45
Stress, Trauma, and Brain Development   48
Early Trauma and Brain Development   50
Studies of Institutionally Deprived Young Children   55

CHAPTER 3. Risk and Protective Factors: The Child, Family,   61
           and Community Contexts

   Research on Risk and Resilience   61
   Protective Factors and Processes   63
   Risk Factors   66
   Conclusion   105
   Appendix 3.1. Summary of Risk and Protective Factors   106

CHAPTER 4. Analysis of Risk and Protective Factors: 109
           Practice Applications

   How to Use Risk Factor Analysis   109
   Prediction of Risk: Assessing Current Risk and Protective Factors   110
   Retrospective Analysis of Risk and Protective Factors   121
   Exercise: Assessment of Risk and Protective Factors   130

PART II. The Course of Child Development

Introduction to Part II: A Developmental Lens on Childhood   133

   Barriers to Understanding the Child's Perspective   133
   Dynamics of Developmental Change   135
   Interactions between Maturation and Environment   135
   Thinking Developmentally in Assessment and Intervention   136
   Organization of Developmental Chapters   136

CHAPTER 5. Infant Development   139

   The Interaction between Maturation and Caregiving   139
   Brain Development: The Importance of Early Experience   140
   Metaphors of Infant–Parent Transactions   140
   Caregivers' Adaptations to Developmental Change   141
   The Neonatal Period: Birth–4 Weeks   142
   Age 1–3 Months   145
   Age 3–6 Months   151
   A Normal Infant and a Competent Parent: A Case Example   156
   Age 6–12 Months   159
   Appendix 5.1. Summary of Infant Development, Birth–12 Months
      of Age   169

CHAPTER 6. Practice with Infants   172

   Assessment Issues   173
   Assessment and Brief Intervention with an Infant and Her Family:
      A Case Example   175
   The First Two Home Visits: Learning about the Family   177
   The Next Two Home Visits   183
   Office Sessions: Videotaping and Interpretive Sessions   186
   Discussion   189
   Observation Exercises   191

CHAPTER 7. Toddler Development   193

Physical Development 194
Attachment and Secure Base Behavior 194
Cognitive Development 200
Language and Communication 201
Symbolic Communication and Play 207
Regulation of Affect and Behavior 211
Moral Development 217
The Developing Self 223
Appendix 7.1. Summary of Toddler Development, 1–3 Years
    of Age 230

CHAPTER 8. Practice with Toddlers   234

Assessment 234
Assessment of Toddler Development: A Case Example 238
Intervention: Parent–Child Therapy 251
Parent–Child Therapy with an Abused Toddler: A Case Example 255
Observation Exercises 257
Interview Exercise 258

CHAPTER 9. Preschool Development   259

Physical Development 260
Attachment 261
Social Development 263
Language Development 270
Symbolic Communication and Play 274
Cognitive Development 277
Regulation of Affect and Behavior 287
Moral Development 294
The Developing Self 300
Appendix 9.1. Summary of Preschool Development, 3–6 Years
    of Age 307

CHAPTER 10. Practice with Preschoolers   311

Assessment 311
Child Care Consultation with a Preschool Child: A Case Example 312
Intervention with Preschoolers: Play Therapy 317
Using Play in the Treatment of Preschoolers 319
Medical Treatment as a Developmental Interference 320
Play Therapy with a Preschool Child: A Case Example 322
Observation Exercise 334

CHAPTER 11. Middle Childhood Development   335

Physical Development 337
The Transition from Preschool to Middle Childhood 338
Attachment 343
Social Development 345
Language and Communication 353
Play and Fantasy 356

Cognitive Development   359
Self-Regulation   367
Moral Development   374
Sense of Self   376
Overview of Developmental Progress in Middle Childhood   385
Appendix 11.1. Summary of Middle Childhood Development, 6 to 11
  or 12 Years of Age   386

CHAPTER 12. Practice with School-Age Children   389

Assessment   389
Intervention   396
Working to Master the Trauma of Repeated Abuse:
  A Case Example   401
Using Developmental Strengths: A Case Example   409
Observation Exercises   418

CHAPTER 13. Conclusion: Developmental Knowledge   419
            and Practice

Applying Practice Knowledge and Skills   420
Ever-Present Complications in Practice   421
Intervention and Developmental Outcome   423

References   425

Index   469

PART I

Contexts of Development:
A Transactional Approach

Introduction to Part I:
Perspectives on Development

Development is the outcome of transactions between the child and her environment. This simple-sounding idea encompasses a complex and dynamic reality. I will briefly introduce some perspectives that help us think about how transactions between the individual child and her multiple relationships and contexts influence development. In Part I, Chapters 1–4 present in some depth the impact of attachment, brain development, and risk and protective factors as transactional contexts of development.

THE MATURATIONAL PERSPECTIVE

Development is founded on the child's innate characteristics, unfolds according to maturational timetables, and moves forward through a series of tasks and challenges of increasing complexity that the child must master in order to extend her ability to function within herself and within her environment. From a maturational point of view, the course of development seems inevitable. Based on the growth of the brain and body systems, new abilities and higher-level capacities for organizing experience emerge across time (Kagan, 1984). For example, between ages 1 and 2, children become capable of rapid language learning as the result of brain maturation (Huttenlocher, Haight, Bryk, Seltzer, & Lyons, 1991). A 6-month-old cannot yet speak words, let alone sentences, because the cognitive systems underlying language are not yet fully developed. Similarly, even a 2-year-old who is very precocious in language does not "get" jokes or understand metaphors because the cognitive abilities required to

3

understand wordplay do not develop until the elementary school years. As the result of maturation, then, a child has very different capacities for action and for understanding the world at ages 2 and 8. Maturational factors determine that any 8-year-old will be much more like other 8-year-olds than like a 2-year-old. Nevertheless, within a group of 8-year-olds, there may be important differences among individual children. Some 8-year-olds will be able to use their social and cognitive abilities more adaptively than others. These differences result from how developmental capacities have been shaped in the history of the child's transactions with multiple environmental contexts.

THE TRANSACTIONAL MODEL OF DEVELOPMENT

From the beginning, the child's transactions with immediate and wider environments influence development. The transactional model suggests that "the development of a child is . . . a product of the continuous dynamic interactions between the child and the experience provided by his or her family and social context" (Sameroff & Fiese, 2000, p. 10). Recent research, for example, has begun to map transactional processes influencing brain development during the first year of life, demonstrating that physical touching, social interaction, and sensory stimulation promote physical brain growth and increase brain functions (Nelson, 1999). Thus, even a process that seems a biological given turns out to be transactional. As development proceeds, quality of parenting, opportunities and stressors in the child's and parents' lives, social circumstances, social institutions, culture, and historical events are all part of a widening circle of influence on who the individual child becomes (Bronfenbrenner, 1979). The younger the child, the more the child's transactions with the environment are mediated through the quality of parenting, which is influenced by the parents' relationship and their individual characteristics, circumstances, and histories. During the early years parents are the conduits through which cultural values shape the child's developmental possibilities.

The transactional model also recognizes that the child, from the beginning, works to organize his experience. Rather than being a passive container into which experience is poured, "The child actively creates his or her own environment, increasingly so with advancing development" (Sroufe, 1990, p. 339). Interactions between caregiver and child are "bidirectional." Infants and young children are shaped by adult behavior, yet their actions also influence how adults respond to them. In turn, the parent's ability to respond adaptively to the child's unfolding development is influenced by immediate circumstantial and more distant social factors that support, or alternatively create stress on, the parent.

DEVELOPMENTAL PATHWAYS AND INTERVENTION

The child's transactions with the environment create alternative paths that development proceeds along. At critical points, determined by periods of developmental change or by external influences, such as trauma or increased opportunity, junctures appear and the child may move off the path she was traveling and onto a different path. At these junctures, the child may proceed in adaptive or maladaptive directions (Bowlby, 1973). A 2-year-old whose parent develops a severe substance abuse problem may suffer neglect and as a result move to a maladaptive pathway characterized by precocious self-reliance and mistrust of relationships. By contrast, a 7-year-old who transfers from an underfunded and poorly equipped school to a school rich in resources—at a developmental point where new cognitive advances increase her motivation to learn—may move to a more adaptive pathway.

How and whether development may be affected by increased risk or opportunity depends on the timing of external factors in relation to current developmental tasks. Developmental capacities that are currently emerging or have very recently been achieved are most vulnerable to disruption by stressors. Capacities that have long ago been consolidated are less susceptible to disruption, although under conditions of severe stress they may also be affected.

> Sara, an 18-month-old toddler, who was unexpectedly separated from her mother when her mother was hospitalized for several days because of a miscarriage, developed symptoms that reflected disturbances in the particular developmental tasks of toddlers, including language acquisition, developing autonomous control of body functions, and practicing independence and mastering separation. She was in a period of rapid language learning, and she stopped talking. Prior to her mother's hospitalization she had begun to be interested in toilet training. She stopped using the potty. She was attempting to master anxiety about separation as a normative developmental issue. In the face of a real separation overlaid by an atmosphere of emotional separation caused by her parents' grief over the loss of a baby, her behavior became preoccupied with strategies for controlling separation, including repetitive symbolic play on separation themes, waking and crying for her parents at night, alternately being demanding and rejecting of her mother in attempts to control and dictate their relationship, and trying to be self-reliant. A short-term intervention helped this child and her parents master these symptoms of developmental interference.

Although the direction of development can change—and be influenced to change—at each stage, change is nevertheless somewhat limited by the pathways already taken. There is less flexibility for change as development proceeds (Hamilton, 2000). A child who has already traversed a long series of adaptive paths is not likely to be easily shifted to a maladaptive path. But similarly, the more maladaptive paths a child has traveled, the more difficult it will be to shift to a more adaptive one if the opportunity arises (Sroufe, Carlson, Levy, & Egeland, 1999). The first 5 years are the most rapid period of development. Opportunity for adequate development during the first 5 years is crucially important because "It sets either a strong or fragile stage for what follows" (Shonkoff & Phillips, 2000, p. 5). The effects of early development, whether positive or negative, cascade into the future, influencing later developmental possibilities (Masten & Coatsworth, 1998). This model creates a strong argument for early intervention as a means of shifting development in positive directions before the path into potential psychopathology is set.

Especially when thinking about children it is important to recognize that many "diagnoses" or "syndromes" represent conditions that are malleable rather than fixed (Bowlby, 1988). Practitioners who work with children frequently sense in their young clients a strong urge to master problems and to move ahead in development. This is consistent with Campbell's (1990) argument that "strong, biologically based self-righting tendencies are assumed to be present in all but the most severely damaged infants; that is, movement is inherently toward normal development" (p. 10).

Intervention plans must take full advantage of the self-righting tendency and of the child's developmental capacities; at the same time, a transactional approach to assessment and intervention looks for ways to help parents respond adaptively to a child's difficulties, to reduce environmental risks, and to increase opportunities for adaptive development (Webb, 2003). Bowlby (1988) pointed out that a child proceeding down a maladaptive or "deviant" pathway could return to the main adaptive pathway if positive influences were strengthened: "the course of subsequent development is not fixed, [and] changes in the way a child is treated can shift his pathway in either a more favourable or less favourable one.. ..It is this persisting potential for change that gives opportunity for effective therapy" (p. 136).

CHAPTER I

Attachment as a Context
of Development

This chapter describes how the early parent–child relationship mediates and influences the course of development. Although parenting is not the only influence on development, it is a critically important one. Attachment theory provides the most useful perspective on early parent–child interactions. John Bowlby formulated attachment theory, and other researchers, particularly Mary Ainsworth, have validated and refined it. Bowlby described attachment as a fundamental need that has a biological basis. The goal of the infant's attachment behavior is to keep close to a preferred person, in order to maintain a sense of security. The motivation to stay close and to avoid separation from an attachment figure can be seen in an infant who wakes up from a nap and begins to fuss and cry, which alerts the parent to come and pick her up.

Bowlby pointed out that attachment serves as a protective device for the immature young of many species, including humans. Babies need the care of adults to survive, and they have many built-in behaviors, such as making strong eye contact, cooing and vocalizing, and smiling, that attract adults to them. Every baby with a normal neurological system develops a focal attachment to the mother or other primary caregiver. The beginnings of the attachment process can be observed in the early weeks of life, but attachment is clearly evident between 4 and 6 months of age. Although the behavioral expression of attachment varies across cultures, attachment is a universal phenomenon in humans (Bowlby, 1969; LeVine & Miller, 1990).

HOW ATTACHMENT DEVELOPS

Infants make attachments with specific people. Although a newborn infant may be comforted by anyone who picks him up, he very quickly differentiates his primary attachment figure(s) from others. During the early weeks of life he learns the particular qualities of his mother (assuming the mother is the primary caregiver). The baby, through repeated interactions, learns to recognize his mother—what her face looks like, what she smells like, what her touch feels like, and how her voice sounds. Through this process the infant's attachment becomes specific and preferential. In most cultures, infants' attachments have an order of preference, usually to mother, then father, and then siblings, although infants who are in care full-time with a single caregiver often develop an attachment to her that is second only to the mother.

FUNCTIONS OF ATTACHMENT

Attachment has four main functions: providing a sense of security; regulation of affect and arousal; promoting the expression of feelings and communication; and serving as a base for exploration.

Providing a Sense of Security

The implicit goal of attachment is to keep the infant feeling secure. When an infant becomes distressed, both parent and infant take actions to restore the sense of security (Bowlby, 1969). For example, an infant becomes upset and communicates this by looking anxious, crying, or moving closer to her mother. The mother moves toward the baby, soothes her with her voice, and picks her up. The baby continues to fuss briefly, then molds to the mother's body, stops crying, and soon begins to breathe more slowly and regularly, indicating a decrease in arousal; her sense of security has been restored. In Bowlby's terms, the infant's distress signal, which is functionally an attachment-seeking behavior, activates the mother's side of the attachment system, and the mother takes steps to calm the baby's distress.

Regulation of Affect and Arousal

A second primary function of attachment, as this example suggests, is to regulate the infant's affective states. "Arousal" refers to the subjective feeling of being "on alert," with the accompanying physiological reactions of increased respiration and heartbeat and bodily tension. If arousal intensifies without relief, it begins to feel aversive and the infant becomes distressed. When this happens the infant sends out distress signals and moves toward the caregiver. In a secure attachment the infant is able to draw on the mother for help in regulating distress. The mother's capacity to read an infant's affects accurately and to provide soothing or stimulation helps the infant modulate arousal (Stern, 1985). Over time, infants and parents develop transactional patterns of mutual regulation to relieve the infant's states of disequilibrium. Repeated successful mutual regulation of arousal helps the infant begin to develop the ability to regulate arousal through his own efforts. Through the experience of being soothed, the infant internalizes strategies for self-soothing. Good self-regulation helps the child feel competent in controlling distress and negative emotions (Cassidy, 1994).

In contrast, "unresponsive or abusive parents may promote chronic hyperarousal that can have enduring effects on the child's ability to modulate strong emotions" (van der Kolk & Fisher, 1994, p. 150). Children who have not been helped to regulate arousal within the attachment relationship tend, as they get older, to feel at the mercy of strong impulses and emotions. They have more behavioral problems because they have not developed effective internal ways of controlling their reactions to stressful stimuli (Solomon, George, & de Jong, 1995). In another type of insecure attachment, parents respond negatively to the infant's expressions of distress. The child learns that in order to maintain the attachment he must inhibit strong feelings, especially negative ones. Over time he internalizes a style of overregulating, minimizing, and avoiding expression of strong emotions (Magai, 1999).

Expression of Feelings and Communication

As the attachment relationship develops during first 6 months of life, it also becomes the vehicle for sharing positive feelings and learning to communicate and play.

> For example, a 6-month-old infant initiates a game of peek-a-boo (which has been previously taught by her father) by pulling a diaper over her face. Her father responds by saying, "Oh, you want to play, huh," and pulls the diaper off, saying "peek-a-boo!" and smiling and looking into the baby's eyes. The baby smiles and begins to wave her arms and kick her feet. The father says warmly, "Oh you like to play peek-a-boo, don't you?" The baby vocalizes, then begins to pull the diaper over her face again in order to continue the game.

This example indicates how attachment is established and how it is perpetuated. Attachment develops out of transactions—the infant expresses a need, to be fed, to be played with, to be comforted—and the parent responds. These transactions, when they are going well, reveal important qualities of the attachment relationship: mutually reinforcing, synchronous behaviors on the part of the parent and infant, a high degree of mutual involvement, attunement to each other's feelings, and attentiveness and empathy on the part of the parent (Stern, 1985).

However, even in the most secure attachment, synchrony is not always present. Parents are not always optimally responsive and attuned, nor do they need to be. Transactions between infant and parent show moment-to-moment variability in the degree of synchrony, attunement, and mutual responsiveness (Nadel, Carchon, Kervalla, Marcelli, & Reserbat-Planty, 1999). Interactional mismatches between baby and parent are commonplace, and they temporarily interfere with the infant's ability to regulate affects. An indicator of secure attachment is the ability of the parent and infant to use interactive coping skills to repair such mismatches when they occur, thus restoring equilibrium for the infant and for the attachment relationship (Tronick and Gianino, 1986b). For example, when a parent is preoccupied or even depressed, the infant watching her begins to feel out-of-touch—that is a minor mismatch. The baby may whine or, alternatively, smile and kick his feet to attract the mother's attention. As the mother responds, the mismatch ends and the feeling of security is reestablished. Siegel notes, "Repair is . . . important in helping to teach the child that life is filled with inevitable moments of misunderstandings and missed connections that can be identified and connection created again" (Siegel, 2001, p. 79).

A Base for Exploration

Later in development, especially from age 1 onward, the attachment relationship becomes *a base for exploration*. Attachment theorists consider the motivation to explore and learn about the world and to develop new skills to be as intrinsic in infants as attachment motivation. Bowlby pointed out that the attachment and exploratory behavioral systems operate in tandem. The confidence with which the child ventures out depends a great deal on her confidence in her attachments. If a toddler has a secure base in her attachment relationship, she will feel free to explore her environment, with the implicit awareness that the caregiver is available if needed (Grossman, Grossman, & Zimmerman, 1999). Since she is not concerned about attachment, exploratory behavior dominates (Bowlby, 1969). Her confidence allows her to interact with her environment in an open and curious way: "Secure children show more concentrated exploration of novel stimuli and more focused attention during tasks" (Grossman et al., 1999, p. 781). A secure 18-month-old playing on her own repeatedly stacks and knocks over blocks. In doing so she exercises motor and cognitive skills and through concentrated practice develops a sense of competence. Exploring from a secure base gives her opportunities to focus on developmental tasks and to feel competent (Meins, 1997). On the other hand, a toddler who is anxious about whether her caregiver will be responsive and protective may be inhibited from exploring, because emotionally she remains focused on making sure her attachment figures are available (Lieberman, 1993).

PATTERNS OF ATTACHMENT

Beginning in the mid-1960s, Mary Ainsworth began to apply Bowlby's attachment theory in a series of studies that would lead to more a specific understanding of the dynamics of attachment and to the identification of three distinct patterns of attachment. First Ainsworth did an anthropological field study of mother–infant interaction patterns of the Ganda people of Uganda through intensive observation. She found that maternal responsiveness and sensitivity and infant reactions to separation were the most important indicators of the quality of attachment behavior of Ganda mothers and infants (Ainsworth, 1967). Her initial observational studies of American mothers and infants confirmed the main findings of the Ganda study and provided beginning support for the validity of attachment theory across cultures. However, Ainsworth also observed cultural differences between the Ganda and American infants' ability to handle stress. The American babies, when observed in the home, seemed less stressed by very brief separations from the mother or by the presence of strangers than did the Ganda infants. Ganda infants were much more likely to initiate attachment behavior (to cry, protest, or try to follow) when the mother left the room than were American babies. The Ganda babies, who were almost always with their mothers, consequently had fewer early separation experiences than American infants.

To take into account the American infants' greater tolerance for separation, Ainsworth devised an experimental procedure called the "Strange Situation" to create a more stressful situation in order to elicit their attachment behavior. This procedure aims to create mild but increasing stress on the attachment relationship, in order to observe the infant's attachment strategies and the degree of security of attachment. In the Strange Situation, the mother and baby (12–18 months old) come into a room the infant has not seen before. After a brief period of play, while the mother sits and watches, a stranger enters the room. After the stranger talks with the mother, the mother briefly leaves the room and returns. The stranger leaves. Then the mother leaves the baby alone for a short time and returns. Ainsworth found that the infant's response to the mother's return was the most sensitive indicator of quality of attachment. Securely attached infants showed characteristic responses when reunited with the mother, and insecurely attached infants also reacted in distinctive ways. In Ainsworth's original study, infants between 9 and 12 months and their mothers were observed for a total of 72 hours at home prior to the Strange Situation procedure. These independent home observations correlated positively with ratings obtained from the Strange Situation procedure. Thus, the validity of the Strange Situation as a research tool for the assessment of attachment in middle-class American samples was established via independent observations.

ATTACHMENT CLASSIFICATIONS

Ainsworth's observational and experimental studies identified the characteristics of secure attachment and delineated two types of anxious or insecure attachment. A third type of insecure attachment has been described by Mary Main (Main & Solomon, 1990). The attachment classifications are:

- Group A: Insecure–Avoidant
- Group B: Secure
- Group C: Insecure–Ambivalent/Resistant
- Group D: Insecure–Disorganized/Disoriented

Infants in each attachment category present distinctly different reactions to the separation and reunion episodes of the Strange Situation procedure. These differences are seen not merely as reactions to the experimental situation but rather as outcomes of the history of attachment qualities and strategies that have developed over time (Ainsworth, Blehar, Waters, & Wall, 1978).

Secure Attachment

The infants rated as secure (B) showed confidence in the attachment relationship, even though they varied in how distressed they became in response to separation. When the mother returned, they tended to greet her positively, to look relieved and happy, and to move close to her. If distressed they wanted to be picked up, and they quickly calmed in response to the parent's attention and soothing. In these securely attached infants, there was an expected pattern of exploratory versus attachment-seeking behavior: "When they were alone with their mothers, they explored actively, showing very little attachment behavior. Most of them were upset in the separation episodes and explored little. All of them responded strongly to the mother's return in the reunion episodes, the majority seeking close bodily contact with her" (Ainsworth, 1982, p. 16). Ainsworth's prior in-home studies of these infants and mothers showed that the mothers of the secure infants were responsive, emotionally available, and loving. These babies coped with the stress of a brief separation because they were confident of their parent's responsiveness. Secure infants were able to express their feelings openly, including positive and negative affects, without the necessity of defending against negative feelings. They showed confidence in their parent's ability to accept their full range of feelings and to help them regulate distressing feelings (Main & Hesse, 1990).

Secure attachments have a positive impact on later development. Children with a history of secure attachment are more confident about exploring their environment and more open to learning. This is first evident in the toddler phase, when the child uses the mother as a base from which to explore, but it persists in later development. Good attachment relationships tend to be generalized to future relationships. Longitudinal studies by Sroufe and colleagues have confirmed that general differences between secure and insecure attachment patterns persist from infancy through the preschool and elementary school years. Children judged as securely attached at 12 and 18 months were seen at 42 months as more flexible and resourceful. They had fewer behavior problems, sought attention from teachers in positive ways, and effectively elicited their teachers' support when distressed. They showed less negative affect and more age-expected control of impulses. They got along with other children well and showed a capacity for empathy. Studies of these children in later childhood showed similar associations between secure attachment history and social competence (Weinfield, Sroufe, & Egeland, 2000).

Children with the benefit of secure attachment *throughout* childhood have the best developmental outcomes. Security in infancy gets development off to a good start, but it should not be considered an "inoculation" against future disruptions of development, which can occur in response to changes in quality of attachment. For example, a preschool child who was securely attached as an infant may move to an insecure attachment—with negative developmental effects—in response to severe stressors on caregivers, such as divorce or the death of a spouse (Thompson, 2000). However, children with histories of secure attachment who move to insecurity can more easily rebound to security as stressors decrease (Weinfield et al., 2000). Overall, ongoing secure attachment is an important protective factor that promotes adaptive development throughout childhood. In contrast to the confidence shown by secure infants, the infants in Ainsworth's other two categories demonstrated anxiety and/or defenses against anxiety in their attachment behavior.

Avoidant Attachment

The infants classified as insecure–avoidant (A) showed very little attachment behavior during the entire Strange Situation procedure. They played independently, did not appear distressed when the mother left, and—strikingly—when she returned they ignored her, showed blank or restricted affect, paid attention to the toys, and actively avoided contact, even when the parent tried to get their attention. They gave the impression of self-reliance, conveying that the attachment was not important. Given the normal importance of attachment for an infant, attachment theorists have described the Avoidant pattern as a defensive strategy. The in-home study suggested why an avoidant defense might be needed: the A babies were frequently ignored and actively rejected by their mothers. Parents spoke of their infants in negative terms, often with inaccurate characterizations of the baby's behavior, such as "He's just crying to spite me." The mothers were seen as angry, both in general and specifically at the infant. They were intolerant of the infant's distress and tended to reject or punish the infant for being distressed. Out of these interactions, avoidant babies develop precocious defenses against feelings of distress. Distress is split off from consciousness, and the defense mechanism of isolation of affect emerges. Avoidant infants tend not to show that they are upset in situations that are distressing for most infants; rather, they appear somber, expressionless, or self-contained. Evidence for these patterns of defensive suppression comes from studies that measured infants' heart rates during the Strange Situation. Both secure and avoidant infants had measurably similar physiological responses to stress during the separation episodes. However, the secure infants expressed their distress, while the Avoidant infants appeared outwardly unconcerned (Spangler & Grossman, 1993). However, the avoidant pattern should not be equated with nonattachment. Rather, the defensive strategy of avoidance is the baby's way of staying close to the parent while protecting herself from overt rejection: "The infant can maximize her proximity to the mother and optimize her felt security by doing nothing and showing nothing" (Stern, 1995a, p. 427). Avoidant infants have learned to expect rejection, and in response, in Bowlby's terms, their attachment behavior becomes "deactivated." They tend not to look to their mothers for help in regulating arousal and affects. Correspondingly, as toddlers, A infants tend to focus their attention away from the parent (and from their own internal states) and toward the outside world. Instead of striking a flexible balance between exploration and attachment as the need arises, they pursue action and exploration in a rigid and self-reliant way (Main, Kaplan, & Cassidy, 1985).

In longitudinal studies, preschoolers judged Avoidant in infancy have higher levels of hostility and unprovoked aggression and negative interactions with other children. They generalize the defenses of avoidance and self-reliance to other relationships. Instead of expressing distress and asking for help with disappointment, they are likely to sulk or withdraw. Because they are emotionally distant and often behave in negative ways, avoidant preschoolers tend to be viewed more negatively and subjected to more discipline by their teachers, thus reinforcing and confirming the child's untrusting assumptions about attachment (Sroufe, 1989).

DYNAMICS OF AVOIDANT ATTACHMENT: A CASE EXAMPLE

The following observation describes interaction that has the qualities associated with avoidant attachment. A teen mother, age 16, and her 8-month-old daughter were videotaped in a free-play session. As Erica plays with a busy box, Ms. Jones leans back against the wall and says, "I'm not going to bother you." Erica picks up an inflated ball, which her mother peremptorily takes away from her. Then her mother points to colors on the ball, saying "Can you say 'red'?" while Erica struggles to get the ball. As Erica crawls onto her mother's leg, she says, "Get offa me." The infant guidance worker suggests, "Maybe she's trying to get close to you." Her mother responds, "No, she's trying to get over here without going around." Erica does not look at her mother, and her face appears impassive throughout the session. Erica knocks over a toy telephone and her mother says, "No! You know better." The worker asks "Do you think she knows better?" and Ms. Jones answers, "Yes." The worker persists: "What is she supposed to know better about?" "Lots of things, like crying for nothing, or beating on stuff." The worker says, "When 8-month-old babies beat on stuff, they're just trying to make noise." Ms. Jones stands up and insists, "Not this little girl. She's destructive." She moves to a corner of the room at a distance from her daughter. Erica does not react to her mother's leaving her side and continues to play with the telephone. Several times her mother calls her to come across the room. Erica looks at her without expression and continues to play. Ms. Jones says, "Bad baby," then goes back and tries to engage her by demonstrating how to press the levers on the busy box. Instead of imitating her mother, Erica puts her fingers in her mouth. Her mother roughly pulls them out. Erica begins to cry and turns away from her mother, who says, "Hey, what's your problem?" The worker asks, "Does she ever just like to be cuddled?" Erica's mother says, "No, not really—maybe when she's sleepy." "Do you hold her then?" "Nope, I give her a bottle and lay her down and shut out the light." The worker says, "You know, it feels pretty good to be held." Ms. Jones responds with a dismissive laugh, turns away from the worker, and, holds up a mirror to Erica, "Want to see the ugly baby?" Then she picks Erica up and puts her at the top of the playroom slide. She says, "Go down!" and laughs when Erica looks apprehensive. Then she helps her slide down. The worker says, "It looked like she was scared." Ms. Jones replies, "It shouldn't have scared her."

The themes in Ms. Jones's view of Erica are dismissal of her needs for nurturance, ignoring her distress, attributing negative intentions to her, and characterizing her in negative terms. Both mother and daughter seem more comfortable when they are disengaged from each other. During the brief times they are engaged, both of them are involved with the toys rather than each other. Ms. Jones puts physical and emotional distance between herself and her baby, as if denying the importance of attachment, and Erica, in a matching response, concentrates on the toys and ignores her mother. Observing their mutual avoidance makes the worker feel sad and anxious, and she focuses her interventions on encouraging closeness. In response, seeming to confirm the attachment pattern, Ms. Jones dismisses the worker's statements and turns away from her.

Ambivalent/Resistant Attachment

Infants classified as insecure–ambivalent/resistant (Group C) showed behavior in the Strange Situation that conveyed a strong need for attachment but a lack of confidence in its availability. Consequently, they reacted intensely to the separation. Ainsworth describes their heightened affect and ambivalence: "These children were anxious even in the pre-separation episodes. All were very upset by separation. In the reunion episodes they wanted close bodily contact with their mothers, but they also resisted contact and interaction with her, whereas Group B babies had shown little or no resistance of this sort" (Ainsworth, 1982, p. 16). The C babies were distressed and angry, and they could not be soothed by contact with their mothers. The in-home study described the mothers of the ambivalent infants as inconsistently responsive to their infants' attachment-seeking behavior: "The conflict of the C babies is a simple one—between wanting close bodily contact and being angry because their mothers do not consistently pick them up when they want to be held or hold them for as long as they want. Because their mothers are insensitive to their signals C babies lack confidence in their responsiveness" (Ainsworth, 1982, p. 18). The infants' heightened affect and ambivalent behavior reflect their anxious uncertainty about how their parent will respond.

The C pattern predicts later disturbances in the infant's capacity for autonomous behavior. Because the child is uncertain of her parent's responsiveness, she tends to focus on the parent's behavior and moods, to the exclusion of other interests. Ambivalent toddlers remain preoccupied with attachment, at the expense of exploration. Their separation worries persist into the preschool and school-age years, long after children with secure attachment histories have mastered normative separation fears. Longitudinal studies have linked the C category with behavioral inhibition and lack of assertiveness in preschool children and with social withdrawal and poor peer interaction skills in early school-age children (Renken, Egeland, Marvinney, Mangelsdorf, & Sroufe, 1989).

AMBIVALENT/RESISTANT ATTACHMENT IN A PRESCHOOLER:
A CASE EXAMPLE

The potential interference of an ambivalent attachment on development is illustrated by the behavior of a 4-year-old at a child care center. I observed Andrew in a scenario that his teachers said was occurring daily. While Andrew's mother talked with a teacher as she was dropping him off, he watched her alertly with a tight, tense expression. When his mother said good-bye, he grabbed her around the legs, beginning to cry angrily. She disengaged from his grasp and passed him to the teacher, who tried to comfort him by holding him. He cried louder as his mother left, then pushed the teacher away and lay on the floor, in a full-blown tantrum. After 2 minutes, he went to his cubby and sat morosely, sucking the hem of his security blanket. Ten minutes later he searched out his favorite teacher and then shadowed her, staying as close to her as possible throughout the morning. His behavior was also notable for what it did not include—active play and involvement with other children. In the pre-school years, play and social interaction facilitate development. This very insecure child remained caught up in attempts to maintain his attachments, which diminished his interest in normal 4-year-old activities that support development.

Disorganized/Disoriented Attachment

Mary Main and her colleagues have identified a third type of inse-cure attachment, which they label as insecure–disorganized/disoriented (Group D). Compared to the other insecure patterns, the D pattern repre-sents a much less organized and consistent approach to dealing with an attachment relationship that the infant experiences as insecure. These infants show contradictory behavior when reunited with the mother after a separation. For example, the infant greets the mother happily and raises her arms to be picked up, then turns away, becomes motionless, and looks dazed. Or the infant shows simultaneous contradictory behavior—walking toward the parent with head averted, or smiling at the parent and looking fearful at the same time. In this pattern, the behavior of the infant appears confused and disorganized, and her attempts to reestab-lish attachment are interrupted by internal conflicts. The infant may also appear afraid of the parent, and instead of approaching the parent may go to the stranger or engage in self-stimulating behavior. D infants appear to lack an organized strategy for eliciting comforting when they are under stress. They do not seem to clearly signal the need for help from the parent in regulating affect. Lacking internal or mutual strategies for regulating distressing feelings, they tend to remain aroused. This per-sistent distress, in turn, contributes to their internal sense of disorder and has an ongoing negative impact on their ability to self-regulate (Barnett, Ganiban, & Cicchetti, 1999).

The source of this dilemma for D infants is behavior by their parents that frightens them. The infant's attempt to use attachment behavior to reduce distress collapses because the parent who is supposed to be a source of security is also a source of fear: "The essence of disorganized attachment is fright without solution" (Van IJzendoorn, Schuengel, & Bakermans-Kranenberg, 1999, p. 226). Two patterns contributing to the development of D attachments have been identified: a history of unresolved trauma in the parent and direct maltreatment by the parent. In the first pattern, the contradictory behavior of D infants is mirrored in the attachment behavior of their parents. A high percentage of parents with disorganized/disoriented infants have histories of unresolved childhood trauma, such as the early loss of a parent, abuse, or witnessing of parental violence (Main & Hesse, 1990; Lyons-Ruth, 1996). They are anxious, fearful people who project trauma-based fears onto the present. Their infants have often been alarmed and frightened by their intense expression of fearful emotions: "Frightening behavior on the part of the still-traumatized parent should lead to a disorganized/disoriented infant, since the infant is presented with an irresolvable paradox wherein the haven of safety is at once the source of alarm" (Main and Hesse, 1990, p. 180).

Other studies have found that very high percentages of abused infants are classified as disorganized/disoriented in the Strange Situation (Barnett et al., 1999). The intense approach/avoidance conflict in the behavior of D infants has been linked to fear of the parent, uncertainty about how a parent will react, and a history of contradictory responses by the parent, ranging from inviting closeness to angry rejection and physical or sexual abuse (van IJzendoorn et al., 1999). Other parental factors associated with the D classification are bipolar depressive illness and active alcoholism or cocaine abuse, conditions that tend to involve extreme and contradictory behavior (DeMulder & Radke-Yarrow, 1991). There is also evidence that disorganized attachment is a symptom of the disintegrative effects that multiple interacting risk factors can have on families. Families characterized by poverty, parental psychiatric disturbance, parental substance abuse, and history of abuse of the parent in childhood have much higher rates of D attachment. Across studies of infants in middle-class families not beset by multiple risk factors, the D classification rate averages 15%, while studies of families in poverty show D attachments ranging from 25 to 34%. In families where infants have been abused, the D rates are much higher, ranging from 48 to 77% (van IJzendoorn et al., 1999). When a family is overwhelmed by many risk factors, the likelihood of family disorganization and child maltreatment is greater.

Research on the impact of disorganized attachment on later development has begun to catch up with data about the other attachment categories. D attachment predicts high rates of controlling behavior toward parents and aggression toward peers in preschool and school-age children (Lyons-Ruth & Jacobvitz, 1999). In school-age children a history of D attachment may predict poor self-confidence and lower academic ability (Moss, Rousseau, Parent, St. Laurent, & Saintong, 1998). D attachment in infancy has also been linked to the use of dissociation as a preferred defense later in development. The altered mental state in dissociation involving "blanking out," or "going somewhere else," is consistent with the frozen, trance-like states observed in D infants (Hesse & Main, 1999).

Multiple Attachments

Although the mother appears to be the primary attachment figure in all cultures, infants can and do establish attachments with multiple caregivers. In two-parent families, the infant's second most important attachment is usually with the father. In Western cultures, at least, father–infant attachment tends to be expressed in play interactions and therefore encourages the infant's exploration (Grossman et al., 1999). In cultures that organize caretaking collectively, infants develop multiple attachments, although preference for the mother tends to prevail (van IJzendoorn & Sagi, 1999; Jackson, 1993). In the Efé culture of Zambia, for example, mothers care for infants collectively, nursing and comforting infants of other mothers (Morelli & Tronick, 1991).

The possibility of multiple attachments raises the question whether an infant can have both secure and insecure attachments. Bowlby argued that the child would develop multiple patterns based on differences in the quality of his relationships with separate significant caregivers. Infants and toddlers do form different types of attachment with different caregivers. In cases where a child has an insecure attachment with a mother, a secure attachment with another important caregiver—father, grandparent, or regular child care provider—may take on a compensatory protective function (Howes & Ritchie, 1998; Howes, 1999).

ATTACHMENT, CLASS, AND CULTURE

Early skeptics questioned whether attachment, as defined by Ainsworth's research, was a middle-class phenomenon. But the link between parental sensitivity and attachment security has consistently been supported in studies of middle- and lower-class samples, including samples that were racially and ethnically mixed and samples that were either primarily African American or white (Ward & Carlson, 1995). However, in the high-risk conditions of poverty and other major stressors, attachment security classifications may be different at different points in time due to the impact of environmental stressors on the parent's ability to maintain responsive attachment behavior (Weinfield et al., 2000). As noted previously, the D category is associated with severe psychosocial risk factors and is more prevalent in maltreating families affected by multiple sources of risk (Barnett et al., 1999).

Cross-cultural studies have yielded different percentages across attachment categories, which have been explained in terms of culturally based limitations of the Strange Situation procedure, rather than in terms of large disparities in the percentages of securely attached infants. Early studies of Japanese infants, for example, assigned very high proportions of infants to the Anxious–Ambivalent/Resistant category, based on their extreme reactions to the separation episode and their inability to become calm when the mother returned. Recall that the Strange Situation was created to induce mild stress in American infants. American infants generally have many experiences of separation from parents, and American culture encourages independence and self-reliance. Japanese culture has very different emphases, as Takahashi (1990) points out:

> The Japanese have long favored child-rearing methods in which a caregiver is always near the infant, such as co-sleeping, co-bathing and carrying the child on the mother's back. . . . Thus Japanese culture treats "being left alone" in striking contrast to American culture. In Japanese culture, it is therefore plausible that the extent of the strangeness of the "Strange Situation," and the accompanying stress go way beyond the bounds of "mild." Some infants, identified as type C babies by the procedure, even if securely attached to the mother, were too disturbed to be pleased at the reunion with her. . . . An objectively identical procedure does not necessarily guarantee applicability to other cultures. (pp. 27–29)

This study of Japanese infants points to a more general idea: different values and practices of caregiving influence the expression of attachment behavior across cultures. Many cultures value interdependence and group affiliation, and these themes are reflected in practices such as "wearing" the infant or keeping her within reach, nursing on demand, nursing as a primary response to distress, and co-sleeping (Morelli & Tronick, 1991; Small, 1998). Such cultures tend to have lower rates of type A attachment (True, Pisani, & Oumar, 2001; van IJzendoorn & Sagi, 1999). By contrast, in Western cultures, the values of independence and self-reliance find expression in caregiving practices such as bottle feeding or early weaning from breastfeeding, expecting infants to "play independently," allowing distressed babies to "cry it out," providing infants with less physical contact with caregivers, and expecting babies to sleep alone and go to sleep by themselves. These cultures tend to have higher rates of A attachment (Isabella & Belsky, 1991; van IJzendoorn & Sagi, 1999).

Studies of very different cultures show rates of secure attachment in the range of 65–70%; rates among the insecure categories vary and may be more influenced by cultural practices. However, the research of Sagi et al. (Sagi, Lamb, Lewkowicz, Shoham, Dvir, & Estes, 1985; Sagi, van IJzendoorn, Aviezer, Donnell, & Mayseless, 1994) on attachment in Israeli kibbutz infants implies there are limits to cultural adaptiveness and that, at an extreme, cultural practices may promote insecurity. The kibbutz philosophy aims to promote collective support and cooperation in children by organizing their lives so that they identify with the peer group equal to or even more than the family. Consequently, in some kibbutz communities, beginning in early infancy children slept in groups in houses separate from their parents. Adult child care providers were present, but the infants had no access to their parents at night. Studies of these children showed an unusually low rate of secure attachment (56%) as well as an unusually high rate of C (ambivalent) attachment (37%). This degree of insecurity was particularly striking because companion studies of Israeli children living *with* their parents in kibbutzim and in Israeli cities both showed secure attachment at a rate of 80% (Sagi et al., 1985; Sagi et al., 1994). Since the children were comparable in background (middleclass, two-parent families), the researchers concluded that "collective sleeping, as experienced by infants as a time during which mothers were largely unavailable and inaccessible, was responsible for the greater insecurity found in this group. Inconsistent responsiveness was inherent in the reality of these infants" (van IJzendoorn & Sagi, 1999, p. 721).

THE UNIVERSALITY OF ATTACHMENT

Although cross-cultural studies identify variations in the forms that attachment behavior takes, as well as differences in approaches to caregiving and expectations of infants, the universality of attachment is not in question (Posada et al., 2002). What factors seem to be universal? A baby needs to have an attachment to a primary caregiver (or, in many cultures, to a set of primary caregivers). Consistency, sensitivity, and contingent responsiveness on the part of the primary caregivers are essential to the baby's psychological development. Across cultures, secure-base behavior—the child's ability to use the caregiver for relief of distress and support for exploration (as defined by each culture)—has been identified as a marker of secure attachment (Waters & Cummings, 2000). When the attachment relationship is pervaded by the caregiver's inconsistency, insensitivity, lack of responsiveness or negativism or rejection of the baby, the baby's psychological development is seriously at risk.

ATTACHMENT AND FUTURE DEVELOPMENT

Sroufe points out that "The dyadic infant-caregiver organization precedes and gives rise to the organization that is the self. The selforganization, in turn, has significance for ongoing adaptation and experience, including later social behavior. . . . Each personality, whether healthy or disordered, is the product of the history of vital relationships"

(Sroufe, 1989, p. 71). Many longitudinal studies have tested this idea. Overall, they have found impressive links between quality of attachment in infancy and later development (Matas, Arend, & Sroufe, 1987; Lyons-Ruth, 1996). Secure attachment in infancy and toddlerhood predicts social competence, good problem-solving abilities, and other personality qualities associated with successful adaptation in later childhood (Sroufe, 1989). Insecure attachment has been similarly linked to problematic behavior and social difficulties in school-age children. Although other factors such as infant temperament and environmental risk factors influence outcomes, *the overwhelming evidence of empirical studies makes clear that quality of attachment is a fundamental mediator of development.*

Internalization of Working Models of Attachment

How are patterns of attachment carried forward as the child develops? Bowlby (1973) pointed out that the child gradually develops a working model of attachment based on how he has been cared for and responded to within the attachment relationship. Over the first few years of life, working models become stabilized as expectations of how relationships work and what one can expect of other people in terms of responsiveness and care. Correspondingly, models of the self in relationships also develop. The young child internalizes assumptions about how effective she is in using relationships, how valued she is, and how worthy of receiving care. The infant whose attachment initiatives have been responded to appropriately over time is likely to develop working models that say, in essence: "I can expect that people will respond to me with interest, concern, and empathy. My actions are effective in communicating my needs and maintaining my attachments." As children get older, parents' ways of communicating about attachment also shape and reinforce working models. Parents who express empathy, talk openly about their child's distress, and balance support with encouragement of autonomy promote secure working models (Bretherton & Munholland, 1999).

A central component of working models is a view of the self within relationships, which contributes strongly to the child's self-representation. The child with a history of secure attachment is likely to develop a positive sense of self, while children with insecure attachments are more likely to develop disturbances in the view of self and in the capacity to maintain self-esteem (Bowlby, 1973). Working models also include a view of one's ability to regulate arousal and cope with stress. Infants who have been effectively helped with regulation of arousal through the soothing and contingent responding of their caregivers develop effective internal and social strategies for regulating affect and arousal and become more competent at coping with stress. By contrast, infants who have experienced high levels of arousal and intense affect, without the help of mutual regulation, are likely to internalize a view of the self as ineffective or out of control and to develop maladaptive coping strategies, such as affective numbing or hyperreactivity, leading to aggression and tantrums.

Working Models as Organizers of Experience

Once established, working models tend to become unconscious. They become filters and organizers of the child's perceptions about relationships. They increasingly guide how the child appraises what is happening in relationships and how he behaves with others (Bowlby, 1980). By the third year, the working models developed through the child's primary attachment relationships have become relatively stable and are now applied to other relationships. The 3-year-old with a history of secure attachment tends to expect that child care providers will be interested, supportive, and responsive. The child with a history of insecure attachment may mistrust the intentions and emotional responsiveness of other adults. In either case, the child unconsciously attempts to organize, shape, and perhaps control new relationships to make them fit his internal working models.

At the same time, assuming that parental behavior in relation to the child remains relatively constant, the child's working models are continually being reinforced through ongoing transactions with parents. Although working models can change through changes in parenting style and experiences in new relationships, this becomes increasingly harder after ages 3–4, when models "become incorporated as stable interpersonal tendencies that endure over time" (Lyons-Ruth & Zeanah, 1993, p. 17). An obvious example is that many children who enter foster care following removal from the parents because of physical abuse behave in ways that seem intended to provoke abusive responses from foster parents. When the child projects working models in this way, the responses of others often reinforce working models, stabilizing them further. For example, if the foster parent reacts negatively (though not abusively) to the abused child's provoking behavior, the child's affective experience with a new caregiver feels consistent with abuse, and his working models are confirmed (Sroufe et al., 1999).

However, many abused children do not continue to reenact old relationships, but instead are gradually influenced by the responsive and empathic behavior of new caregivers. Although working models tend to be powerful and persistent, they can be changed through good care. Working models can be altered in negative directions as well by family changes such as divorce or a parent's illness, and even by such normative events as the birth of a second child (Teti, Sakin, Kucera, Corns, & Das Eisen, 1996). My next door neighbors' new baby was born as I worked on this chapter. Their 18-month-old son, an alert and easygoing toddler, began to cry frequently. I saw his father carrying him around the backyard while he cried inconsolably. His father told me, "His mom is busy with the baby, and he just wants her. I can't seem to calm him down like usual." It was easy to suspect that the child's previously secure working model, which may have included the feeling "I am the only one they love," was challenged by his observations of his mom's attention to the baby. These sensitive parents responded with empathy to this toddler's sense of loss, which helped restore his sense of security and prevented a negative change in his working models.

As these examples suggest, there are qualifications to the idea that attachment classifications and working models are stable over time. When Bowlby tied the concept of developmental pathways to attachment theory, he was explicitly leaving room for the possibility that life experiences could alter working models of attachment (Bowlby, 1980). He argued that significant new relationships, new opportunities, or new risks could change an individual's working models, either positively or negatively. The idea that attachment style would be consistent over time has been supported by longitudinal studies of middle-class children. These children, who grow up in relatively protected circumstances, demonstrate high rates of continuity in attachment styles (Waters et al., 2000). Children first assessed as infants were reevaluated at ages 19–20. There was significant continuity of security of attachment at the time of the second assessment. However, 28% of these middle-class children changed attachment categories, mostly from secure to insecure. Nearly every individual moving to an insecure rating had encountered negative life events, such as a parent's death, parental divorce, life-threatening illness, psychiatric disorder in a parent, or physical or sexual abuse by a family member (Waters et al., 2000).

By contrast, studies of lower-class children, who as a result of poverty often experience many negative life events, show much less continuity in attachment patterns (Weinfield et al., 2000). In these children, early secure attachment more often gives way to insecure patterns because of the ongoing multiple risks associated with poverty. These results "emphasize the nature of risk in the lives of children who grow up in poverty and chaotic environments" and make clear that "Difficult life experiences take their toll on children despite possible avenues of resilience," such as early secure attachments (Weinfield et al., 2000, p. 701).

PARENTAL MODELS OF ATTACHMENT

Research on the parent's side of the attachment has identified three major factors affecting the caregiver's capacity for responsiveness: (1) the caregiver's internal working models of caregiving, assumed to be derived from his or her own early experiences with being cared for (Main et al., 1985); (2) parental risk factors such as mental illness or substance abuse; and (3) whether the caregiver is receiving outside support from other adults. In this section, I will focus on the first issue and will discuss the issues of parental risk factors and support for parents in Chapters 3–4.

Bowlby argued that working models of attachment tend to persist throughout life and that they are particularly activated by parenthood, thus setting the stage for transmission of attachment patterns across generations (Bowlby, 1988). This theory has been confirmed by a number of studies showing the direct effects of the mother's family of origin relationships on her parenting practices (Lyons-Ruth, Zeanah, & Benoit, 2003).

Mary Main and her colleagues have explored the persistence of working models into adulthood and their effects on parenthood. Main did studies of attachment patterns of middle-class children at ages 1 and 6 and found a high rate of consistency. Children assessed as securely or insecurely attached at age 1 were almost always classified the same at age 6. The parents of these children were also interviewed using the Adult Attachment Interview, a protocol designed to elicit information about their working models of attachment through a discussion of memories related to attachment and past and current relationships with their parents. Finally, the results of the Adult Attachment Interview were matched with the attachment classifications of the children. The representations of attachment by the parents strongly correlated with the attachment classifications independently assigned to the children (Main et al., 1985). This matching of adult and child attachment classifications has been repeatedly replicated in research (Hesse, 1999; Riggs & Jacobvitz, 2002). Prospective studies using the Adult Attachment Interview with pregnant women have found that the parent's adult attachment classification prior to the baby's birth *predicts* the infant's attachment classification at 1 year of age in about 70% of infants (Benoit & Parker, 1994; Ward & Carlson, 1995). These studies present a striking demonstration of the power of parental working models in shaping attachments.

Characteristics of Secure Adults

The parents who were rated from the Adult Attachment Interview as having secure working models had five primary characteristics. They (1) valued attachment relationships; (2) believed that their attachment relationships had a major influence on their personality; (3) were objective and balanced in describing their relationships; (4) showed a readiness of recall and ease in discussing attachment, which seemed to suggest that they had reflected on their experience; and (5) took a realistic rather than an idealistic view of their parents and their attachment experiences (Main et al., 1985).

Many of the secure adults described good early experience and relationships with parents, but some described difficult histories that included trauma and loss. What distinguished the adults who were judged secure was not their actual experiences but rather how well they had remembered, understood, and integrated their early experience. The quality of their discourse distinguished them from the adults judged insecure. Their accounts of their attachment relationships tended to be fluent, coherent, and organized, and they were easily able to include negative and positive feelings about their experiences. This matches Ainsworth's finding that securely attached infants are able to openly express a full range of emotions. Talking about their attachment experiences did not seem to make them overly anxious or cause them to resort to obvious defense mechanisms. This finding is consistent with findings about trauma. People who have experienced trauma but are able to recall and understand what happened are less likely to suffer from post-traumatic stress disorder or other trauma-related problems.

Characteristics of Insecure Adults

Adults whose working models reflected insecure attachments generally felt less positive about attachment relationships, tended to deny the influence of attachment experiences on their personality, and did not seem objective in their descriptions. Beyond these general considerations, the insecure parents fell into three main patterns, which tended to match the Ainsworth attachment classifications of their infants.

Dismissive Adults

Parents in this pattern "dismissed attachment relationships as being of little concern, value or influence" (Main et al., 1985, p. 91). They did not have vivid memories of attachment experiences and tended to describe current relationships with their parents as distant or cut-off. The parents who dismissed the importance of attachment were likely to have avoidant infants, who tend to turn away from parents and to depend on themselves rather than seeking attachment.

Preoccupied Adults

In the second insecure pattern, "the parents seemed preoccupied with dependency on their own parents and actively struggled to please them" (Main et al., 1985, p. 91). They tended to hold themselves responsible for difficulties in their attachment relationships and to idealize their parents.

They showed anxiety about their current relationships and tended to worry about how others perceived them. The infants of these parents most often were classified as ambivalent, the pattern in which infants are anxious about the availability of their caregivers.

Unresolved Adults

These parents had histories of unresolved trauma in childhood, including physical and sexual abuse. Many had experienced the death of a parent during childhood and showed ongoing symptoms of disordered mourning. They continued to be fearful about loss and had irrational views, such as blaming themselves for being abused or for "causing" the death of a parent (Main & Hesse, 1990). Their accounts of attachment were disorganized and lacked coherence. If they started to describe childhood traumatic experiences (such as the death of a parent or physical or sexual abuse), they often lost track of what they were saying, fell silent, or abruptly switched topics without showing any awareness that the quality of their discourse had disintegrated (Main & Morgan, 1996). The infants of these fearful parents were most often classified as disorganized/ disoriented.

Defensive Processes in Insecure Parents

The characteristics of the discourse of all three types of insecure parents also distinguished them from the secure parents: their discourse was hard to follow, self-contradictory, apparently irrational, or shifted without clear transition from topic to topic. Many seemed unaware of contradictions, particularly between the general and the specific. For example, a parent might state that her mother was "wonderful and understanding" but then go on to describe severe beatings or times she lied to avoid her mother's wrath—without noting the difference between the two representations of her parent. These stories suggested a defensive idealization of the parent(s) that was not integrated with the specific realities of the relationship (Hesse, 1999).

Alternatively, many of the parents of insecurely attached children insisted they had almost no memory of their childhood and in particular claimed they could not recall much about attachment relationships, again suggesting defensive processes were at work. Bowlby labeled such memory problems "defensive exclusion of information" (Bowlby, 1980). Defensive exclusion is motivated by the wish to avoid painful memories and stems from painful and negative attachment experiences. An aversive attachment leads to early emotional detachment, which in turn diminishes the salience of memories of the attachment relationship (Bowlby, 1980).

In summary, parents with secure relationships with their children give coherent descriptions of positive and negative elements of their childhood without strong defensiveness. Parents with insecure relationships with children either dismiss the importance of attachment or are preoccupied with attachment issues. Main emphasizes the influence of defensive processes on insecure working models and current attachment behavior: "Where the parent's own experiences and feelings are not integrated, restrictions of varying types are placed on attention and the flow of information with respect to attachment. These restrictions appear in speech in the form of incoherencies and in behavior as insensitivities" (Main et al., 1985, p. 100). These defense-based working models interfere with the parents' ability to perceive the child's attachment signals accurately, may cause them to ignore attachment cues, or may cause them to distort the child's signals to make them fit with their own attachment preoccupations.

ATTACHMENT THEORY AND FAMILY SYSTEMS THEORY

There is significant overlap in attachment and family systems theories. Both emphasize the transactional nature of relationships. Both accept ideas of circular causality and multigenerational transmission of relationship patterns. Minuchin's typology of interactions in family systems—adaptable, disengaged, enmeshed, and chaotic—closely parallels the attachment patterns of secure, avoidant, ambivalent, and disorganized/disoriented, as well as the Adult Attachment classifications of Autonomous, Dismissive, Preoccupied, and Unresolved (Minuchin, 1974; Byng-Hall, 1999).

In the clinical situation, a multigenerational approach to understanding current interactions in a family typically finds repetition of patterns of relationships, conflicts, and modes of coping with conflict or distress. The concept of working models suggests why these intergenerational repetitions occur. For example, family therapists have identified the common pattern of the "parental child," a child who is implicitly assigned the job of taking care of a parent, often a parent who is depressed. Bowlby has described this concept, using different terms, from the perspective of working models of attachment. When a parent inverts the parent–child relationship by requiring the child to take care of him or her, the child may learn that the only reliable way to receive love is to bestow care. Bowlby labeled the working model of attachment that develops out of this inversion as "compulsive caregiving" (Bowlby, 1978). When a person who has learned to be a compulsive caregiver becomes a parent, he or she may be possessive and protective of a child, but also re-enact the inversion of the parent–child relationship. The child is unconsciously viewed as the person who "should" at long last provide the parent with love. When there is more than one child, the parent may choose the child he or she most identifies with to become the caregiver.

Byng-Hall (1999) illustrates the usefulness of integrating attachment and family systems perspectives with his description of the "too close— too far" couple relationship. This relational system is conflictual and maladaptive because one partner has an avoidant/dismissive style of responding to attachment concerns, while the other partner has an ambivalent/preoccupied style. Byng-Hall notes: "Their strategies for the same thing—how to maintain secure attachments—are directly opposite" (Byng-Hall, 1999, p. 634). Their differing working models set the stage for escalating "pursuer–distancer" interactions when either is feeling anxious regarding their attachment. The avoidant partner (in Byng-Hall's example, a male) withdraws emotionally, and the Ambivalent partner reacts by pursuing him with clinging or demanding behavior. The cycle of pursuit and distancing creates ongoing conflict in the couple's relationship, which inevitably affects the attachment security of their children.

Attachment dynamics between parents become a context of their children's development. Two parents with secure/autonomous attachment styles present their child with an experience of the family system as a secure base (Cobb, 1996; Byng-Hall, 1995). By contrast, a child of the avoidant–ambivalent parents described above can easily become triangulated into his parents' conflictual dynamics. As the tension between his parents decreases his feelings of security, he goes to the ambivalent parent. She comforts him but then clings to him, ignoring his cues that his attachment needs have been assuaged, restricting his autonomy because she needs him.

THE ATTACHMENT PERSPECTIVE IN THE ASSESSMENT OF YOUNG CHILDREN

For practitioners the utility of the research findings that have validated attachment theory is that they orient us to observe interactional sequences and to look for congruency between parental working models of attachment and infant/child attachment patterns. Like family systems theory, attachment research teaches us that parent and child behavior tend to be complementary. Parents with working models derived from histories of secure attachment are responsive to their children, who in turn tend to develop secure attachments and positive working models. In contrast, parents who dismiss the importance of attachment are likely to dismiss their children's needs for comforting and nurturance. When these negative attitudes carry over into caretaking transactions, such children are likely to adopt the avoidant pattern.

Although research contributes to our clinical understanding, it is important to distinguish between research instruments and clinical assessment. The Ainsworth Strange Situation and Main's Adult Attachment Interview reliably reveal attachment patterns when applied to individuals in a research setting. However, they are not directly transferable to practice. Research procedures require adherence to protocol, while clinical practice requires the flexibility to adapt assessment strategies to the needs and manner of presentation of the client. Assessment depends on careful observation of interactions, usually across two or more interviews, as well as on a broad exploration of family history, developmental history, and ecological contexts (Zeanah, Larrieu, Heller, & Valliere, 2000). Nevertheless, knowledge of attachment patterns derived from research allows the social worker to observe for interactions and behavior that suggest a particular type of attachment. For example, on a home visit a worker notes that a parent treats her baby roughly while changing his diaper and seems frustrated over having to care for him. At the same time, the baby does not look at his mother, turning his head away when she comes near. These observations, which must be supported by future observations, suggest an Avoidant attachment. Similarly, a parent's inconsistent and disjointed discourse when he is asked about memories of his parents suggests that his "state of mind with respect to attachment" reflects insecure models that affect his relationship with his child (Hesse, 1999, p. 421). The following extended case example demonstrates the application of attachment concepts in an assessment.

KELLY AND HER MOTHER: A CASE EXAMPLE

Referral: Background Information

Kelly Keeney's mother referred her 21-month-old daughter for evaluation at the recommendation of the staff at an infant and toddler center, which cared for her full-time while her mother attended a community college in a large city. Ms. Keeney was a 20-year-old Irish American single parent. They lived in a small apartment near the urban campus. Ms. Keeney's income was derived from Aid to Families with Dependent Children (AFDC) and student loans. She was a competent student and had plans to transfer to a 4-year college and get a degree in nursing. Kelly's father had broken off his relationship with Ms. Keeney during her pregnancy with Kelly. He had seen Kelly briefly two times but was not involved in her care and provided no financial support.

The center director's sophisticated knowledge of infant development and attachment was reflected in the way she framed the staff's concerns about Kelly. Even though she had attended the center for nearly a year, Kelly was not demonstrating attachment to any single caregiver, and the staff reported feeling out of touch with her. She did not make eye contact, did not initiate many interactions, and often ignored their directions even though she seemed to understand them. She did not interact much with other children, though it is important to note that she was one of only two children over 1 year of age attending the center. She seemed reckless and impulsive in her movements and often fell, but she usually did not cry or seek comfort when she hurt herself. The director said that Ms. Keeney was a concerned parent but that she also seemed self-preoccupied, and speculated that she did not provide stimulation appropriate to a toddler.

Parent Interview

Ms. Keeney said she was worried about Kelly's development. She had recently taken a child development course and phrased her concerns in developmental terminology: Did Kelly's short attention span mean she was behind in cognitive development? She was not speaking very much, and did this signal a language delay? Ms. Keeney agreed that there might be an attachment problem. She said that Kelly had not been a cuddly baby and that she wouldn't hug or kiss her when she dropped her off or picked her up at the center. She explained that Kelly had been born pre-maturely and had to be hospitalized for 2 weeks after birth: "I was still in classes, and I couldn't spend a lot of time with her when she was in the hospital, so maybe she didn't bond to me." Ms. Keeney also wondered if Kelly was a lot like herself. Her mother had told her that she was never a cuddly baby, and she felt she had been an unhappy and withdrawn child. She did not want to have Kelly repeat her unhappy childhood but was worried that this was already beginning to happen. Ms. Keeney was eager to receive help and was open in reporting Kelly's history and her own childhood history.

Interacting Histories

Ms. Keeney reported the details of her pregnancy and Kelly's birth in an even, matter-of-fact manner that seemed incongruent with the emotion-ally difficult circumstances she was describing. During her first year in college she became involved with Kelly's father. Just before she learned she was pregnant, he broke up with her and dropped out of school. When she told him she was pregnant, he told her he did not want to resume the relationship. Her mother was furious that she was pregnant and insisted that she get an abortion. However, Ms. Keeney realized in retrospect that she had delayed the abortion decision until it was too late because she had continued to hope that Kelly's father would come back to her. As the pregnancy progressed, her mother shifted to insisting she give the baby up for adoption at birth. When she said she intended to keep the baby, her mother threatened to cut off all contact and, once, threatened to kill herself. Ms. Keeney summarized this period in a bland tone: "Yeah, it was a hard time, but by the time Kelly was born, I wanted her."

The stress on Ms. Keeney caused by these losses and betrayals during pregnancy was intensified by the difficult circumstances of Kelly's premature birth. Ms. Keeney had enrolled in the winter term, hoping she would be able to complete the term. This was unrealistic and evidenced a denial of the impact of the coming baby on her life, since her due date was a full month before the end of the term. When Kelly was born 5 weeks prematurely, she felt totally unprepared. She had not bought a crib or taken childbirth classes. She had been concentrating on her school-work rather than thinking about the baby.

A Premature and Ill Infant and an Unprepared Parent

Although Kelly weighed nearly 5 pounds at birth, her lungs were immaturely developed. She was diagnosed with severe respiratory distress and placed in a neonatal intensive care unit (NICU). Shortly after birth her lungs collapsed and her condition became grave. She was placed on a ventilator. Five days later her lung condition had improved sufficiently for the ventilator to be removed. She made steady progress until she was discharged 2 weeks after birth.

Ms. Keeney recalled the period of Kelly's hospitalization as chaotic and painful, although when she reported the following events there was again a discrepancy between her bland affect and the painful content. Up to Kelly's premature birth, the pregnancy had been "easy." Ms. Keeney was alone during the birth. When she called her parents, her mother threatened suicide if she did not give the baby up for adoption. In contrast, her father was supportive and concerned about the baby's condition. When Kelly's lungs collapsed, Ms. Keeney was told that she might not survive. She called her mother again, who said that it "might be for the best if she died." She recalled feeling frightened and numb during the few days Kelly's condition was critical. Ms. Keeney's account of the period after she was discharged and Kelly remained in the NICU suggests loneliness and a sense of disorganization. She visited Kelly nearly every day but recalled that there were some days when "there was no one to take me." With the encouragement of the nursing staff, she began to nurse Kelly when she was about 2 weeks old. Her mother called her several times urging her to give the baby up. When she refused, her mother told her she was ruining her life and then cut off contact. When she called Kelly's father, he was neutral and unwilling to visit the hospital. Ms. Keeney recalled this conversation as extremely painful because she had fantasized that he would come back to her when the baby was born.

Ms. Keeney remembered Kelly's first year as increasingly stressful as she tried to manage full-time schooling and the care of an infant. In the early months, Kelly had been a quiet and undemanding infant who could be taken everywhere, including to class, and so hardly disrupted her life. But as she became more active and mobile, Ms. Keeney felt more and more intruded upon by the baby's presence. She found a full-time sitter when Kelly was 6 months of age. Ms. Keeney began encouraging her daughter to play by herself and spent as much time as she could studying when they were at home. She was often frustrated by Kelly's increasingly demanding behavior. The pattern of expecting Kelly to play on her own persisted up to the time of the evaluation.

Parental Background

Ms. Keeney described her growing up primarily in terms of a difficult relationship with her mother and a supportive but somewhat distant relationship with her father. Her parents' marriage had been conflictual for as long as she could remember. Her mother had often threatened divorce and suicide as a means of controlling her father. Ms. Keeney remembered that she had been very frightened by her mother's frequent threats to leave the family or to kill herself. Bowlby (1973) has described how parental threats of abandonment or suicide cause separation anxiety and a focus on the moods of the parent because the child is confronted with the possibility of losing a primary attachment figure.

Ms. Keeney's memories of her childhood overlapped with her concerns about Kelly. She was worried that Kelly would grow up too distant from others, and noted she had been that kind of child. She herself had been a premature and ill infant. Her mother told her she had been a baby who didn't like being held; this attribution rang true for her because she remembered never wanting to be hugged or kissed when she was a child. She was withdrawn in school and did not remember having many friends. She said, "I was the kid no one liked because I was always whining and crying."

Observations of Attachment

I observed Kelly in three settings: my clinic office, the family's apartment, and the child care center. During the first part of the office visit Ms. Keeney's mood was upbeat, and she spoke and played with Kelly in an animated way. Kelly appeared happy about her mother's responsiveness. As they played together with a toy house, Ms. Keeney put a mother and baby in bed together, and Kelly laughed happily. When Ms. Keeney suggested putting the baby in the play pen, Kelly's affect became solemn. Ms. Keeney put the baby in the play pen and said it was time for her nap. Kelly became distressed. She whined irritably and jerked away from her mother. She moved away from her and crawled behind a chair. A moment later, she began playing peek-a-boo, and Ms. Keeney joined in.

Then she asked Kelly if she was sleepy and went over to hug her, but Kelly pulled away from her angrily.

After repeated observations of their interaction, I realized that this first observation had contained some important themes in their attachment. They could enjoy each other. Kelly was delighted when her mother was playing with her. However, when her mother introduced themes of disengagement into the play by suggesting the baby be put in the playpen and put down for a nap, Kelly withdrew from the joint play and became fussy. She reengaged her mother with peek-a-boo, but became angry and fussy again when Ms. Keeney suggested she might be sleepy. The pattern of their interactions suggested that Kelly wanted her mother's attention and that Ms. Keeney tended to set limits on how much she would respond to Kelly's bids for attention. Kelly became irritable but kept trying to engage her mother. Kelly was both intensely focused on the attachment and angry because she expected rejection and lack of attunement. Their interactions seemed to approximate Ainsworth's C category, insecure–ambivalent/resistant.

These attachment themes were more clearly presented during the home visit. Ms. Keeney seemed preoccupied and depressed. She told me that the evaluation had stimulated many sad feelings about her loss of Kelly's father and that she had been feeling down for the last 2 days. Kelly looked somber, and I was struck immediately that her affect mirrored her mother's. Kelly was pleased when I gave her my attention. However, her mother wanted to talk to me and suggested that she play in the bedroom, which was blocked from the living room where we sat by a wooden gate. I said that one reason for my visit was to see Kelly in her home and that I would like to be able to observe her. Ms. Keeney told her to play with her toys. As Ms. Keeney became engrossed in describing her own distress, Kelly became provocative and aggressive. She threw toys in her mother's direction and against the walls. Her behavior seemed angry, yet her expression was more blank than angry. Ms. Keeney seemed perplexed by her behavior. She asked Kelly if she was thirsty and got her some juice, which she accepted but did not drink. She continued to throw toys, and her mother decided she must be tired. She took her into the bedroom and put her in her crib. I was struck that Ms. Keeney could not read her affects or perceive her wish for attention. Rather, her caretaking focused on controlling Kelly's intrusions into our conversation. She did not seem aware that what she was saying might be distressing to Kelly. Affectively, she seemed remote from her and preoccupied with her own memories. Over the two sessions I noticed how attuned and reactive Kelly was to her mother's moods: when Ms. Keeney was serious, Kelly was somber; when Ms. Keeney was depressed or preoccupied, Kelly protested with aggressive behavior; when her mother was cheerful and animated, Kelly would mirror her positive affect and try to engage her.

At the child care center, I observed Ms. Keeney say good-bye to Kelly. She hugged her and Kelly returned the hug, but her face was blank and she looked away from her mother as she left. She seemed to withdraw emotionally. Yet I did not think this indicated, as suggested by the child care staff, that she was "unresponsive." Having previously observed Kelly's ambivalent behavior toward her mother, which seemed to express her need for more attention and more attunement from her, I believed her withdrawal was a defensive response to the distress of separation. Over the next 45 minutes I noticed that Kelly was acutely interested in the comings and goings of adults. She greeted each adult who came into the room and said good-bye when anyone left. The day I observed her, she was the only toddler at the center. She played by herself. Although there were caregivers present, they did not actively join in her play. In fact, they were preoccupied with caring for the infants and tended to leave Kelly to her own devices. It appeared that the staff, like her mother, tended to expect Kelly to be independent and self-reliant. On Kelly's side, she made few approaches to the teachers. It appeared that she might be generalizing to other caregivers an expectation that she could not count on responsiveness if a caregiver was preoccupied.

Clinical Hypotheses Based on an Attachment Perspective

Prior to Kelly's birth Ms. Keeney experienced her pregnancy as the cause of significant losses. Both her boyfriend and her mother rejected her because she was pregnant. She went through the pregnancy without support and without the affirmation of anyone who could share her normal excitement and apprehensions. Understandably, her attitude toward pregnancy was ambivalent. On the one hand, she acknowledged the reality of the coming baby by seeking prenatal care and by imagining what the baby would be like. On the other, her positive attitude toward the pregnancy was primarily supported by the fantasy of getting back together with her boyfriend and forming a family. When he avoided her and refused her overtures, the fantasy could not be sustained, and she increasingly felt intruded upon by the pregnancy. The pregnancy became subsumed under her grief. Her attempts to avoid grief by continuing in school influenced her denial of the impact of the pregnancy on her life. She registered for a full schedule of classes even though her due date was 1 month before the end of the term.

The crisis of Kelly's premature birth brought together forces that served to deepen Ms. Keeney's ambivalence. She faced the possibility of her infant's death. When it became clear that Kelly would survive, Ms. Keeney had to relate to her in a context, the NICU, where caregiving and decisions about the baby were controlled by medical personnel. Studies of ill and premature babies suggest that parents often feel like visitors and onlookers and find it difficult to feel close to their baby, with the result that their confidence as a parent is compromised (Minde, 2000). Ms. Keeney had little opportunity to hold and care for Kelly until she was nearly 2 weeks old. This is not an unusual circumstance for the parents of ill, premature infants, but it added to Ms. Keeney's sense of distance from Kelly that had already been established by her preoccupation with grief and denial of grief during her pregnancy.

After Kelly was discharged, Ms. Keeney continued going to class, often taking the baby with her. Consonant with her own needs, she saw her as a quiet, undemanding baby who could be taken anywhere and who hardly disrupted her life at all. Her early caregiving, while well intentioned, was somewhat mechanical and attuned more to her needs than to Kelly's. Her lack of attunement was not merely the result of her attempts to go on with her life as it had been before Kelly's birth—she was also depressed. A chronic dysthymia had been made more severe by losses, rejection, and an internalization of her mother's blame for having and keeping Kelly. Ms. Keeney's depression led to inconsistent responsiveness to Kelly.

Parental Depression and Attachment

In attachment studies, psychological unavailability over time due to maternal depression is linked with insecure attachments, particularly Ainsworth's C classification, insecure–ambivalent/resistant (Teti, Gelfand, Messinger, & Isabella, 1995). If a parent is unavailable emotionally for long periods of time during infancy and early childhood, the child is likely to develop working models that are consistent with depressive symptoms. That is, the child's working model of attachment is that attachment figures are unavailable and uncaring, and the working model of the self is that I am unlovable and unworthy of love (Bowlby, 1988). By 3–6 months infants of depressed mothers look depressed themselves, showing less positive affect and lower activity level than normal infants. They mirror their mother's affects (Field, 1992). Kelly's "quietness" as an infant was strongly influenced by her mother's depression. Her masked expression, irritability, and limited range of affect as a toddler suggested she might be internalizing a depressive style. Toddlers of depressed mothers look more sad, speak less, and show less exploratory behavior (Radke-Yarrow, McCann, De Mulder, Belmont, Martinez, & Richardson, 1995).

Infants of depressed mothers are likely to develop difficulties in regulating feelings. Because the mother is preoccupied with depression, she frequently fails to respond to the infant's distress signals. In consequence, the infant does not receive her help in regulating affects and is likely to withdraw from the interaction (Tronick & Gianino, 1986a). Kelly's stoic, withdrawn appearance suggested she had adopted a defense of with-drawal, which she now generalized to other relationships. However, another trend in Kelly's handling of affects was also clear—she could become very angry, particularly at her mother. Ms. Keeney acknowledged that she had felt intruded upon by Kelly's increasing mobility and activity level as she moved toward toddlerhood. She responded by developing new expectations for Kelly. Instead of expecting her to be quiet and adaptable, now Ms. Keeney required her to be more "independent," to play by herself. In response to these expectations, to her mother's attempts to limit their interaction, and to her mother's continuing depression, Kelly began to react with aggression. Unable to draw on her attachment relationship or on her own meager internal controls, Kelly tended to react to disappointment in her mother's responses to her with angry behavior.

Projections of Working Models

The quality of attachment was also influenced by Ms. Keeney's projections of her working models onto Kelly and her relationship with her. Although she wanted to see Kelly as a happy child, her perceptions of her were strongly influenced by her self-perception as a silent, withdrawn child. Her view of Kelly was further complicated by the merging of these negative self-images with her thoughts about Kelly. Kelly was associated with her rejection by her mother and boyfriend. Her mother's near-explicit message was, "Since you will not give Kelly up, I want nothing to do with you; if you had not had her, I would still love you." She also had fantasized that her boyfriend would have returned to her if she had not become pregnant. Thus, her view of Kelly was linked to her model of herself as the unworthy child who "caused" others to reject her.

The parental side of her working models was also evident. Based on these models, it seemed "right" to think that Kelly should not make emotional demands on her and that she should push Kelly toward precocious autonomy and separation, as her mother had required of her. Further evidence of the carryover of her early working models was her difficulty in seeing Kelly's distress as attachment-related. Instead, she tended to displace the distress away from the relationship by misattributing it to Kelly's internal states—hunger or sleepiness. Ms. Keeney was working hard to avoid her loneliness and neediness, which were rooted in a childhood sense of deprivation in attachment relationships, her recent losses, and the current absence of supportive people in her life. Kelly's neediness threatened her defensive attempts to deny and avoid such feelings in herself. Instead of responding contingently and accurately to Kelly's signals of distress, she conveyed to her daughter that she should shut down her feelings, as she herself had learned to do.

Research and Practice

The case of Kelly and Ms. Keeney illustrates both the uses and limitations of research knowledge in clinical work. By specifying which variables are relevant and which are excluded from examination, research approaches both clarify and simplify the lives of people being studied. Attachment research is remarkable in its exploration of the complexity of parent–infant interactions. Because of this, many practitioners find attachment research useful in their work (Stern, 1995a; Lieberman & Zeanah, 1999). Knowledge of infant and adult attachment patterns provides us with valuable lenses for viewing real behavior and understanding clients' histories. Nevertheless, when we evaluate individuals and families, we always find their lives are more complicated than research findings might indicate. For example, if we ask which attachment classifications fit Kelly and Ms. Keeney, we might argue that Kelly presents qualities of both Avoidant and Ambivalent attachment, while Ms. Keeney seems to embody aspects of Preoccupied and Unresolved adult attachment.

In practice, establishing the exact attachment pattern is far less important than understanding the specific dynamics of the attachment of a parent and child. Understanding these dynamics both in the present and as a function of Ms. Keeney's working models pointed the way to an intervention plan, which combined individual therapy for Ms. Keeney and parent–child sessions. In the individual therapy Ms. Keeney explored the impact of her working models on her view of self and her view of Kelly in the context of a supportive relationship with the social worker. The parent–child work emphasized positive play activities that aimed to strengthen the parent–child relationship.

Although organizing the treatment using attachment concepts led to a successful intervention, there were clearly other factors to consider besides attachment in formulating the case and designing a treatment plan. Ms. Keeney demonstrated a number of strengths that are not obvious in an account that is sharply focused on attachment. She was bright, determined to complete her education, able to be warm and loving toward Kelly, and very eager to receive help for her and for herself as a parent. Several other factors were affecting the quality of attachment. Ms. Keeney was poor, relatively isolated, and lacked the support of other adults for her parenting. She was still struggling with grief over several recent losses. It was necessary to view Kelly's attachment difficulties in the broader context of these parental and environmental risk factors in order for intervention to be successful.

CHAPTER 2

Brain Development

The infant of a European American mother and a Costa Rican father is spoken to in English and Spanish. Through constant exposure, he learns to speak both languages. Another child with two English-speaking parents learns only English and does not begin to study Spanish until she reaches high school. The second child may become proficient in a second language by the time she finishes college. However, it will be with great effort and practice that she learns to think in the second language, and she is very unlikely to develop a perfect accent. The bilingual child does those things without effort because circuits in his brain have literally been wired by early and constant exposure to the language to make him fluent in it. The child who learns two (or more) languages demonstrates how adaptable, or plastic, the young brain is. The brains of both children are genetically endowed to allow them to learn multiple languages, but experience determines whether that potential will be used. Recent research on brain development stresses that the brain is both "experience-dependent" and "use-dependent." Genes form the foundation of the brain's potential, but experience shapes emerging brain organization through the individual's transactions with the world. A child spoken to in two languages learns them both. What experience offers, the brain takes.

Brain cells or neurons develop, organize in groups that carry out special functions, and these special functions become interconnected through the elaboration of brain circuitry. Genetics provides the template and timetable for this process. Experience shapes the particular ways a child's brain learns to respond to the world. In neuroscience, as in child development, the nature–nurture dichotomy has been integrated into the question "How does nurture selectively influence the expression of nature?" (Levine, 2002, p. 1)

Research has begun to clarify interconnections between levels of organization in the brain—cellular, neurochemical, structural—and child development as it is observed in behavior. For example, the prefrontal cortex has been identified as the area of the brain associated with logic, step-wise problem solving, and other "higher" cognitive abilities; when the prefrontal cortex begins to mature at about age 7 or 8, these abilities begin to appear in children's thinking. An exact, tight chain of causality extending from what happens in brain neurons to what happens in ordinary behavior has not yet been established for more complicated brain functions. But research made tremendous strides during the 1990s "decade of the brain" in understanding general processes of how a child develops in relation to how his brain grows and organizes. As the review of research in this chapter will suggest, mental health practitioners need to integrate an understanding of brain development into their knowledge of child development.

This chapter will describe the basic processes of brain development, emphasizing the role of experience in shaping the brain, and risk and protective processes that influence brain organization and, by extension, the overall development of the child. For a more detailed review of brain anatomy, see Nelson (2000b).

SEQUENCE OF BRAIN DEVELOPMENT

The brain develops "from the bottom up." The "primitive" areas of the brain—the brainstem and systems in the midbrain (diancephelon)—develop during gestation and in the early months after birth. These parts of the brain regulate body functions, including respiration, heart rate, blood pressure, sleep cycles, and appetite. The limbic system, which is associated with emotional processing of experience and emotion regulation, and the cortical areas, associated with cognitive and executive functions, develop over the first 3 years. The neocortex and its prefrontal lobes continue to develop through adolescence. Both anatomically and functionally, the brain has a hierarchical organization. The functions of the brainstem and midbrain are more patterned and less complex than the limbic and cortical areas, which carry out more intricate tasks and perform them with more flexibility, as exemplified by abstract thinking in the cortical areas. The cortical areas, as they develop, exert a modulating influence on the more primitive parts of the brain. Perry notes: "With a set of sufficient motor, sensory, emotional, cognitive, and social experiences during infancy and childhood, the mature brain develops in a use-dependent fashion, a mature, humane capacity to tolerate frustration, contain impulsivity, and channel aggressive urges" (Perry, 1997, p. 129).

EARLY BRAIN GROWTH:
SYNAPTOGENESIS AND MYELINATION

Although the brain continues to develop throughout childhood and adolescence, the period between the 7th month *in utero* and age 2 constitutes
a time of "exuberance" in the growth and organization of synapses in the
brain. At birth the brain weighs 25% of its eventual adult size; by age 2 it
has attained 75% of adult weight. During these two years the brain's
development contributes not just to increased weight but more impor-
tantly to increasing elaboration and complexity of central nervous system
functioning. The brain is composed of two basic types of cells, neurons
and glia. Neurons send and receive messages and store information. Glial
cells nourish and provide supportive tissue for the neurons. Specialized
glia called myelin cells provide insulation for brain circuits.

The development of the whole range of human functioning, including motor abilities, sensory capacities, emotional response, and cognitive
skills, is based on the rapid synaptogenesis, or linking of neurons that
predominates during this period. Synaptogenesis is the "wiring" process
that occurs when neurons, and groups of neurons connect by sending out
dendritic axons (long nerve fibers). When the axon reaches the target neuron, a synapse or connection is established that allows neural impulses to
be transmitted from one group of neurons to another. Neurons produce
chemical messengers called neurotransmitters, such as serotonin, adrena-
line, noradrenaline, and others, that concentrate at one end of the neuron.
Neurotransmitters facilitate the transfer of neural impulses across synapses. When they are released into the synaptic cleft, they bind to a receptor
protein on another neuron, which in turn causes a chemical signal in
the receiving neuron. Neurotransmission activates (or deactivates) neurons and areas of the brain, causing the brain's "actions" that result
in thoughts, emotions, internal regulation, and outward behavior. The
dense branching, or arborization, of dendrites allows neurons to communicate in a coordinated way across multiple synapses, creating a control
system that mediates and regulates all aspects of human behavior.

As these connections are established, fatty myelin cells form around
the dendritic axons, insulating them in a way similar to the plastic coating
on electrical wires. This insulates circuits from others, reducing "static"
and allowing faster transmission of neural impulses. The speed and
efficiency of brain neural processing increases gradually until mid-
adolescence. Processing speed improves as pruning of synaptic circuits
streamlines them and myelination insulates the circuits, allowing them to
function more efficiently (Nelson, 2000b). As myelination proceeds, new
functions develop. For example, walking becomes possible when nerve
pathways in the spinal cord become myelinated.

SYNAPTIC OVERPRODUCTION AND PRUNING

The brain is genetically programmed to overproduce synapses or connections between neurons during its early growth period. This dense branching of connections between neurons accounts in part for the brain's rapid increase in size from birth to age 2. Synaptic production is also influenced by use. Neurons that are frequently stimulated by neurotransmitter activity in the circuits connecting them grow denser dendritic branches, strengthening those connections that are regularly used. Those synapses that are not stimulated—not used—gradually are "pruned away" throughout childhood and into adolescence (Huttenlocher & Dabholkar, 1997).

Pruning organizes and specializes brain circuitry. Animal studies suggest that there are "critical periods" for the development of some brain functions. If experiences that stimulate the development of synaptic connections do not occur, pruning can cause potential functions to be lost. A clear example is the case of infants born with cataracts. If the cataracts are not surgically removed by age 2, the child's vision does not develop, because the unused synapses in the visual cortex are pruned away, resulting in blindness even if the cataracts are removed later. Other functions, such as memory and learning, are less influenced by sensitive periods and continue to develop throughout life (Nelson, 2000a).

Synaptogenesis and myelination occur at different rates as different brain regions with particular functions develop. Motor reflexes and sensory abilities, including hearing and vision, are fairly well developed at birth and undergo rapid maturation during the first half-year of life. Production of synapses in the visual and auditory cortexes peaks at about 3 months, and then a pruning process begins. The circuits that control the ability to understand and communicate via language continue to be overproduced until near the end of the first year. But at that point there is evidence that pruning has already been occurring. A 3-month-old has the capacity to distinguish between the full range of sounds in human languages; by age 1, sound recognition has increasingly become restricted to the sounds in the language or languages the infant regularly hears, and she tends to assimilate unfamiliar sounds with sounds that are part of her language rather than being able to hear the contrast. However, the window on sound recognition remains open into middle childhood, as evidenced by the school-age child's ability until about age 10 to learn to speak another language without an accent (Kuhl, 1993; Cheour et al., 1998). Synapses in the neocortex, which controls higher cognitive functions, continue to be overproduced, pruned, and myelinated through the years of middle childhood and do not attain their final organization until late adolescence (Huttenlocher & Dabholkar, 1997).

PLASTICITY AND EXPERIENCE

While in some species brains are mature at birth, the human brain matures over many years. This means that as the brain develops it can be influenced in subtle and profound ways by the quality of the individual's transactions with the environment (Nelson, 2000a). During the early years when it is growing most rapidly, the brain shows a great deal more plasticity than during later years. Children with brain injury affecting one hemisphere during the first 5 years often recover full function because the brain is able to reroute damaged circuits. For example, children with early damage to the left cerebral cortex—the site of language ability—can go on to normal language development because the brain compensates by relying on the right hemisphere (Bates et al., 2001). Because of this plasticity, risk and opportunity factors during the early years have more influence on how the brain will ultimately function (Nowakowski & Hayes, 1999).

During the early part of brain development, up to ages 3–4, the brain is more reactive to environmental influences than in later development. (Perry, 2002a). Positive influences such as responsive caregiving, appropriate stimulation, and learning experiences support optimal brain development. But the plasticity of the young brain also makes it vulnerable to negative factors such as neglectful caregiving, abuse, trauma, and malnutrition.

BONDING, ATTACHMENT, AND BRAIN DEVELOPMENT

The brain of the infant "is designed to be molded by the environment it encounters" (Thomas et al., 1997, p. 209). Since human infants are not independent at birth but instead need a very long period of protection and care, the caregiver's responses to the infant shape brain development. Mothers are biologically primed to become the infant's "environment." The mother's and infant's initial orientation to each other is influenced by built-in complementary endocrine reactions. Hormones released at birth promote intense alertness in the infant, which allows her to respond to her mother's initial touches and emotional overtures. Right after delivery a corresponding release of hormones in the mother creates feelings of well-being and openness to bonding with the infant. The infant's first suckling at the breast stimulates the mother's secretion of oxytocin, a hormone associated with caring and social interaction (Eisler & Levine, 2002).

The infant's senses mature rapidly during the first few months of life, allowing her to "take in" the qualities of her environment directly. Recognition of the mother begins at birth through smell and touch, and evolves into an attachment through interactions involving skin-to-skin contact, mutual gaze, and sharing of emotions. As the mother touches, soothes, and feeds the infant, she "creates a set of specific sensory stimuli which are translated into specific neural activations in areas of the developing brain destined to become responsible for socio-emotional communication and bonding" (Perry, 2002a, p. 95).

Research on skin-to-skin touching between parent and infant following birth shows that it contributes to better regulation of arousal, more organized sleep–wake cycles, longer periods of restful, calm sleep, and overall calmness in the young infant (Hofer, 1995). These findings have been used as the model for an intervention with premature infants, who not only "lose" the intrauterine environment before they are ready but also may be isolated from touch because they are in incubators. Premature infants in "kangaroo care"—being placed with skin-to-skin contact against their mothers' breasts for at least 1 hour each day—showed better self-regulation and attentiveness and a greater amount of calm sleep at 3 and 6 months, as compared with premature babies who did not receive regular skin-to-skin contact (Feldman, Weller, Sirota, & Eidelman, 2002). These results are consistent with research on the positive effects of regular massage of infants (Field, 2000).

Face-to-face engagement is a particularly potent vehicle for the interactional stimulation essential for early brain development. Primates, including humans, have a sophisticated array of facial muscles. This complex musculature makes possible a large range of facial movements that convey a corresponding range of emotional expressions. Looking at another person's facial expression enables us to intuit her emotional state and to follow changes in how she is feeling as her face changes. Corresponding to the ability to convey emotion through facial expression, "Primates have neuronal groups in the brain that are specialized to respond to faces and also to particular facial expressions! . . . We are hard-wired to have emotion and meaning shaped by the perception of eye contact and facial expression" (Siegel, 1999, p. 150). Human infants clearly begin to respond to face-to-face contact by 3–5 weeks. Very young infants study their caregivers' faces, focusing especially on the eyes. Concentration on the face and eyes intensifies over the next few months and is one of the foundations of attachment (Simpson, 1999).

The attachment relationship is the infant's most significant environment during the first year of life, the period of the most rapid brain growth, and therefore has a powerful influence on the development of brain systems. A secure attachment provides the experiences, through face-to-face interaction, emotional attunement, and playful exchange, that encourage optimal brain development. Equally important, a secure attachment provides a protective source of mutual regulation that supports the gradual development of self-regulation. Siegel summarizes this transactional process: "Coherent interpersonal relationships produce coherent neural integration within the child that is at the root of adaptive 'self-regulation' " (Siegel, 2001, p. 86).

CAN PARENTS BUILD BETTER BRAINS?

As knowledge about the transactional context of brain development and plasticity has grown, the following question has been raised: Can parents increase their children's brain power by providing intensive stimulation during the early period of brain growth? The answer depends on what is meant by stimulation. For example, in a materialistic and object-oriented culture such as the United States, research findings that very young infants are more interested in highly contrasting patterns of black-and-white stripes have been translated into the production of cloth books and toys that replicate that pattern. Advertising encourages parents to buy these products and many others, with claims that they increase brain development. Young infants do like boldly contrasting patterns, as evidenced by the fact that they will stare at them for longer periods. But the implicit message that stimulation is provided primarily by the toy is misguided. The stimulation provided by parents through responsive, active, playful, attuned caregiving is what infants really need. So far, at least, there is little evidence that extra stimulation will lead to denser brain circuitry or smarter children, though it is clear that brain functions maintain vigor through use and practice (Nelson, 2000a).

However, language development is enhanced by a certain type of stimulation. Infants and toddlers who are spoken to regularly by parents in the context of direct interaction tend to learn more words by age 2 and to be more verbal than other children whose parents speak to them very little. Verbal stimulation "exercises" and increases brain circuitry related to language, which translates into greater language ability (Huttenlocher et al., 1991). However, not all "stimulation" is equal: children exposed to language via television or overhearing other people speak to one another receive little benefit to language development. Children who become more verbal have parents who engage them directly and take pleasure in face-to-face interaction (Tamis-LeMonda, Bornstein, & Baumwell, 2001). In early childhood especially, it is positive relationships with caregivers that offer the best environment for optimal brain development.

RISK AND PROTECTIVE FACTORS INFLUENCING BRAIN DEVELOPMENT

Brain development is protected by the overall health of the mother during pregnancy, adequate nutrition pre- and postnatally, and full-term gestation. After birth, brain growth is enhanced by secure and stimulating relationships. By contrast, there are a number of biological and environmental factors that lead to compromised brain development. These include genetic disorders, exposure to toxic substances, poor nutrition, prematurity, and exposure to stress, deprivation, or trauma.

Genetic Disorders

The most common genetic disorders are based on chromosomal abnormalities, where there is an extra or missing chromosome or chromosomes are arranged abnormally. The most common chromosomal disorder is Down syndrome (1 per 600 live births). Down syndrome includes significant mental retardation, poor muscle tone, distinctive facial and hand characteristics, and, sometimes, serious heart and gastrointestinal defects (Shonkoff & Marshall, 2000). Rarer chromosomal disorders include the fragile-X, Prader–Willi, Angelman, Turner, and Klinefelter syndromes. The first three involve a range of physical anomalies and moderate to severe mental retardation. Children with Turner and Klinefelter syndromes tend to have normal IQs but significant learning disabilities (Shonkoff & Marshall, 2000).

Prenatal Exposure to Alcohol

Prenatal alcohol exposure is the most common and most studied example of developmental neurotoxins: "Alcohol use during pregnancy continues to be the leading preventable cause of birth defects" (Maluccio & Ainsworth, 2003, p. 512). Heavy alcohol exposure during gestation can cause fetal alcohol syndrome or significant effects even when the full syndrome does not appear. Fetal alcohol syndrome has an incidence of 2 in every 1,000 live births, while neurodevelopmental effects short of the full syndrome are estimated at over 20 per 1000 births (Shonkoff & Phillips, 2000). Fetal alcohol syndrome includes head and face anomalies, delays in reaching developmental milestones, attentional problems and hyperactivity, and, in about half of the cases, mental retardation. Alcohol-exposed children without physical deformities nevertheless show a range of brain dysfunctions. While heavy alcohol use (either as constant or sporadic binge drinking) by the mother is a risk throughout pregnancy, the most serious effects on brain development occur in the third trimester, when neuronal cells are being produced at their highest rate (Shonkoff & Phillips, 2000).

Nutrition and Brain Development

Brain development is dependent on adequate nutrition, most crucially from the second half of pregnancy through age 2. Malnutrition causes underproduction of neuronal and glial cells, slower myelination, and poor overall brain growth, resulting in lower IQ and other cognitive deficits that can have a lasting impact (Shonkoff & Marshall, 2000). However, these effects can be reversed if adequate nutrition is provided during the early years (Nelson, 2000b). A specific correlate of malnutrition, iron deficiency, has negative effects on cognitive and motor development. Iron is essential to several aspects of brain development, including neurotransmitter production and myelination (Rao & Georgieff, 2000). Long-term studies of children who were iron-deficient in infancy show continuing lower scores on tests of cognitive and motor functioning (Lozoff, Jimenez, Hagen, Mollen, & Wolf, 2000).

Breast feeding provides the nutrients needed for good brain growth, including a high concentration of fat, which is required during the first 2 years to promote myelination. Pediatricians also recommend iron supplementation for the mother during pregnancy and for the child during infancy.

In the United States, as in other countries with significant numbers of children in poverty, poor nutrition is associated with growing up in an impoverished environment. Federal food programs attempt to address this problem through the Special Supplemental Nutrition Program for Women, Infants, and Children (WIC)—and "food stamps." Mothers' prenatal participation in WIC reduces the risk for prematurity and low birth weight and contributes to higher cognitive functioning in early childhood (Tanner & Finn-Stevenson, 2002).

Prematurity

Normal or full-term gestation is 38–40 weeks. About 40% of infants born at the edge of viability—24 weeks—survive. With each subsequent week of gestation, survival rates increase (about 69% at 25 weeks and 80% at 26–27 weeks). Infants born between 28 weeks and full-term have a 95% chance of survival. The risks to brain development associated with premature birth are more marked the earlier the gestational age and the lower the birth weight. Younger premature infants (24–28 weeks) have high rates of serious intracranial hemorrhage, which causes motor and cognitive deficits, including cerebral palsy and mental retardation. Less serious intracranial bleeding contributes to later behavioral, attentional, and memory problems (Shonkoff & Phillips, 2000). A second, more generalized effect of prematurity on brain development is that the fetus is removed from the ideal gestational environment at a time when the brain is developing rapidly and transferred to the less-than-ideal environment of the neonatal intensive care unit (Huppi et al., 1996). Illnesses that often accompany prematurity can compromise nutritional intake, resulting in temporary malnutrition during a period of rapid brain growth.

STRESS, TRAUMA, AND BRAIN DEVELOPMENT

Chronic exposure to stress unmediated by caregivers or directly resulting from poor caregiving has significant effects on brain development in young children. These effects have not yet been definitively mapped in studies of humans, and therefore the evidence remains fragmentary. However, converging findings from animal studies and research on children who have experienced severe early deprivation in caregiving, abuse, or trauma suggests that early exposure to stressors leads to neurochemical changes that promote stereotyped and maladaptive responses to future stressors and may interfere with normal development. These responses can be observed in behavior and have begun to be explored at the level of hormonal and neurotransmitter alterations in the brain/endocrine "stress response systems."

Stress Response Systems

The function of biological stress response systems is to secrete hormones and neurotransmitters that provide adaptive responses to external stressors and to modulate internal stress. The brain system operates in tandem with the endocrine system, specifically the hypothalmic–pituitary–adrenal (HPA) system. When there is an "environmental challenge," the HPA system secretes and releases neurohormones called catecholomines, which in turn trigger increases in the amount of cortisol in the bloodstream. Catecholomine release underlies the familiar "fight-or-flight" response, in which the individual's alertness, concentration, appraisal of the environment, and physical energy intensify in the face of danger. Cortisol release allows for continuation of these responses. In reaction to stressors, "cortisol levels raise rapidly . . . initiating the peripheral catabolic processes required for mobilizing energy reserves to meet the metabolic demands imposed by the stressor" (Lupien, King, Meaney, & McEwen, 2001, p. 657). In both human and animal studies, cortisol is "one of the best markers of altered physiological states in response to stressful situations" (p. 657).

When faced with threat, the stress response system focuses brain activity on dealing with the threat and temporarily inhibits other functions. Animal studies have shown that the release of cortisol promotes the freeing of energy so that the individual can take action, but at the same time suppresses the immune system, physical growth, and emotions and memory (Shonkoff & Phillips, 2000). The hippocampus, a brain area that plays a central role in learning and memory, can atrophy if it is bombarded by high concentrations of stress hormones, resulting in memory impairments (Nelson & Carver, 1998).

Prolonged Stress Alters the HPA System

Infant rats and monkeys exposed to the chronic stress of maternal deprivation show elevated concentrations of cortisol and corticotropin releas-
ing hormone (CRH), a neurohormone that sets the stress response system
in motion (Kaufman & Charney, 2001). Behaviorally they appear anxious
and constantly on alert. The biochemical and behavioral evidence suggests that in these maternally deprived animals the brain circuits that regulate response to stress "get locked in the 'on' mode and have trouble
shutting off [and] . . . because the stress system functions to put growth-
oriented processes on hold, frequent or prolonged periods of stress may
negatively affect development" (Shonkoff & Phillips, 2000, p. 213). In animal studies, these negative effects have been largely reversed when the
animals are returned to a good caregiving environment, even when the
caregivers are "foster mothers" rather than their own mothers (Kaufman
& Charney, 2001). But animal studies have also established that there is a
sensitive period for normal development of the HPA system in rats; animals who have been subjected to deprivation beyond this sensitive
period do not recover (Gunnar, Morrison, Chisholm, & Schuder, 2001).

A sensitive period for the development of the HPA system in
humans has been hypothesized. Evidence for this possibility comes from
recent human studies, which have begun to establish links between early
chronic stress and persistently higher cortisol levels later in development.
For example, elevated cortisol has been found in 7- and 8-year-olds
whose mothers had been depressed during the child's first 2 years. These
children also showed higher-than-expected incidence of internalizing
problems such as depression and anxiety disorders. The authors argued
that the higher cortisol levels and internalizing problems in middle childhood reflected the early establishment of a more reactive hormonal stress
response system (Ashman, Dawson, Panagiotides, Yamada, & Wilkinson,
2002). These biological studies are consistent with earlier research that
demonstrated links between persistent maternal depression in infancy
and children's development of depression and anxiety disorders (Field,
1998). Both types of studies hypothesize that the mother's unavailability
due to depression is the chronic stressor that mediates the development
of biological and psychological dysregulation.

A Canadian study showed that late adopted Romanian orphans,
who had spent their first 2 years in extremely deprived conditions, had
higher cortisol levels across the day, as compared with early-adopted
Romanian orphans and Canadian children raised in their families. Even
though they had been living in their adoptive families an average of 6½
years, the children who had spent the longest time in the orphanages still
had abnormal cortisol levels (Gunnar et al., 2001). This persistent abnor-

mality suggests that the long-term stress of severe deprivation caused alterations in the HPA axis. More studies are needed to confirm the hypothesis that the HPA system may be permanently dysregulated in children subjected to long-term deprivation; however, it is consistent with behavioral observations of regulatory problems reflected by inattention, overactivity, impulsivity, and aggression in late-adopted Romanian children and other children who have grown up in depriving institutions (Kreppner, O'Connor, Rutter, & the English and Romanian Adoptees Study Team, 2001).

EARLY TRAUMA AND BRAIN DEVELOPMENT

Recent research suggests that early chronic trauma negatively affects brain development and body stress response systems (DeBellis et al., 1999a, 1999b). Some beginning studies using magnetic resonance imaging have shown that children traumatized in the first few years have smaller brains overall, and other brain abnormalities (DeBellis et al., 1999b). Chronic trauma causes the stress response system to become more sensitive to future stress (Perry, 1994). As noted previously, evidence is growing that early chronic stress alters the HPA system. Children with histories of chronic abuse and trauma have greater concentrations of stress hormones than nontraumatized children. The longer the exposure to trauma, the higher were the abnormal concentrations of stress hormones and neurotransmitters (DeBellis et al., 1999a) These biochemical changes mean that the stress response systems of traumatized children are activated much of the time, even when no stressors are present, and also that they become more active when stress is mild. Essentially, the nervous system responds inappropriately, as if severe stressors are present. Behaviorally, this biochemical overactivity translates into symptoms of posttraumatic stress disorder (PTSD): hyperarousal, hypervigilance, high anxiety, and difficulty in sleeping. In a highly reactive child these symptoms may appear so often that he appears to have attention-deficit/ hyperactivity disorder (ADHD) (Perry, 1997).

The necessity of being constantly on alert to respond to expected traumatic stress has the potential to interfere with development in many ways. It appears that maladapted stress responses systems have especially negative impacts on the regulation of arousal and emotion. The individual's ability to appraise environmental cues and respond in a modulated way is impaired by the automatic and overreactive quality of the stress response (Schore, 2001). A traumatized child who has witnessed violence or been abused spends a great deal of energy scanning the behavior of others for signs of threat. She becomes attuned to nonverbal cues that signal the potential for violence. High arousal overshadows and interferes with other brain activities, such as curiosity, concentration, and motivation to learn. IQ testing of a group of children who were exposed to chronic trauma showed a significant split between verbal and performance subscales, with low verbal ability and at least average performance scores. Chronic threat causes the young brain to overemphasize nonverbal skills, with a corresponding diminishing of verbal skills (Perry, 2002b).

Perry (1997, 2002b) has argued that early neglect or trauma causes overdevelopment of functions in the lower and midbrain areas and underdevelopment of the limbic and cortical structures. Broadly, the parts of the brain that develop earlier are more primitive in their reactions to stress. If stress occurs much later in childhood, the child will be better prepared to cope with it adaptively rather than reactively because higher brain functions are now available. But when chronic stress or trauma occurs in infancy, before processes of regulation and cognition associated with limbic and cortical areas have developed, the lower brain areas cope with threat by means of emergency measures that in the long run are maladaptive and that interfere with future development. Perry states: "The more any neural system is activated, the more it will modify and build in the functional capacities associated with that activation. . . . And the more threat-related systems are activated during development, the more they will become built in" (Perry, 2002b, p. 193).

Early Chronic Trauma and Memory

In treatment of trauma-based hyperarousal in older children and adults, the therapist relies on the client's ability to remember traumatic events sufficiently to describe them. An explicit memory can be located in time, allowing the client to understand that his current arousal responses are triggered by associations with the past and not by what is actually happening in the present. Explicit memory refers to memory that can be called to mind, expressed in words, and assigned to a historical time frame. This kind of memory develops as representational abilities for language and other symbolic activities emerge beginning at age 1 and continues to mature through the preschool years. Because the brain circuits and cortical systems involved in explicit memory are still developing during this period, explicit memories of events before age 3 are rare (Nelson & Carver, 1998).

Implicit memory involves registration and storage of perceptions below the level of consciousness. Before an infant can conceptualize an event, she can demonstrate that a preverbal or implicit memory has been registered through reacting behaviorally when the event is repeated (Rovee-Collier & Hayne, 2000).

A child who had been neglected and frequently abused by her mother and was removed from her care at age 6 months became highly distressed when she saw her mother again at 14 months. She rushed over to her foster mother and clung to her. After a short time she stopped crying but withdrew, looking at the floor with a blank expression, all the while holding on to her foster mother's blouse. This child had become increasingly secure in her foster home and did not typically have distressed reactions to strangers. Her mother had not done anything overtly to provoke her fearful crying. Her reaction was an example of a type of implicit memory called "priming," "whereby an exposure to a stimulus at one point in time increases the probability of 'recognizing' (albeit covertly) that stimulus at a later point in time" (Nelson & Carver, 1998, p. 799). From the perspective of trauma theory, it is likely that this toddler recognized her mother and reacted in a conditioned manner with hyperarousal, associating her with abuse and pain, even though she probably did not have a conscious memory of being abused. Explicit memories are "stored" in the cortex, but this child's response was mediated by the primitive parts of the brain that encoded the response to the original stressor.

Early Trauma and Dissociation

In the above example, this little girl responded to threat, or more precisely the expectation of threat, through hyperarousal and distressed attachment-seeking behavior. The second aspect of her response, affective withdrawal, was also significant. Traumatized infants cannot act on the fight-or-flight response, and when hyperarousal does not elicit a protective response from a caregiver, the infant will shut down affectively or dissociate. Even though her foster mother did comfort her, it is likely that this child's sequences of response all related to implicit memories of experience with her mother, when dissociation was the only escape route possible.

It is likely that chronic neglect is a particular pathway to reliance on a dissociative response. An infant who becomes aroused because of distress cries out. If crying repeatedly brings no response, the infant shuts down emotionally and her brain learns to respond to arousal by dissociating (Perry, 2002b). In animal studies, as well as in observations of neglected, institutionalized infants, the individual appears passive, apathetic, lethargic, and defeated. This description matches behavioral characteristics of children subjected to chronic abuse and neglect beginning in infancy (Spitz, 1945; Chisholm, Carter, Ames, & Morison, 1995). In animal studies, defeat responses involve a different set of neurochemical reactions than does hyperarousal. Rather than overactivation of the HPA axis, the brain relies on the secretion of dopamine and endogenous opioids, which blunt pain and dull consciousness of external reality. Human studies of the neurochemical basis of dissociation are just beginning, but given the behavioral similarities in responses of neglected animals and infants, Perry hypothesizes that similar hormonal and neurotransmitter changes occur in both (Perry, 2002b).

At the level of brain functions, the effect of early trauma or emotional neglect is to interfere with the development of explicit memory as well the capacity for empathy and modulation of impulses. Depending on how long trauma continues, cognitive and social development may also be affected. In severe cases of persistent abuse and neglect, pervasive developmental disorders may result (Perry, 1997; Nelson & Carver, 1998).

PERSISTENT SYMPTOMS IN A TRAUMATIZED CHILD: A BRIEF CASE EXAMPLE

Deonte Moore was a 6-year-old biracial child (white and African American) who was referred for outpatient evaluation because of aggressive behavior toward his younger sister and other children in his foster home. He also appeared depressed and had symptoms of traumatic stress, including hyperarousal, nightmares, hyperactivity, and sleep difficulties. Deonte was exposed to chronic trauma during his first 3 years. He was physically abused and witnessed frequent domestic violence, as well as other violent incidents. Both parents were crack cocaine users, and they severely neglected Deonte and his younger sister. When Deonte was a bit over 3, his parents abandoned the children in a supermarket parking lot.

When he entered foster care, he was "in a shell," not speaking at all, and showing minimal reactions to people in his new home. He avoided contact with his foster parents and hoarded food in his room. As he began to develop attachments with his very competent and caring foster parents, he demanded their full attention and became aggressive toward his sister and other foster children in the home. This aggression diminished somewhat over the next year. One and one-half years after abandoning the children, the parents received permission for visitation, with the possibility of reunification. Visits were supervised at first, and then the children began spending weekends in unsupervised visitation. Before visits Deonte would have tantrums, refuse to get dressed, hide his shoes, and run away. His posttraumatic symptoms and intense aggression returned. When his foster parents went on vacation, he and his sister stayed with their parents for 10 days. During this time, Deonte was physically abused by both mother and father. Visiting was stopped and ultimately parental rights were terminated.

I began treatment a few months after Deonte was reabused. Although he became engaged at a superficial level by playing board games, he attempted to keep me at a distance, often by literally turning away from me or refusing my help in getting a toy down from a high shelf. He was very anxious and hyperalert. Whenever our play seemed to refer, however indirectly, to his history of abuse, he would shut down affectively. He would become silent, avoid eye contact, and would not respond to my words, even when I empathized with his feeling afraid to think about the scary things that happened to him and told him he could choose to wait to talk about them. This boy's dilemma—and mine as his therapist—was that he seemed to be constantly reliving his traumatic memories and behaviorally reenacting them, yet was terrified to explore them in play therapy. Any allusion, accidental or direct, to his traumatization seemed to evoke a fight-or-flight arousal response. At home or at school, he would become aggressive or hyperactive. In therapy, he would show the signs of arousal—fear in his eyes, muscle tension, and increased activity, but then would seem to dissociate. I suspected that his arousal and shutting down reflected dysregulation of the stress response system. At home, he was not able to relax enough to go to sleep. His foster mother would find him wandering the house in the middle of the night.

Deonte continued to resist exploration of his traumatic memories in therapy, and was increasingly aggressive at home and school. He attacked his younger sister and another young foster child, and was attacking classmates every day at school, apparently in response to his own intense anxiety rather than provocations by other children. He threatened to kill himself and once tried to jump out of a moving car. I referred him to our inpatient unit, and he was hospitalized for 12 days. During the hospitalization he was very guarded and sad, but did not act out aggressively. Deonte clearly felt more secure in the hospital, and he seemed less depressed when he was discharged.

After this brief hospitalization, Deonte was able to tell me some memories of abuse by his parents. He described how his dad had "stepped on my face" when he was 2, and recounted witnessing his father stab his uncle. But after these disclosures, he withdrew again, and his foster mother reported that he was becoming more aggressive and out of control. This behavior may have been stimulated by talking about memories of abuse and violence, but may also have been an anniversary reaction, since the increase in symptoms coincided with the period a year previously when he had been returned to his parents and reabused.

He was hospitalized again, this time for nearly a month. As his time in the hospital lengthened, his mood became brighter and more relaxed and his aggression was more controlled. Again, the predictable and safe world of the hospital seemed to reduce his hyperarousal. Significantly, when he was told he would be discharged, he threatened to kill himself and began hitting staff.

After discharge, his depressive and trauma-based symptoms escalated very quickly. He was expelled from school until a plan was established to control his aggression. His foster mother was committed to Deonte, but no longer felt she could keep his sister and two other young foster children safe from him. At this point I decided to recommend residential treatment. In my letter to the foster care agency, I wrote: "Deonte needs more intensive treatment than is possible in an outpatient setting. We are recommending a long-term residential placement where he will have the opportunity to work on his deep feelings of rage and sadness. To do this work, he will need to have around-the-clock support, both to provide him with security and consistency and to help him control his aggression."

Deonte was placed in a long-term residential setting. Because of his early and chronic traumatization, his prognosis was guarded. However, a safe, predictable, secure long-term setting offered the best chance for him to gradually reduce his dependence on the fight-or-flight mechanism as a means of coping with reality. Deonte's early traumas had activated a stress response system organized around survival, and he was at risk for remaining at that level of functioning, much to the detriment of his future development.

STUDIES OF INSTITUTIONALLY DEPRIVED YOUNG CHILDREN

Although systematic (and cruel) deprivation allows for experimental rigor in animal studies, these methods cannot, for ethical reasons, be applied to human subjects. However, children in "natural experiments" who have been exposed to severe deprivation, neglect, abuse, and trauma show brain effects that parallel those demonstrated in animal studies (Perry, 2002a). Summarizing a number of studies, Perry (2002a) notes:

> When early life neglect is characterized by decreased sensory input (e.g. relative poverty of words, touch, and social interactions) there will be a similar effect on human brain growth as in other mammalian species. . . . Sensory–motor and cognitive deprivation leads to underdevelopment of the cortex in rats, nonhuman primates, and humans. (pp. 92–93)

Institutional Deprivation: Two Children's Stories

For nearly 2 years, I worked as a part-time volunteer in an state-run orphanage in a Middle Eastern country. This orphanage housed children from birth to age 4. Care provided was custodial. Children were fed and bathed regularly but had little opportunity for attachment to caregivers, who worked in shifts and frequently moved to other jobs. There was little chance for the kind of interactional stimulation that is known to advance brain development in the first 2 years. It was common for infants to be placed in the orphanage immediately after birth. However, some children had spent part or all of their first year in their biological families. To provide some images of the effects of institutional care and variables related to age at placement, I will contrast two 3-year-old girls, Yasmin and Zuzan.

Yasmin. Yasmin was placed at birth and had spent her entire 3½ years in orphanage care. She was a quiet child who rarely spoke. Her dead eyes and persistently blank expression conveyed a dull and tenuous connection with her surroundings. She noticed people but did not attempt to interact. Most striking to me was how little she reacted to experiences that ought to be either pleasurable or distressing. She did not show enjoyment when she had the rare chance to eat ice cream, when the orphanage celebrated a visit by the queen. Rather, she ate the ice cream as methodically as she typically ate the daily meal of rice porridge. She had no reaction to the pleasure a few of the other children showed. When a caregiver yelled at her for urinating in her pajamas, she showed no distress and simply moved away. This child seemed deeply dissociated from life, more withdrawn than depressed. In retrospect Yasmin seems to have been a child who had given up on the possibility of human connections, except on a need-satisfying basis. Few of the children in this orphanage were adopted, but Yasmin's global withdrawal based on deprivation of human stimulation would not have drawn prospective parents to her.

Zuzan. Zuzan had been placed at age 1 by her parents who had been too poor to support her. Where Yasmin was noticeable only by her blankness, Zuzan was noisy, demanding, and vivacious. Although she was intensely anxious about attachment, certainly because her attachments to biological parents had been severed at age 1, Zuzan constantly made efforts to engage adults. She smiled, complained, cried, and physically moved toward adults. She competed with other children for adult attention. Because of her strong social skills, she often succeeded. Zuzan was a favorite of the caregivers and sometimes received physical and emotional affection from them. Unlike most of the children, who had been deprived from birth, Zuzan knew from her experience in her biological family how to connect with adults. She would reach out to any new adult visiting the orphanage. Although such behavior is often labeled "indiscriminate friendliness," and seen as a symptom of lack of attachment, from Zuzan's perspective it was a survival skill, a means of gaining caring responses no infant or toddler can do without. Zuzan's brain had been wired during her first year to make her a social being. Although she had been damaged psychologically by losing her parents and spending her second and third years in poor institutional care, she probably had a strong potential for rebound because her brain had been relatively protected during her first year of life. She was one of the few children who were adopted.

These images of Yasmin and Zuzan hopefully will provide some grounding for the reader as I discuss the data on effects of deprivation on children institutionalized since birth. Unfortunately, the experience of most Romanian orphans was much more like Yasmin's than Zuzan's.

Conditions in the Orphanages

Children adopted from Romanian orphanages after the fall of the Ceaucescu regime in 1989 spent their early months and, in many cases, years in state-run institutions that provided minimal stimulation and interaction, and little opportunity for attachment. Instead infants were left in their cribs, underfed, and severely neglected in their physical and medical needs: "The picture that emerged from institutions was of babies and toddlers packed tightly together in rows of cots, of constantly wet clothing and bedding, and of prop bottle feeding. . . . There was little crying, but some children would rock, bang their heads on the sides of the cot, or slap their legs and heads. There was virtually no individual attention" (Castle et al., 1999, p. 427). Caretakers worked in shifts, and caretaker–child ratios ranged from 1:10 to 1:20. Most of the children had been placed in orphanages at under 1 month of age, primarily because Romanian families were reacting to a severe economic depression, social disorganization, and to policies of the oppressive Ceaucescu dictatorship, which encouraged increases in population by outlawing birth control and abortion. Romanian women had thousands of babies they could not care for, and saw the orphanages as their only alternative (Castle et al., 1999). When Ceaucescu was deposed, it was discovered that approximately 65,000 children were living in state orphanages. Many of these children were adopted in the early 1990s by parents from Western countries (Gunnar, Bruce, & Grotevant, 2000).

Outcomes of Severe Institutional Deprivation

Studies of these children provide a systematic look at the neurodevelopmental and behavioral effects of early global deprivation, as well as a test of the resiliency of young children to recover from extreme neglect. At adoption, Romanian orphanage children almost universally showed severe effects of deprivation, including growth failure and psychosocial dwarfism, malnutrition, health problems, global developmental delays, cognitive delays, difficulties in self-regulation, and social/attachment problems, and in some children "quasi-autistic symptoms" (Morison, Ames, & Chisholm, 1995; Rutter, Kreppner, & O'Connor, 2001). A small number of children had consistently received some individual attention from staff. These children were less delayed at adoption and showed better overall adaptation after adoption, suggesting that individualized caregiving was a protective factor for orphanage-reared children (Castle et al., 1999).

Overall, these studies found a clear "dose–response" association between developmental delays and length of time in the orphanage. Those children who were institutionalized longest, from birth to age 2 or more, showed the most persistent effects of deprivation. If deprivation persists beyond 2 years, the capacity to recover becomes increasingly limited (O'Connor et al., 2000; Morison & Elwood, 2000). This is likely due to the effects of long-term deprivation on brain development during the years of fastest growth, and reflects a decline in brain plasticity after the first 2 years (Perry, 2002a).

The longitudinal study of Romanian adoptees demonstrates that many, especially those adopted before age 6 months, have made strong recoveries as the result of adequate care provided in their adoptive homes, even though assessments immediately after the children were removed from the orphanages showed that *all* the children, regardless of age, were severely delayed. This capacity for rebound from the effects of horrendous conditions provides evidence that the brain remains plastic during the early years and also suggests that humans have a fairly long "sensitive period" for brain development (Gunnar et al., 2000). However, significant numbers of Romanian orphanage children, compared with adopted children reared in families from birth, continue to have moderate to severe problems.

Length of deprivation—in this case, length of time in the orphanage—is the major influence on the child's capacity to resume a more normal developmental trajectory. The early-adopted children, who spent less than 6 months in orphanages, had the best outcomes in terms of catch-up development; the late-adopted children (adopted between 24 and 42 months), while showing considerable catch-up, showed the least recovery and continue to have significant delays in cognitive development, head circumference, and physical growth (O'Connor et al., 2000). Late-adopted children showed much higher rates of serious attachment and self-regulation problems; these types of problems often coexisted.

Self-Regulation Difficulties

In children adopted by families in the United Kingdom, severe problems of inattention and hyperactivity were very common in assessments done at age 6: 13.6% of children adopted before 6 months, 32.1% adopted between 6 and 24 months, and 38.6% adopted after age 2 were rated by teachers and parents as having severe problems of inattention/overactivity. By comparison, epidemiological studies show the rate of ADHD is 3–7% in school-age children (American Psychiatric Association, 2000). These researchers concluded that the high rates of inattention/overactivity were the direct result of prolonged deprivation, and noted that deprivation is an atypical pathway to ADHD, which is generally assumed to be based on inborn neurological impairments (Barkley, 2003). That many Romanian adoptees have severe attentional disorders whose symptoms are the same as a biological disorder suggests that prolonged deprivation changed brain circuitry in these children, leading to disinhibition and poor self-regulation, which are the basis of symptoms in biologically based ADHD.

Attachment Disturbances

In the orphanages, Romanian infants received little or no responsive care and had no chance to establish preferential attachments with one or a few caregivers (O'Connor & Rutter, 2000). Chapter 1 described attachment patterns of infants who have the opportunity to form selective attachments. The secure and even the insecure types reflect the general features of attachment, in that the infant develops strategies of staying close to a preferred attachment figure, even one who may be inconsistent, rejecting, or abusive. The Romanian orphans did not have this opportunity. Therefore, when they were adopted, nearly all showed behavior that reflected a lack of experience in an attachment relationship, as well as extreme self-reliance, suggesting that their experience in the orphanage had taught them that others could only be counted on minimally and that they had to take care of themselves. They did not attempt to relieve distress through attachment-seeking behavior (O'Connor & Rutter, 2000).

When the Romanian children were assessed at age 6, nearly 80% showed either no attachment problems or very mild ones. They had established attachments with their adoptive parents. However, consistent with other aspects of development assessed in this study, those children who had spent 2 years or more in orphanages had much higher rates of severe attachment problems. Even in this group, the apparent resiliency of late-adopted children was amazing, in that only 30% of those who spent 2 years or more in institutional care showed severe attachment disorders at age 6. Yet, the effects of deprivation are sobering when the late-adopted group is compared with the "control group" of U.K. children adopted before 6 months: only 3.8% of these children had attachment problems (Rutter et al., 2001).

Attachment Disturbance and Self-Regulation Problems

A striking finding was that children with attachment disturbances often had inattention/overactivity problems. It is likely that children with severe attachment difficulties will also have difficulties with self-regulation (Kreppner et al., 2001). In Chapter 1 I pointed out that one of the primary functions of attachment is to help the infant regulate arousal and emotions. A responsive caregiver helps the infant modulate arousal or distress. Gradually, through experiences of dyadic regulation, the infant learns how to self-regulate. The Romanian orphanage infants received little or no help with regulation. It is not surprising that an absence of attachment would lead to regulatory problems (Rutter et al., 2001).

Summary

The studies of Romanian adoptees provide an unusual opportunity to understand the effects of severe deprivation in humans. Although the Canadian and U.K. studies did not attempt to map brain changes in the Romanian children, their findings are consistent with experimental studies that have shown changes in brain structure, circuitry, and chemistry in animals in response to deprivation and lack of caregiving. They also support recent findings about the effects of chronic trauma. I have discussed the research on Romanian orphanage children in detail because it suggests a bridge between animal and human studies and offers plausible human evidence for several important ideas about brain development:

- Environment shapes early brain development.
- The young brain, especially up to age 2 years, has a great deal of plasticity, and has a strong capacity to recover from deprivation and neglect.
- There are relative limits to brain plasticity. The children who spent longer than 2 years in institutions showed much less recovery and had more enduring and pervasive developmental problems.
- Some areas of functioning are more vulnerable to early assaults on the brain's development. For example, the capacity for self-regulation was affected much more strongly than cognitive development, as reflected in high rates of inattention/overactivity as a persistent disorder in Romanian adoptees.

CHAPTER 3

Risk and Protective Factors: The Child, Family, and Community Contexts

Development unfolds in individual, family, and community contexts that influence its course. To understand a particular child's development we must attend to the transactions between that individual child and the layers of ecological context that surround him. In Chapters 1 and 2 we saw how variations in the organization of attachment and the development of the brain contribute to the creation of different developmental pathways. In this chapter and the next we broaden the discussion of transactional contexts to include individual qualities of the child, parental and familial factors other than attachment, and social/environmental factors, and discuss how these factors may protect and enhance the developmental process or, alternatively, may increase the risk of compromised developmental outcomes.

RESEARCH ON RISK AND RESILIENCE

During the 1960s researchers studying psychosocial risk noticed that children exposed to the same risk factors, such as growing up in chronic poverty, were affected differently. Some children developed serious disturbances, some were moderately or only mildly affected, and some even seemed to use the challenge of the stress to become stronger. Those children who had good outcomes in spite of exposure to risks to development were called "resilient." Resilience has been defined in a number of ways, including the following:

- The ability to function competently under threat or to recover from extreme stress or trauma quickly (Masten, Best, & Garmezy, 1990)
- "The capacity . . . to meet a challenge and use it for psychological growth" (Baldwin, Kasser, Zax. Sameroff, & Seifer, 1993, p. 743)
- Good developmental outcomes and adaptive abilities in spite of growing up in high-risk situations (Masten & Coatsworth, 1998)

Each of these overlapping definitions captures important aspects of the concept. These definitions, however, imply that resilience exists primarily *in* the individual. Early studies emphasized the apparent inherent "invulnerability" of children who seemed to succeed developmentally in the face of serious risks. Recent conceptualizations recognize that the existence and development of children's resilience is a transactional process dependent on supportive factors in the environment, especially responsive, protective parenting. Resilient children tend to have had "environments that are supportive in critical ways [and] . . . the capacity for resilience develops over time in the context of environmental support" (Egeland, Carlson, & Sroufe, 1993, p. 518). Resilience is also now seen as a normative process rather than a special attribute that promotes adaptation only in high-risk conditions: "Resilience is an integral part of development that every child must achieve" (Baldwin et al., 1993, p. 743). Of course, it is harder to become resilient in adverse environments, and in such environments ongoing support is critical. Consequently, research has focused on intervening processes that serve to protect children's development in spite of their growing up under conditions of risk (Werner, 2000).

This research has practical applications consistent with traditions in social work intervention, which emphasize promoting resilience through ecological *and* individual interventions (Fraser, Richman, & Galinsky, 1999). The identification of risk and protective factors and processes is a critical part of any assessment (see Appendix 3.1 at the end of this chapter). From this assessment we are guided toward interventions that seek to increase protective factors and mitigate risk factors.

The following sections review findings on protective and risk factors. For the purpose of clarity, child, parental, and community/environmental factors are presented separately, though in reality all three levels of risk and protective factors interact to influence the development of the child. Even though they are presented separately, it is important to understand that risk and protective processes have a transactional relationship. Poor outcomes and resilience should be seen as a continuum of possibilities, based on the balance of risk and protective factors across development and on the timing of new stressors or opportunities in the course of a child's life (Egeland et al., 1993; Sameroff, Bartko, Baldwin, Baldwin, & Seifer, 1998). Given this continuum of possible outcomes, it is important to examine the balance of risk and protective factors, since the presence of protective factors tends to offset risk: "The greater the risk factors, the worse the outcomes; the more promotive factors, the better the outcomes" (Sameroff & Fiese, 2000, p. 141). It is also necessary to consider the duration and timing of risk and protective processes. At-risk children who are subject to protective processes over time are more likely to develop resilient traits and adaptive coping mechanisms.

PROTECTIVE FACTORS AND PROCESSES

Protective factors, either in the child or environment, mitigate risk by reducing stress, providing opportunities for growth, or strengthening coping capacities. Recent research on resilience has increasingly recognized the ongoing transactional process of development and protective factors. Children who are resilient tend to have experienced consistent, responsive parenting over time. While secure attachments in infancy and early childhood predict adaptive functioning in later childhood, most resilient children have actually had adequate parental support *throughout* their development (Egeland et al., 1993). It may be more appropriate to refer to protective factors *as protective processes,* since to be truly effective in promoting resilience they must be present across many years of the child's development (Luthar, Cicchetti, & Becker, 2000).

Child Protective Factors

Factors "in" the child that influence vulnerability and resilience include biological conditions, genetic inheritance, and personality characteristics. "Inherent" protective factors noted in resilience studies have included good-natured temperament, good health, good self-regulation, and above-average intelligence. Certain personality characteristics are associated with resilience, such as positive self-esteem, an active style of responding to stress, the ability to elicit positive attention from parents and other adults, believing in one's ability to solve problems, and the ability to balance autonomous functioning with help seeking when necessary (Masten & Coatsworth, 1998).

In long-term studies of high-risk children, Emmy Werner found characteristics associated with resilience at each developmental stage. In infancy, these resilient children were good-natured, active, and responsive, and did not have feeding or sleeping problems. As toddlers and preschoolers, they were somewhat advanced in the areas of "alertness and autonomy, their tendency to seek out novel experiences, and their positive social orientation" (Werner, 1993, p. 504). In middle childhood, they demonstrated the ability to get along with peers, good communication abilities, good cognitive and reading skills, a reflective rather than impulsive cognitive style, effective use of academic skills independent of level of intelligence, use of flexible coping strategies in response to stress, many hobbies and interests, and the ability to find emotional support outside the family and to use other adults as role models. They also demonstrated an ability to find niches that allowed them to utilize their talents and gain positive feedback (Werner, 1993, 2000). Other developmental accomplishments associated with resilience include the capacity for empathy and the development of a conscience (Turiel, 1998).

An advanced developmental level is a protective factor, since the older the child, the better able he will be to appraise, interpret, and cope with distressing events (Rutter, 1985). Children who have a previous history of mastering the tasks of development are more resilient. The feedback that one has coped successfully with a difficult situation (coming from within as well as from others) serves to improve both appraisal and coping abilities and thus helps the child become more resilient in the face of future stressors. Children who have coped successfully also tend to develop an "internal locus of control," which means that they believe they can take active steps to master difficult situations, as opposed to feeling that external events control them (Werner, 2000).

Parental Protective Factors

In general, the effectiveness of intrinsic protective factors is mediated by developmental level. The younger the child, the less effective such qualities as a positive attitude will be in mitigating risk and the more the child will need external protective factors that come from family support. Other internal protective factors, such as cognitively based coping skills or internal locus of control, are by definition not available to young children because they require developmental capacities the child has not yet attained. The very designation of child factors as "internal" or "intrinsic" is misleading because it obscures how they are influenced by the child's transactions with the environment from birth. As described in Chapter 1, resilient personality traits are linked to a history of secure attachment, responsive parenting, and positive working models of relationships and self (Egeland et al., 1993).

In addition to secure attachment, other parental protective factors have been identified: parental warmth, good caregiving after the child has been through a stressful experience, modeling of competent behavior and coping skills, appropriate expectations of the child, household rules and structure, and monitoring of the child's behavior (Masten, Best, & Garmezy, 1990). Werner (1993) found that the expectation of prosocial behavior, such as taking care of siblings or helping relatives or neighbors, was associated with resilience: "At some point . . . the youngsters who grew into resilient adults were required to carry out some socially desirable task to prevent others from experiencing distress or discomfort. Such acts of *required helpfulness* can also become a crucial element of intervention programs that involve high-risk youth in community service" (p. 511; emphasis in original).

In turn, positive parenting abilities have been linked to the level of the parent's education and particularly to the quality of support the parent receives. A positive relationship between parents supports the parenting function. So does shared caregiving by parents and other relatives. The parents' involvement with kin and neighbors, family religious faith and participation, and access to health and social services also support parenting (Werner, 2000). Religious faith modeled by parents and internalized by children provides a sense of stability in the face of adversity, "a conviction that their lives have meaning, and a belief that things will work out in the end, despite unfavorable odds" (Werner, 2000, p. 125). Ongoing involvement with supportive extended family is a particularly important protective factor for teen parents and their children. Many studies have found that children of teenage parents (who are also more likely to be single parents) are at risk for poor long-term outcomes, including lower IQ, poorer academic performance, and higher dropout rate, delinquency, and adolescent parenthood. Children of teenage parents have much better outcomes when grandparents and other relatives are involved in supportive ways (Wakshlag & Hans, 2000).

Protective Factors in the Broader Context

Although quality of parenting is the most important mediator of risk for children, other relationships can be protective. An ongoing positive relationship with a nonparental adult such as a grandparent, teacher, or friend's parent promotes resilience even when parenting ability is impaired (Werner, 2000). For children growing up with a severely mentally ill parent, warm relationships with other adults, either in or outside the family, contribute to more adaptive functioning (Radke-Yarrow & Sherman, 1990). Supportive grandparents are a particularly potent protective factor. Secure attachments and consistent relationships with grandparents tend to offset parental risk factors such as psychopathology, substance abuse, and insecure attachment (Werner, 2000). Positive experiences and feedback at school can also offset a stressful family environment (Werner, 2000). At-risk children particularly benefit from classrooms that provide clear rules, strong organization, and predictability, as well as high expectations and strong encouragement from teachers. A recent study found that classrooms with these qualities supported good self-regulation and school adjustment in poor African American children exposed to multiple stressors. The most adaptive children had parents who provided support and monitoring of behavior, so that home and classroom were mutually reinforcing (Brody, Dorsey, Forehand, & Armistead, 2002). Mentoring programs also provide important supportive relationships for school-age children, particularly when the mentoring relationship lasts more than a year. Studies of well-run mentoring programs have demonstrated positive effects on children's academic achievement, school attendance, prosocial behavior, and refusal of alcohol or drugs (Thompson & Kelly-Vance, 2001).

At a broader level, consistent parental employment, adequate housing, home ownership, high-quality child care and schools, living in a safe neighborhood, and having adequate financial resources are all protective factors, which tends to become obvious only when these conditions are not present. In this context, social privilege, based on middle-class status and the absence of barriers such as racism, is at the root of many protective factors. Similarly, social inequality and disadvantage, based on structural lack of opportunity, inadequate social policy, and racial or ethnic discrimination, is at the root of many risk factors (Conger, McLoyd, Wallace, Sun, Simons, & Brody, 2002).

RISK FACTORS

Conditions that create developmental risk include the following:

- Vulnerabilities in the child, such as mental retardation or chronic illness
- Impaired parenting
- Socioeconomic and institutional factors, such as lack of access to medical care or chronic exposure of the family to poverty and social disadvantage

Risks that are chronic, such as being reared by a schizophrenic parent, have more far-reaching effects on development than do acute risks, such as the parent's experiencing a brief psychotic episode followed by recovery of normal functioning. Risk factors are increasingly dangerous as their number goes up because their effects interact with and potentiate one another, increasing the level of stress and making the child increasingly vulnerable. One or two risk factors can generally be coped with, but when there are three or more the child and parents are more likely to become overwhelmed, resulting in developmental or psychiatric disorder in the child. Sameroff and colleagues' (1987) initial study of the effects of risk factors on cognitive ability dramatizes this point. Four-year-olds from low-income families who had been exposed to 0–2 risk factors had IQs averaging 115. The IQs of children exposed to 4 risk factors averaged

94, and those confronting 7–8 risk factors had IQs in the mid-80s. *Accumulation of risk accounted for a 30-point difference in IQ in otherwise similar children* (Sameroff, Seifer, Barocas, Zax, & Greenspan, 1987). A more recent study documented the same link between the number of risk factors and psychological adaptation, self-competence, problem behaviors, involvement in positive activities, and academic performance (Furstenberg, Cook, Eccles, Elder, & Sameroff, 1999). The most insidious and destructive scenario occurs when risk accumulates, both over time and in the number of factors, and when there are few countervailing protective mechanisms (Sroufe et al., 1999).

Child-Based Vulnerabilities

Biological Factors

Children's development is put at risk by a range of biological conditions, including genetic syndromes, *in utero* exposure to teratogens (e.g., infectious diseases in the mother transferred to the fetus, or chemicals toxic to the fetus, such as alcohol or cocaine), prematurity and low birth weight, birth injury or anoxia, and chronic illnesses. Genetic risks range from specific medical syndromes, such as the fragile-X and Prader–Willi syndromes, to more general risks for certain types of mental disorders. Psychiatric research has identified familial patterns, assumed to be based on genetic transmission, for a number of disorders, including autism, attention-deficit/hyperactivity disorder, mood disorders, Tourette's and other tic disorders, and schizophrenia (American Psychiatric Association, 2000; Rende & Plomin, 1993). However, many people with genetic risk do not develop psychiatric diagnoses, because they are protected by opportunity and supportive environments.

Growing knowledge of general features of gene expression, combined with the clear evidence of genetic transmission in certain conditions, suggests that genes influence all aspects of human behavior. This leads to theorizing about genetic explanations of apparently social phenomena. For example, do genetically inherited characteristics, such as irritability, occurring in a parent and child influence the negative interactional dynamics that evolve in their relationship? It is logical that genetic predispositions would have a significant influence on how this particular parent and child would come to respond to each other (Reiss & Neiderhiser, 2000).

On the other hand, no measureable genetic chain of causality has been established for such complex forms of behavior, and it remains easier to analyze how behavior is shaped by observing parent–child interactions. Further, the expression of genetic potential is strongly influenced by environmental quality, particularly as mediated by quality of parenting (Collins, Maccoby, Steinberg, Hetherington, & Bornstein, 2000). This evidence comes from adoption studies. For example, adopted children whose birth mothers were schizophrenic were studied longitudinally to see if they would develop schizophrenia. In terms of genetic risk, children of a schizophrenic parent are 10 times more likely to develop the disorder than members of the general population (American Psychiatric Association, 2000). Quality of family environment had a clear influence on whether or not the child's potential for schizophrenia was realized: "Virtually no cases of schizophrenia in the offspring were detected when the adoptive family was rated as healthy (i.e., well organized and with little conflict among members). However, the genetic risk for schizophrenia was fully expressed in adoptive families rated high on conflict and disorganization" (Reiss & Neiderhiser, 2000, p. 364).

Epidemiological studies have distinguished between the causes of severe versus mild developmental disorders that have a biological component. About 75% of severe disorders, including severe mental retardation, multiple physical anomalies, and severe neurological disorders, have biological causes related to damage to the fetus during the first 6 months of pregnancy. These include chromosomal anomalies, inadequate nutritional supply to the fetus *in utero*, adverse drug effects and prenatal infections (Kopp & Kaler, 1989). Less severe disorders—mild retardation, minor neurological and sensory difficulties—by contrast, have exclusively biological causes only about 20% of the time and instead "are linked to deleterious social and economic circumstances or to a combination of biological and social vulnerabilities" (Kopp & Kaler, 1989, p. 227).

Biological Conditions and Attachment. Biological vulnerabilities at birth have the potential to affect attachment (McFadyen, 1994). Infants born with biological damage are frequently harder to relate to. They may be less responsive than normal infants, or they may be irritable or constantly distressed. Parents may not know how to respond to an ill, premature infant and may at first resist investing emotionally in an infant who may die or be seriously compromised. Parenting risk factors, such as depression or a history of insecure attachment, may compound the parent's difficulties in relating to the infant. Finally, the environmental risk of being in a neonatal intensive care unit (NICU) for an extended period interacts with these child and parent factors (Minde, 2000). All of these risk factors were at play and affected quality of attachment in the example of Kelly and Ms. Keeney in Chapter 1.

Transactional Effects of Biological Conditions over Time. Biological conditions frequently compromise future development because they may have ongoing sequelae, such as mental retardation, neurological disorders such as cerebral palsy, congenital anomalies requiring surgical correction, behavioral and attentional disorders, and difficulties in the development of self-regulation (Rutter, 1989; Minde, 2000). These ongoing effects can also contribute to difficulties in attachment, or may, for understandable reasons, lead the parents to emphasize the child's "sick" or "delayed" qualities over areas in which her development is adequate. Often parents who have babies who are very ill in infancy or are diagnosed with chronic illnesses in early childhood have had to constantly monitor the child's physical states. Hyperattentiveness and protectiveness may persist as a generalized style of relating to the child they continue to perceive as fragile. Parents may constantly run interference for the child and limit her choices, limiting the acquisition of autonomous skills that are within her developmental abilities (Thomasgard & Metz, 1996). The child may internalize the parents' view of her and begin to restrict herself inappropriately. This may evolve into a form of "secondary gain," in which the child begins to use the illness or disability as a means of avoiding responsibilities and expectations (Feinstein & Berger, 1987). From the perspective of intervention, it is important to discuss with parents the need to develop appropriate expectations for what their child can accomplish and to encourage them to set limits on the child's using her disability to avoid doing things she is capable of. The intensive and invasive medical treatment of chronic or serious illnesses such as cancer can also pose developmental risk, especially during early childhood when the child's coping mechanisms are not well developed. Multiple hospitalizations in infancy and early childhood, especially those involving surgery, may interfere with the child's developmental tasks and compromise the parent–child relationship because of ongoing stress on the parents (Minde, 2000).

Risk for maltreatment also increases when a child is physically or mentally disabled. Children with mental retardation, health-related disabilities, or sensory deficits, such as blindness or deafness, are 3–4 times more likely to be maltreated. One explanation for this finding is that parents who have some degree of risk for abuse may become overtly abusive or neglectful in response the stress of caring for a child with significant difficulties (Sullivan & Knutson, 2000).

Secure Attachment as a Protective Factor against Biological Risk. Research on children with biological conditions suggests that secure attachment and responsive caregiving over time have more impact on developmental outcome than the particular biological deficit. Biological conditions obviously impact development, but responsive parenting ameliorates the risks and helps the child develop adaptive coping mechanisms (Sameroff & Chandler, 1975). Summarizing research on this issue, Lyons-Ruth et al. (2003) note: "Most parents may be able to compensate even for severe deviations in the infant's behavior and development, although infants are not similarly able to compensate for parental disturbance" (p. 613).

Temperament

Temperamental factors constitute another child-based vulnerability. Temperament refers to biologically based personality traits that affect the child's orientation to the world. Thomas and Chess (1977), studying infants beginning at 3 months of age, identified three patterns of temperament—"easy," "difficult," and "behaviorally inhibited," or "slow to warm up." Temperamentally easy children have a positive mood, moderate activity level, adaptability to change, regular biological patterns, good attention span and persistence, mild-to-moderate intensity and sensitivity, and positive responses to new situations. Resilience research has identified this type of temperament as a protective factor.

The other two patterns—"difficult" and "behaviorally inhibited"—have been implicated as potential risk factors. Children with difficult temperaments contrasted with the easy children. Their moods tended to be negative, and they were very active, "negatively" persistent, overly sensitive, intensely reactive, and resistant to change. Their biological rhythms were irregular, and they tended to withdraw in new situations. Behaviorally, these traits translate into a restless, irritable, hard-to-soothe baby who wakes up many times at night. Children with difficult temperaments are less rewarding for parents. Parents may quickly feel inadequate when they are unable to comfort an infant who is constantly fussy or, later, a preschooler who is negative and demanding (Wachs & Kohnstamm, 2001).

Compared with both the easy and difficult temperaments, children described as "slow to warm up" tend to be less reactive, less overtly emotional or intense, and less active. They are inhibited in novel situations, although they may participate actively if they have had enough time to size up a new experience. Behaviorally inhibited children seem cautious and shy, and respond to stress, especially in unfamiliar situations, by withdrawing emotionally.

Temperament, Parental Factors, and Goodness of Fit. Difficult temperament has the potential to interfere with the development of adequate self-regulation. These children have more difficulty soothing themselves and responding to parents' attempts to soothe them. Because they are so reactive and hard to comfort, they may have frequent experiences when parents cannot help them calm down; consequently, they are less able to generalize from the experience of mutual regulation to self-regulation. Such interferences may contribute to later difficulties in sustaining attention and maintaining selective attention (Posner & Rothbart, 1994). Strong behavioral inhibition has also been associated with potential psychiatric risk. Very inhibited children are much more reactive to new situations, as documented by physiological measures, including increased bodily tension, blood pressure, and heart rate (Kagan, Resnick, Clark, Snidman, & Garcia Coll, 1984). These physiological responses are characteristic of anxiety disorders, and later studies of these same children with high behavioral inhibition showed that they had higher rates of anxiety disorders in middle childhood (Rubin, Burgess, Kennedy, & Stewart, 2003).

Nevertheless, it appears that temperament is a risk factor primarily in combination with parentally based risk factors. Although it is widely believed, for example, that difficult temperament constitutes a risk factor for abuse, research studies show that parental personality characteristics and psychopathology, often exacerbated by external stressors, are the determinants of abuse, and that child factors, including temperament, are not significant factors (National Research Council, 1993). Similarly, studies of the family context of behaviorally inhibited children suggest that parents of these children have high levels of anxiety themselves and that they reinforce the child's inhibited behavior through overprotection and restriction of autonomy (Messer & Beidel, 1994). Although a few studies make links between irritable temperament in infancy and the development of avoidant attachment, overall research has not implicated temperament as a direct causal factor in insecure attachment. Infant irritability is primarily a risk factor when parents are subject to stress from other risk factors (Vaughn & Bost, 1999).

Thomas and Chess (1977) proposed the bidirectional model of "goodness of fit" to explain the interaction between child temperament and parenting behavior. For example, a parent who tends toward self-reliance and prefers a "cool" interactional tone may feel frustrated and overwhelmed by an infant or toddler whose temperament inclines him toward high activity, intense emotions, and strong need for interaction. The fit here would not be a good one, whereas a parent with a more active, involved, and "warm" style would more easily adapt to the child's temperament and create a better interpersonal fit. The impact of temperament on development is best understood from a transactional perspective. When the parent of a "difficult" child is able to provide consistent empathy and limit setting while avoiding natural tendencies to overreact, withdraw from, or take personally the child's behavior, the parent provides a "holding environment" for the child that encourages adaptive development (Sanson & Rothbart, 1995).

Temperament as a Transactional Process. Identifying temperamental characteristics is a useful way of understanding how a child responds internally to his experience. However, since temperament does not exist in isolation from the parents' styles of responding to the child, it is only one piece of the puzzle in clinical evaluation. Recent research has raised questions as to whether what appears to be temperament is more the result of parental working models and early caregiving interactions (Crockenberg

& Leerkes, 2000). Given that temperament is assumed to be inherent, it was expected that it would be stable over time. However, research findings offer only modest support for the stability of difficult temperament and somewhat stronger support for the persistence of behavioral inhibition (Rothbart & Bates, 1998). In the original research of Thomas, Chess, and Birch (1968), difficult temperament in infancy did not increase risk for behavior problems, but difficult temperament at age 3 did predict later behavior problems. This suggests that there is a strong association between caregiving and temperament, since the link between difficult temperament and behavior problems was only evident after the child had been in a caregiving relationship for 3 years. Many studies have found correlations between the way parents describe themselves and the way they characterize their infants' temperaments. Highly emotional parents describe their infants as like themselves, and parents who view themselves negatively or who have significant depression or anxiety are likely to see their children as "difficult" (Rothbart & Bates, 1998). Lyons-Ruth and Zeanah (1993) point out that in infancy "adverse temperamental attributes have weak links with subsequent maladaptation unless contextual influences [the caregiving relationship] support the link" (p. 19). Parents' working models of attachment also shape their perceptions of temperament. Several studies using the Adult Attachment Interview found that the mother's adult attachment classification during pregnancy *predicted* the child's attachment classification at 1 year of age in 70% of cases (Lyons-Ruth, Zeanah, & Benoit, 2003). The infants' behaviors were consistent with their mothers' expectations before birth.

These studies raise questions about the utility of thinking about temperament in isolation from the transactional context of the attachment relationship. What is perceived solely as temperament is influenced by the parent's working models or the degree of stress a parent experiences. Research matching infant temperament characteristics and parent personality style has shown that irritable or "distress-prone" infants develop insecure attachments and poorer self-regulation when their mothers are either rigid in personality or slow to respond to distress (Crockenberg & Leerkes, 2000). Parents under stress may have difficulty helping a child feel secure. The child may react with fussiness or aggression, which increases the parent's stress and leads him or her to perceive the child as "difficult."

In clinical evaluation, however, it is very useful to explore the parent's perceptions of the child's temperament and to assess goodness of fit (Chess & Thomas, 1986). Parents often need help understanding why their regular styles of comforting do not work as well with a child with difficult temperament, and they need support for the exhausting work of parenting such a child (van den Boom, 1994). Whatever the "origins" of temperamental qualities, extremes of temperament, such as strong negative reactivity or intense inhibition, increase risk for developmental, social, and behavioral problems (Rothbart, Posner, & Hershey, 1995).

Parental Risk Factors

The functions of parents are to protect the child, promote adaptive development and self-esteem, model and support the child's movement toward self-regulation, provide encouragement and opportunity for growth, and convey cultural values to the child. These functions begin in the attachment relationship and persist throughout development, both through direct parental influence and the child's internalization of working models. Winnicott (1965) pointed out that parents do not need to be perfect but rather "good enough." Although "good enough" parents make mistakes and may at times be inconsistent, overall they carry out the normal functions of parenthood. "Good enough" parents are able to see their children realistically, have expectations of the child that are consistent with her actual developmental level, and have the capacity to empathize with the child's point of view.

Parenting that heightens developmental risk involves relative failure or inability to carry out the normal functions of parenthood. Galdston (1979) suggests that "the parenting process can be described as dysfunctional when the welfare of the child is sacrificed to the needs of the parent" and when the parent acts on a distorted, unrealistic view of the child (p. 582). Parental risk factors derive from direct behavior toward the child, such as maltreatment, and from parental difficulties, such as substance abuse or psychopathology, that impair parenting ability. Other factors related to familial or parental status may increase parenting vulnerability. These include teenage parenthood, single parenthood and father absence, paternal unemployment, family disruption or divorce, large family size (four or more children), and low level of education for mothers (Coley & Chase-Lansdale, 1998).

Positive parenting behavior buffers stress in childhood. The presence of parental risk factors reduces the parent's ability to mediate stressors, making the child more vulnerable to other risk factors (Osofsky & Thompson, 2000). In general, the lack of parental support and mediation of stressors leaves children to cope on their own. The younger the child, the less he will be able to cope on his own and the more likely he will develop maladaptive patterns of coping in response to stress. For example, the child who has been traumatized at age 3 or 4 by witnessing domestic violence frequently faces an impossible task at this level of development. He must master the trauma without the support of his mother, who has herself been traumatized by being beaten and consequently is unable to provide emotional support and explanations to her child. In this and analogous situations, the child may develop emergency-based coping strategies, such as hyperaggression and emotional numbing, which are understandable responses to the trauma but which, if they persist, become inappropriate and maladaptive coping mechanisms that impede development (Davies, 1991; Webb, 2002). When parents help their children cope with stressful experiences, both directly and by modeling adaptive coping, the child's coping ability and stress resistance are augmented. When parents, because of their own difficulties, are not able to buffer children from stress, children do not learn adaptive coping and are more vulnerable to future stressors and psychopathology (Osofsky & Thompson, 2000).

The following discussion of parental risk factors provides brief descriptions of parent–child dynamics and developmental impacts associated with each risk factor. Although each factor is described separately for clarity's sake, it should be noted that parental risk factors often occur in clusters. Two substance-abusing parents may neglect and abuse their children, and expose them to intense conflict and domestic violence. In such a situation it is not possible to sort out the impacts of the separate risk factors.

High Parental Conflict, Family Disruption, and Divorce

Ongoing parental conflict is associated with a higher degree of developmental risk. Marital relationships that are full of anger and conflict, and (to a lesser degree) distancing, create insecure environments for the child (Davies, Harold, Goeke-Morey, & Cummings, 2002). Young children exposed to chronic anger between parents show behavioral and affective disorganization and increased aggression. Some children exposed to frequent parental fighting take on a caregiver role to the parent with whom they are aligned. Conflictual couples, whether overtly hostile or hostile and alienated, are more likely to have different values regarding child rearing and discipline (Katz & Woodin, 2002). Parental conflict is especially difficult for the child when the parents triangulate the child into the conflict, by arguing about her or requiring her to take sides in the conflict. Fighting that puts the child in the middle predicts more behavior problems, as well as shame and guilt, in children (Kelly, 2000). Research suggests that children do better in adequately functioning single-parent families or stepfamilies than in high-conflict two-parent families (Amato, 2001). Even children who are distressed by their parents' divorce often answer the question "Is there anything good about divorce?" by saying, "Yes—they're not fighting all the time!"

Parental separation and divorce spawn a number of stressors impacting children: disruption associated with the period before and after parents separate; frequently, the sense of loss of one parent; changes in residence and school, resulting in loss of prior friends and support systems; downward economic mobility; the mother's return to work or increase in work; depression and self-absorption in one or both parents; and later, parental dating, remarriage, and stepfamily relationships. In the first year or two, children's reactions to separation and divorce often interfere with normal development. Anxiety about the security of their attachments, depression, and negative, oppositional, aggressive behavior are common symptoms. School performance may drop. In spite of these expected reactions, many children within a 2-year period seem to cope with their parents' divorce and resume their normal developmental progress (Hetherington & Kelly, 2002).

Factors that buffer the child's reactions to divorce include the following: ongoing emotional availability and consistency in parenting, often reflected in joint-custody arrangements; in sole custody, an ongoing relationship with the noncustodial parent; minimizing disruption of the child's home/school environment; the parents' ability to establish a healthy postdivorce adjustment; and, particularly, the parents' ability to move beyond previous conflicts and to shift into the new role of cooperating to support the child's needs and development (Emery, 1999; Whiteside & Becker, 2000).

In high-conflict marriages, children's symptomatic behavior has been in evidence long before the actual separation. Children exposed to intense and frequent conflict between parents before divorce have the same symptoms as children in high-conflict divorces. Children who have observed years of conflict often exhibit self-regulation problems consistent with hyperarousal of the stress response system (Cummings & Davies, 1994). Further, in some families, divorce is best seen as a crisis that exacerbates existing risk factors. Risk to development created by parental alcohol addiction or significant psychopathology will only intensify when that parent becomes the primary caretaker following divorce (Kelly, 2000; Pruett, Williams, Insabella, & Little, 2003).

In recent years, many states in the United States have passed laws promoting joint custody. Children benefit from joint custody when parental conflict is low, when parents can communicate and cooperate on behalf of the child, and when the parents prefer, or at least accept, joint custody as a means of each parent's maintaining a significant relationship with the children. Under those conditions, joint custody is superior to sole custody in promoting children's adjustment, because the child benefits from consistent relationships with *both* parents (Bauserman, 2002).

By contrast, joint custody in situations where the parents continue to fight—both in front of the children and through the legal system—tends to keep the child in the middle of the conflict and is associated with higher rates of psychiatric symptoms and ongoing enmeshment in the parents' conflicts. When parental conflict remains intense, sole custody buffers the child from ongoing conflict, because one parent is the child's primary caretaker and is in charge of decisions about the child (Johnston, 1995). Some research shows that school-age children do better in the custody of the same-sex parent (Clarke-Stewart & Hayward, 1996). This is consistent with psychoanalytic theory, which asserts that school-age children's development is promoted by identification with the same-sex parent.

Two parental factors after divorce present the most risk for children. The first is when the parent the child lives with suffers a decline in parental functioning after the divorce, often because the stress of divorce precipitates a serious depression, which lasts for several years. When parenting is impaired over a long period of time, the child has to struggle with divorce and loss issues on his own, without parental buffering, and is likely to develop ongoing symptoms (Kelly, 2000). The second factor is ongoing hostility, fighting, recriminations, and court battles between parents. The effects of ongoing conflict on the child may be profound, because he is continually exposed to parental fighting, to put-downs of one parent by another, and to implicit or explicit requirements that he ally with one parent against the other.

In situations where the mother has sole custody, another risk factor associated with high postdivorce conflict is the withdrawal of the father from the child's life. The loss of the father's involvement can be particularly problematic for boys, though girls suffer as well (Amato, 2001). Relocation by a custodial parent that makes contact between the child and the other parent also holds risk, especially for younger children, who are more affected by long separations from the noncustodial parent (Kelly & Lamb, 2000, 2003).

Harsh Parenting, Corporal Punishment, and Coercive Family Process

Harsh, punitive, and inconsistent parenting influences the child's working models, so that the child comes to expect interactions with parents to be negative and aversive. A child's difficult temperament may create the conditions for harsh parenting, but ineffective parenting behavior and corporal punishment, often based on the parent's working models, plays the major role in creating a pattern of negative interactions (Dishion, Patterson, & Kavanagh, 1992). Parents who use harsh discipline tend to see their children negatively, often from infancy. They also unrealistically attribute abilities of self-control, understanding of intentionality, and awareness of right and wrong, when children are too young to have attained these abilities. A parent who slaps his 10-month-old's hand for reaching for a glass figurine, saying "she *knows* she's not allowed to play with things that are breakable," illustrates such inappropriate expectations. Parents who attribute negative qualities to their children and use corporal punishment often have histories of having been treated harshly or abused as children and have internalized a view that children must be controlled through coercive, physical means (Nix, Pinderhughes, Dodge, Bates, Pettit, & McFadyen-Ketchum, 1999).

Parents' negative working models are likely to be strongly activated in response to children's autonomy-seeking behavior during the toddler period. Patterns of conflict beginning in the second and third years often lead to long-term behavior problems. Parents who react with anger and physical punishment to toddlers' assertive and limit-testing behavior encourage the child to use aggression, modeling her behavior after the parent's (Shaw, Gilliom, Ingoldsby, & Nagin, 2003). Patterns of mutual anger and aggression and coercive interactions develop, setting the stage for the development of oppositional behavior and conduct disorder (Broidy et al., 2003).

Patterson and colleagues have summarized the literature on family variables related to antisocial behavior as follows: "Families of antisocial children are characterized by harsh and inconsistent discipline, little positive parental involvement with the child, and poor monitoring and supervision of the child's activities" (Patterson, DeBaryshe, & Ramsey, 1989, p. 329). Demanding, negative behavior is reinforced because parents pay much more attention to it than to prosocial behavior. Interactions between parents and children come to be dominated by coercion, threats, and aggression by both parent and child. The child internalizes the notion that aggression is a means of escaping or exerting control over aversive events (Patterson, 1982a). Over time the characteristics of the interactions—coercive behavior, escalation of anger, reactivity, negative affect—shape the child's working models of relationships as well as the parent's view of the child. The expectation of conflict and coercion becomes solidified, and both parent and child become perpetually "ready for trouble" (Nix et al., 1999).

Children with disruptive behavior tend to internalize negative views of self based on how they are viewed by their parents. The child who has been treated negatively begins to see himself negatively. His expectations of relationships involve punishment, conflict, and rejection. He projects these working models and meets the world with mistrust, expecting to be aggressed against. As the child generalizes aggressive behavior and coercive strategies to relationships outside the family, he is likely to be rejected by peers and identified by teachers as having behavior problems. Their negative reactions, however, will feel consistent with his working models. The child's aggression often does provoke retaliation or punishment, which tends to confirm his working models.

Children with disruptive behavior often view themselves as victims and blame others for "causing" them to be aggressive. Because they feel victimized, they believe that their aggressive behavior is justified, and this short-circuits feelings of guilt or remorse. Their self-image, as a victim who is hurt or treated unfairly and therefore has to be tough, contrasts with the ways others perceive them. For many children with disruptive behavior disorders, the self-image as a victim is accurate, because many have been abused or subjected to cruel punishments. The working model of self and others that develops out of coercive family processes interferes with moral development, distorts peer relationships, and—because of the child's aggressive stance—tends to foreclose opportunities to receive positive feedback. By middle childhood conduct problems often take on the status of traits, or typical patterns of response (Broidy et al., 2003).

Child Maltreatment

Maltreatment by parents, including neglect and physical, sexual, or psychological abuse, has serious and ongoing effects on children's development. Although it is useful to separate the different types of maltreatment for purposes of definition and study, in reality neglect and the separate forms of abuse often overlap. A sexually abused child is often being emotionally abused via threats of retribution or catastrophe if she discloses the sexual abuse. Case reports of children removed from their parents commonly state that they were left without supervision *and* that they bear scars and bruises indicating physical abuse. Research also suggests that there is a large overlap—as well as some differences—in the developmental effects of the different types of maltreatment. Maltreatment that is *early* and/or *chronic* has the most detrimental effects on development (Bolger & Patterson, 2001).

Psychological abuse is a common denominator across all types of maltreatment, and this may account for the common developmental effects. When parents are hostile toward their children, attribute negative qualities to them, exploit or corrupt them, or expose them to chaotic experiences, many of the foundations for adequate development are affected, including self-regulation, self-esteem, sense of competence, and sense of security (Hart, Binggeli, & Brassard, 1998). Another factor that may explain similar effects is that maltreatment is frequently traumatizing, so that a child's immediate and long-term responses to repeated maltreatment reflect posttraumatic symptoms and adaptations (Ford & Kidd, 1998). Because this discussion of maltreatment must be brief, I will concentrate on commonalities in parenting behavior, interactional dynamics, and developmental effects across the different types of maltreatment.

In general the parenting style of maltreating parents has been described as less flexible, more punitive, and characterized by unrealistic expectations of the child's abilities. Maltreating parents deny or undervalue the child's needs and abuse the power they have over the child

(Glaser, 2002). The majority of neglected and physically abused children develop insecure attachments, ranging from 70 to 100% across studies (Crittenden, 1992b). Sexually abused children often develop insecure attachments, though it is not clear whether this is primarily based on early caregiving patterns or on the traumatic disruption of attachment and a shift in working models caused by exploitation of the child by an attachment figure (Briere, 1992). Many sexually abused children, rather than having experienced chronically poor parenting, face in sexual abuse a trauma of betrayal, which compromises their ability to trust others and to perceive their intentions accurately (Freyd, 1996). Neglectful parents tend to ignore or simply "not see" the child's needs. They provide little stimulation, do not monitor the child's behavior, and do not establish routines for the child (Glaser, 2002).

Trauma and Maltreatment

Many children who have been physically or sexually abused show symptoms and adaptations consistent with posttraumatic stress disorder (PTSD) (Briere, 1992; Putnam, 2003). The essence of trauma is an overwhelming feeling of helplessness, often accompanied by physical or psychic pain, terror, and horror. In response to a traumatic stimulus, such as being severely beaten by a parent, the child experiences the physiological and affective arousal of the fight-or-flight response and finds that no action is possible and no help from outside is available. In the midst of the traumatic event, the child feels powerless and alone. From a cognitive point of view, in trauma horrified affect overcomes thinking. Being unable to get help, to act, or to use cognitive strategies to avoid the horror, the child falls back on a more primitive defense, affective shutting down or numbing. The severity of trauma increases when the perpetrator is a parent or other close person on whom the child must depend. This is damaging because the child's trust is betrayed. His expectations are reversed—a person who is supposed to protect him becomes the victimizer (Finkelhor, 1995).

Child Abuse Trauma and Developmental Interference. Once a maltreated child has been traumatized, and especially if the traumatization has been repeated, defensive adaptations occur that interfere with later development. The abilities to appraise reality accurately and to regulate arousal are compromised. Instead of being able to attend realistically to what is happening, the hyperaroused and hypervigilant traumatized child begins to view most events through the lens of trauma in an effort to avoid a repetition of the maltreatment. As described in Chapter 2, recent research has identified that early physical or sexual abuse causes physiological changes in the HPA (hypothalmic–pituitary–adrenal) axis, and the secretion of endogenous opioids, resulting in either persistent hyperarousal or dissociation (Putnam & Trickett, 1997; DeBellis et al., 1999a).

Chronic traumatization tends to create rigid defenses. The child acts in an all-or-nothing fashion, either with acts of aggression, frantic attempts at escape, or intense psychological withdrawal and affective constriction. Dissociative and numbing defenses are particularly likely to develop in response to chronic physical or sexual abuse, although the child may also become enraged and aggressive when she feels under threat (Pynoos, Steinberg, & Goenjian, 1996). Defensive behavior becomes automatic in situations that evoke memories or affective reminders of the trauma. Eventually, coping strategies such as affective constriction may become so generalized that the child's opportunities for cognitive and affective development are compromised (Terr, 1991).

Chronic traumatization interferes with the development of a young child's reality testing and even ability to symbolize. Abused toddlers who are in the early phase of language development may show delayed or impoverished language (Cicchetti & Beeghley, 1987). The toddler who does not yet have language as a reliable vehicle for encoding his experiences is hampered in processing trauma. The younger the child, the more likely the trauma will be registered nonverbally as affectively charged, fragmented imagery, which makes the child more reactive to similar affects and imagery (Perry, 2002a). The ability to think about and understand an experience is a potent defense against traumatization (van der Kolk, 1987). Older school-age children and adolescents may fare better following trauma because they can use their cognitive abilities to master the stress. Younger children have more difficulty cognitively processing trauma because their ability to understand reality is not yet mature (van der Kolk & Fisher, 1994).

Developmental Effects of Maltreatment. Maltreatment interferes with many areas of development. The developmental effects of abuse show up in infancy in the form of depression, poor affect regulation, high arousal, and anger. Severely abused infants show retardation in all spheres of development (Zero to Three, 1994). Maltreated toddlers show high levels of aggression and anger, and are hostile in situations that do not seem to call for hostility (Crittenden, 1992a). Maltreated preschool children have poorer social and interactive play skills, and are impulsively aggressive or disruptive, which causes peers to avoid them (Darwish, Esquivel, Houtz, & Alfonso, 2001). Physically and sexually abused preschoolers also rely more on dissociation as a means of dealing with stress, compared with nonmaltreated children. Dissociation tends to persist and interferes with learning during the school years (Macfie, Cicchetti, & Toth, 2001). In school-age children chronic maltreatment has been linked to maladaptive problem-solving abilities, cognitive disorganization, poorer language development, and lowered academic performance (Eckenrode, Laird, & Doris, 1993; Kurtz, Gaudin, Wodarski, & Howing, 1993).

Maltreated children tend to have histories of insecure attachment, with high rates in the Disorganized/Disoriented category. The absence of a secure base in attachment has in turn been related to less exploratory behavior and less behavior oriented toward developing competence (Barnett et al., 1999). Insecure attachment makes maltreated school-age children mistrustful and less ready to learn from new adults. Both physically abused and neglected children have been found to develop a more self-centered orientation and have less capacity for empathy than normal children. They show disturbances in the development of the self, which in school-age children shows up as a sense of personal inadequacy (Kinnard, 2001).

Socially, maltreated children have more difficulty appraising what others intend and what is happening in interactions (Finkelhor, 1995). Because they anticipate aggression and rejection, they may misread the behavior of others and take defensive actions that are not appropriate to the situation (Weiss, Dodge, Bates, & Pettit, 1992). These problems, combined with impairments in ability to trust others, lead to ineffective relationships with peers. Peers tend to reject and isolate them because they are more aggressive and negative in interactions (Dodge, Pettit, & Bates, 1994).

Developmental Effects of Neglect. Neglected children who have not also been abused show the effects of lack of stimulation and mutual interaction and support. They are more passive, depressed, and easily frustrated. As preschoolers they tend to give up more easily on cognitive tasks. They have higher rates of language delays. Consistent with the long-term lack of parental warmth and support in their experience, neglected children tend to view themselves negatively, expect others to see them in a negative light, and feel helpless and hopeless in situations of interpersonal conflict. By early elementary school, they test lower in IQ than abused children, tend to withdraw from classroom expectations, perform worse academically than abused children, and isolate themselves from peers (Waldinger, Toth, & Gerber, 2001; Hildyard & Wolfe, 2002).

Maltreatment and Future Psychopathology. The developmental effects on maltreated children can, over the long run, evolve into a wide range of psychopathology. Epidemiological surveys of adults maltreated as children show higher risk for antisocial disorders, PTSD, dissociative disorders, depression, personality disorders, and drug and alcohol dependence. In addition, sexually abused girls have higher rates of bulimia in adolescence and adulthood (Cicchetti & Toth, 1995; Putnam, 2003; Johnson, Smailes, Cohen, Brown, & Bernstein, 2000).

Foster Care as a Secondary Risk Factor

As an outcome of maltreatment, placement in foster care is associated with serious risk. The number of children entering foster care has been rapidly increasing since 1980, with an even more accelerated increase in the 1990s due to the crack cocaine epidemic (Maluccio & Ainsworth, 2003). Welfare reform in the late 1990s is another contributing factor. Maltreatment has increased in the years since welfare was drastically reduced (Fein & Lee, 2003). Between 1998 and 2002, the number of children in foster care nationally increased by over 100,000, to 581,000 (Children's Defense Fund, 2002).

Most children placed in care have been maltreated and judged to be at developmental risk due to the effects of abuse and neglect. When they enter care, however, they suffer a loss of parent, family, and a familiar environment. Once in care they face problems of adaptation. Finally, given the inadequacies of the foster care system, they frequently must cope with disruptions of new relationships and environments as they are moved from one foster home to another. Although high percentages of foster children are referred for mental health treatment, many children do not receive treatment they require. Instead, the underfunded child welfare system too often fails to provide mental health services and responds to children's behavioral problems by moving the child to another foster home (Leslie, Landsverk, Ezzet-Lofstrom, Tschann, Slymen, & Garland, 2000). Compared with children who remain in single foster homes, children who have been frequently moved show poorer attachment to foster parents, poorer school performance, more self-defeating behaviors, and more conduct problems (Newton, Litrownik, & Landsverk, 2000; Leathers, 2002).

For large numbers of children in foster care, the disorganizing effects of substance abuse on parenting guarantee that their preplacement lives have been chaotic. They enter care with serious developmental problems (Maluccio & Ainsworth, 2003). They often have been severely neglected, show disorganized attachment, are used to fending for themselves, may have "disorderly" habits such as eating whenever they are hungry or hoarding food, and will tend not to look to others for help, guidance, or structure. When these precociously self-reliant and undersocialized children enter a foster family in which the adults hold authority and take responsibility for family functioning, they may resist the new structure, in part because their sense of control and autonomy has been usurped and in part because their early experiences of abuse and neglect have made them terrified of being dependent (Fanshel, Finch, & Grundy, 1990). These characteristics in turn make it difficult for foster parents to engage with them.

Disrupted Attachment and Foster Care. Disruption and loss of attachments are central to the experience of the foster child. Even if the child's attachment to the biological parent or parents fits one of the insecure categories, removal to foster care represents a disruption of attachment and a loss of an attachment figure. Although Protective Services often removes siblings at the same time, they are frequently placed in separate foster homes. This adds to the children's sense of loss, particularly because in neglectful homes siblings have come to depend on one another more than on the parent. Children coming into foster care should be seen as grieving children, even when they are relieved to have been removed from the abuse (Folman, 1998). The child welfare system tends to keep only minimal information about children's preplacement histories (Fein, 1991). Caseworker turnover and multiple placements reinforce the foster child's feeling that "nobody really knows me." When traumatized children enter care with people who do not know about the traumas they have experienced, the sense of being alone may be intensified.

Not knowing about the child's earlier traumas leaves the foster parent without any context for interpreting or empathizing with the child's ongoing symptomatic behavior (Folman, 1995). In clinical evaluation, it is important to recall that a foster parent's view of a child may represent only a current snapshot, and that her symptoms may reflect the crisis of entering care. A clinical evaluator may learn more about the child's history from the child, and then can convey information to the foster parent that contextualizes and makes sense of the child's symptomatic behavior. This clarification of connections between a a child's current behavior and her preplacement history helps foster parents become more empathic toward the child, which increases the chances that a mutual attachment can be established (Dozier, Albus, Fisher, & Sepulveda, 2002).

Threats to Continuity for Children in Foster Care. Foster children must cope with many changes and secondary stressors over which they have no control: replacement (change of foster home); caseworker turnover; conflicts between workers and foster parents; conflicts between foster parents and biological parents; inconsistency in parental visiting; return home, followed by reentry into foster care; and failed adoptions. Consequently, many foster children live with an uncertain sense of the future. Length of time in care—sometimes in multiple placements, with no resolution of either being returned, parents' rights being terminated, or being adopted—increases the child's sense of a lack of permanency (Kaufman & Zigler, 1996). Uncertainty about whether the child will be returning home may limit the foster family's ability to invest in the child, which further conveys to the child how tenuous his status is.

Many children who move through multiple placements, or are returned home only to be removed to foster care again, adapt to these discontinuities in relationships and environment by detaching and becoming self-reliant (Kates, Johnson, Rader, & Streider, 1991). This is particularly likely to occur when a child's working models of attachment involve the expectation of neglect or maltreatment (Penzero & Lein, 1995).

Risk in Foster Care as a Function of Early Experience. Although this review of research on risk in foster care has highlighted risk factors of the foster care system and the discontinuities between the child preplacement and placement experiences, children's functioning in foster care is fundamentally predicted by their preplacement experiences in their families of origin (Fanshel et al., 1990; Folman, 1995). Many children with histories of insecure attachment, severe maltreatment, and early trauma and loss, along with a corresponding absence of protective factors, may enter foster care already on a seriously maladaptive pathway that shapes the child's behavior in care regardless of the quality of care.

Given this background, it is unrealistic to anticipate that foster parents will always be able to meet the needs of disturbed and deeply hurt children. Placement "failure" often reflects a mismatch between unrealistic system expectations and the actual capabilities of foster parents, who are too frequently asked to care for children who require much more intensive treatment. The frequency of placement disruption is paralleled by the high rate of foster parents who stop fostering, often citing as reasons lack of adequate training to deal with difficult children and lack of support from social service agencies (Denby, Rindfleisch, & Bean, 1999). These issues, in turn, reflect that the foster care system is seriously underfunded.

Witnessing Family Violence

Children who witness their mothers being attacked by fathers or male partners are at risk for traumatization, impediments to development, and mental health problems (McClosky, Figueredo, & Koss, 1995). Child witnesses of domestic violence have problem profiles similar to those of abused children, showing clinical symptoms at rates two to four times higher than those in children in the general population (Johnson et al., 2002). The overlap between domestic violence and maltreatment, particularly physical abuse, ranges from 40 to 60% across studies (Edleson, 1999b). A recent study found that child abuse is 5 times more likely in families where spouse abuse is occurring (Rumm, Cummings, Krauss, Bell, & Rivara, 2000).

Witnessing Violence and Trauma. Like physical abuse, witnessing violence tends to be traumatic. Hyperarousal, fearfulness, reactivity to posttraumatic reminders, and posttraumatic play and defenses are common in children exposed to chronic domestic violence (Lehmann, 2000). Children in violent families witness a great deal of psychological abuse, often as the prelude to overt violence. It is not surprising that witnessing violence should be traumatic, given that the child, at close range and in the midst of overwhelming emotions, sees her mother being brutalized. The sensory impressions of witnessing violence—hearing screams and crying, observing intense emotion and behavior, seeing blood—intensifies the child's terror. The fact that it is the child's primary caregiver who is attacked intensifies the impact of trauma (Fick, Osofsky, & Lewis, 1997).

Trauma may be further heightened by events that follow domestic abuse: police presence, arrest of the abuser, hospitalization of the mother, and periods of living in a domestic violence shelter, often followed by a return home to live with the abusive parent. Another aspect of trauma, which is often also explicitly enforced by the batterer, is social isolation. Battered women may not have access to social support, and this has a negative impact on their ability to provide the understanding the young child needs to cope with reactions to witnessing violence. The mother may not be able to make connections between the child's symptomatic behavior and the experience of witnessing violence. This is particularly likely when the child is under age 6 and has difficulty articulating her worries, or when the mother defends against recognizing the child's posttraumatic symptoms because they remind her of her own traumatization. The mother may become more punitive rather than understanding. The child may experience this as a failure of attachment and become even more symptomatic. Boys may be more at risk for the combined effects of traumatization and attachment failure because the mother may interpret the boy's symptomatic aggression as indicating that "He's just like his father" (Davies, 1991).

Such mother–child dynamics add a relational element to trauma. Adults who are traumatized themselves are less sensitive to their child's experience of trauma. Exposure to domestic violence in infancy has been linked to disorganized/disoriented attachment. One of the pathways to D attachment is a history of unresolved trauma in the parent. It is logical that a *currently* traumatized parent would have difficulty promoting secure attachment in her baby (Scheeringa & Zeanah, 2001; Zeanah, Danis, Hirsgberg, Benoit, Miller, & Miller, 1999). If chronic exposure to violence occurs in infancy and the caregiver is unable to provide mutual regulation of the child's distress, brain development may be skewed either toward hyperreactive or dissociative patterns of responding to stress (Perry, 2002b). Over time, in addition to the direct traumatic effects of witnessing violence, children are secondarily affected by their mother's less competent parenting: "The experience of chronic abuse depletes one of the ability to give emotional support to others, including one's children" (Levendosky & Graham-Bermann, 2000, p. 90).

Other Consequences of Witnessing Violence. Living with a violent parent may also affect moral development. Not only does the child see violence as a means of controlling relationships and responding to stress, he may be explicitly taught by the batterer that violence is "justified." Children, particularly boys who identify with their fathers, may internalize this moral logic.

Children who have witnessed violence show higher rates of aggression toward peers, and generalized externalizing behavior problems (Moffitt & Caspi, 1998). This behavior has been explained in terms of the posttraumatic defense of identification with the aggressor and as the result of imitation of and identification with a parent who models violence as a means of domination or tension reduction (Edleson, 1999a). Because of same-sex identification and cultural sanctioning of male aggression, boy witnesses are particularly likely to behave aggressively. School-age girls, for similar reasons of identification and socialization, show higher rates of depression and anxiety (Henning, Leitenberg, Coffey, Turner, & Bennett, 1996). Children of both sexes exposed to chronic psychological abuse and violence may adopt dissociative defenses and develop a sense of powerlessness, because they cannot stop the violence. Children commonly minimize or deny violence. These avoidant defenses of "wishing violence away" help them regulate emotion and arousal, allowing them to cope in a family where violence regularly occurs (Edleson, 1999a; Lee, 2001). However, establishment of such emergency "all-or-nothing" defenses may reduce a child's success in later developmental tasks.

Moderating Factors. The risks of exposure to domestic violence may be moderated if the mother is able, in spite of being victimized herself, to maintain a positive and supportive relationship with the child. This is possible, but not easy to accomplish. Other supports for the mother such as the extended family, domestic violence shelters, and legal aid services may serve as protective factors, since their support may allow the mother to leave the violent relationship (Osofsky, 1996).

Emerging Issues in the Protection of Children and Women. Evidence of the overlap between domestic violence and child abuse raises the issue of how Children's Protective Services (CPS) should intervene in reports of children's exposure to domestic violence. A few states have codified witnessing domestic violence as a basis for reporting to CPS. Other states have defined the problem as "neglect," or "failure to protect," which can have the effect of holding the abused parent responsible for children's witnessing violence (Kaufman Kantor & Little, 2003). Assessing risk to children in the context of spousal abuse is often a difficult task for child protection workers, who may lack expertise in domestic violence (Koverola & Heger, 2003). The goals of CPS and the domestic violence movement historically have been at odds: "When domestic violence was identified, CPS workers have often misunderstood its dynamics and held battered mothers responsible for ending it. . . . The domestic violence movement has focused primarily on the needs of battered women, and been slower to address the needs of these women's children" (Finlater & Kelly, 1999). The challenge of protecting children and supporting abused women is an emerging area of practice. Several states provide domestic violence training for CPS workers and have integrated domestic violence consultants into CPS units. Long-term collaboration between women's and children's advocates is needed to develop interventions meeting the needs of children and their mothers (Fleck-Henderson, 2000).

Death of a Parent

The death of a parent in childhood may create developmental risk, depending on a number of circumstances. Earlier research suggested that parental loss during childhood heightened the risk for psychiatric disorder, particularly depression (Bowlby, 1980).

These studies, however, were drawn from clinical populations. Only a small number of parentally bereaved children in the general population develop clinically significant depression (Dowdney, 2000). But bereaved children do have a wide range of grief reactions, including crying, depressive affect, concentration problems, separation anxiety, and worry about the surviving parent. Many go through a period of poorer school performance and more difficult peer relations. Since longitudinal studies have not been done, the course of children's grieving is uncertain. Grief symptoms diminish over time, but may wax and wane in response to stress or developmental transitions (Dowdney, 2000).

Heightened Risk: Stigmatized and Traumatic Deaths. Deaths from suicide or murder carry more risk because of their traumatic nature (Cerel, Fristad, Weller, & Weller, 1999, 2000). When the death carries a stigma, as in murder or suicide, in crime-related circumstances, or from AIDS, the child's risk increases because the family's shame, guilt, and need for secrecy may prevent open mourning and lead to distorted understandings about the death and the child's relationship with the deceased (Telingator, 2000). Children confront a more complicated grieving situation and severe developmental risk when the circumstances of death are violent and especially if the child witnessed the death, including the extreme of witnessing one parent murder the other. The child experiences such losses as traumatic and will show symptoms of posttraumatic stress, including hyperarousal, emotional numbing, intrusive thoughts about the way the parent died, memories of hearing shots or seeing blood, and fears about personal safety and dying that lead particularly to sleep problems and nightmares (Dowdney, 2000). In interventions with traumatizing losses, the trauma work must precede the grief work. A child caught up in the horror of what happened must be helped to understand and cope with posttraumatic symptoms before moving on to exploring the loss (Shapiro, 1994).

Variables Influencing Ongoing Responses to Parental Death. Recent formulations, while acknowledging that parental death is a severe stressor, focus on transactional factors that may heighten or decrease risk. Important factors to consider include the quality of the child's attachment relationship with the parent before death, whether the death was unexpected or traumatic, the surviving parent's or caretaker's ability to provide emotional support and facilitate the child's mourning, and the degree of overall disruption in the child's life (Worden, 1996). A child whose parent dies usually is being cared for by an adult who is also grieving—the spouse, partner, or parent or other relative of the person who has died. It is not easy for an adult to grieve his or her own loss and remain a responsive caregiver. Surviving parents have high rates of psychiatric symptoms the first 1–2 years after bereavement (Dowdney, 2000). Children may feel a double loss, because their remaining parent is emotionally less available and may have trouble maintaining predictability in day-to-day routines. Similar concerns apply when a parent with a terminal illness requires care over many months or years before dying. The stress imposed on the healthy parent may compromise his or her parenting ability, leaving the child in the position of watching one parent deteriorate while the other is less available to support the child (Saldinger, Cain, Kalter, & Lohnes, 1999).

Adults who receive support while they are grieving are better able to respond to children's grief. The critical variables that decrease risk following the death of a parent are responsive caregiving, the surviving caregiver's maintenance of consistent routines and a stable home life, the caregiver's ability to facilitate the child's mourning by talking and reminiscing about the dead parent, and cultural practices that support mourning (Nickman, Silverman, & Normand, 1998; Shapiro, 1994).

Permission to mourn and open discussion about the deceased parent help the child maintain an internalized image of the parent, even as the intensity of grief diminishes. Positive identifications with a deceased parent contribute to the child's sense of personal identity, promote internalization of values, and provide an image of the attachment relationship that the child can draw on when under stress (Silverman, Nickman, & Worden, 1992).

Parental Psychopathology

Individuals with serious mental illness are at higher risk for unemployment, poor self-care, exploitation, homelessness, and life disruptions due to psychotic episodes. The children of the mentally ill, by extension, can also be exposed to these risks. Children may also experience discontinuity of caregiving, at times when their parent is hospitalized or when they are removed from the parent due to neglect. Children of severely mentally ill parents have high rates of exposure to abuse, neglect, and bizarre behavior. Parents suffering from poorly controlled schizophrenia and manic depression often behave inconsistently and lack emotional attunement (Powell, 1998). The risk for being the object of inappropriate parental behavior is especially great when the child is viewed as a fantasy object or has been incorporated into the parent's delusional system. For example, a schizophrenic father wanted his infant son to become an opera singer and played loud opera music 24 hours a day in the baby's room. In rare cases the child may be terrorized, injured, or even killed by a parent who has delusionally turned the child into a persecutor or identified him with the parent's wish to die (Anthony, 1986). Children of severely disturbed parents may grow up feeling isolated from peers and the community because of the parent's illness. They may develop a confused sense of reality as a result of the parent's bizarre behavior. Sometimes the parent's strange actions and psychotic episodes have not been explained or discussed within the family, creating a sense of their "normality," which, as the child grows older, becomes increasingly dissonant with the larger social reality (Dunn, 1993). Children often become caretakers for their parents and siblings. They may develop strong feelings of guilt and disloyalty about differentiating themselves from the psychotic parent, as well as about their "failure" to change the parent (Dunn, 1993).

Studies of Maternal Depression. Maternal depression may have serious impacts on attachment and later development. Mothers with severe and chronic depression have insecurely attached children in the range of 55–87% across studies (Teti et al., 1995). Compared with nondepressed controls, depressed parents show less physical affection, play less with their infants, and provide less stimulation. Children experience frequent and long periods of disengagement from the parent preoccupied with depression (Field, 1992, 1998). Infants of depressed mothers are likely to develop difficulties in regulating feelings because of the parent's inconsistency in mutual regulation (Cummings & Davies, 1999). Depressed parents are more critical and more likely to view the child negatively. Children exposed repeatedly to such negative attributions often internalize them as self-representations that are critical, self-deprecating, and self-blaming. This creates vulnerability to depression in themselves (Goodman & Gotlib, 1999).

Some depressed parents, rather than ignoring or rejecting their children, require their children to take care of them, establishing an enmeshed relationship that restricts the development of autonomy (Radke-Yarrow et al., 1995). Depressed mothers who behave in this way foster the seemingly paradoxical combination of children who are securely attached yet function poorly outside the attachment relationship (Radke-Yarrow et al., 1995). Because of their strong identification with a severely depressed mother who lovingly demands that they remain totally involved with her, their movement toward autonomy, independent competence, and ability to relate to peers is compromised. Although secure attachment is almost always seen as a protective mechanism, in the special circumstances just described above a more distant relationship with the depressed parent can be deemed protective (Radke-Yarrow et al., 1995). This is also likely to be true of children of psychotic parents—lack of identification and distancing become protective factors. The most salient protective factor for children of mentally ill parents is an ongoing positive and developmentally appropriate relationship with another adult (Werner, 2000).

Parental Substance Abuse

Parental substance abuse presents a risk for large numbers of children. Approximately 11% of children in the United States, or 8.3 million, "live with at least one parent who is in need of treatment for an alcohol or illicit drug problem" (Maluccio & Ainsworth, 2003). Most substance-abusing parents have multiple risk factors, including child maltreatment, psychiatric disorders, marital conflict, or domestic violence. Drug or alcohol dependence is associated with maltreatment, particularly neglect. Addicted parents frequently fail to supervise their children or respond to their basic caregiving needs. Parental substance abuse is one of the most salient factors predicting that children will repeatedly come to the attention of Child Protective Services (Fuller & Wells, 2003). Although substance abuse cuts across all social classes, it is more common for low-income and impoverished people (Osofsky & Thompson, 2000).

Studies of prenatal exposure to cocaine, heroin, methadone, or marijuana have been inconsistent in documenting long-term defects that are clearly attributable to drug exposure. Additionally, there have been so few long-term studies to date that the effects on development beyond the first 3 years are unclear (Lester, Boukydis, & Twomey, 2000). Observations of jittery, inconsolable, disregulated "crack babies"—born addicted to cocaine because of prenatal exposure—led early researchers to predict serious ongoing neurological effects. Later studies showed that these initial effects were not permanent, leading to conclusions that minimized the effects of cocaine. More recently, a growing consensus suggests there is a range of effects that affect development in subtle rather than devastating ways (Lester, LaGasse, & Brunner, 1997).

The most common effects of prenatal drug exposure are intrauterine growth retardation, which causes low birth weight, and regulatory problems, such as decreased responsiveness or irritability after birth, as well as attentional problems and difficult temperament later in development. Studies of cocaine exposure have also shown subtle effects on IQ and more significant effects on language development (Lester, LaGasse, & Seifer, 1998; Bennett, Bendersky, & Lewis, 2002).

In spite of these effects, the consensus of studies seems to be that quality of caregiving after birth is a better predictor of developmental outcome (Zuckerman & Bresnahan, 1991). If caregiving is adequate, the effects seen soon after birth tend to gradually disappear. However, a parent who remains drug-addicted after the child's birth is unlikely to be a good caregiver. For a seriously addicted parent, the addiction takes priority over the needs of the children. Such a parent tends to be neglectful of physical and nutritional needs and emotionally uninvolved with the infant. Poor caregiving increases the negative effects of prenatal exposure (Black, Nair, Schuler, Keane, Snow, & Rigney, 1997). Further, substance-abusing parents are far more likely than other parents to physically or sexually abuse their children. Parental substance abuse is a contributing factor to 50% of all cases of substantiated child neglect and abuse and is therefore a significant factor in children's placement in foster care (Child Welfare League of America, 1998). Compared with parents who do not abuse drugs, parents with serious substance abuse are 4 times as likely to neglect their children, and these children are likely to enter foster care at a younger and more vulnerable age (National Center for Addiction and Substance Abuse, 1998; Semidei, Radel, & Nolan, 2001). Clinically, it is common to learn that children came to the attention of protective services because they were left alone while parents were away procuring drugs. As noted previously, the crack cocaine epidemic of the mid-1990s led to a large increase in foster placements of young children (U.S. Department of Health and Human Services, 1999). A study of children raised by mothers addicted to crack cocaine during the first 3–4 years of their lives showed much higher rates of emotional and behavioral disturbance, compared with a group of children reared by drug-free mothers. Problems with aggression, emotional regulation, and poor peer relationships characterized these children as preschoolers (Hawley, Halle, Drasin, & Thomas, 1995).

The effects of prenatal alcohol exposure are well established. Fetal alcohol syndrome, resulting from prenatal exposure to extremely heavy drinking by the mother, has long-term developmental sequelae (Institute of Medicine, 1996). Family interactions when one or both parents are alcoholics are characterized by inconsistency in the parent and uncertainty in the child, lack of parental warmth, and coercive parent–child dynamics, which other research has linked to behavior disorders in children (Steinglass, 1987; Campo & Rohner, 1992). The disruption of the parents' relationship due to one parent's alcoholism often leads to poorer parenting in the parent who is not an alcoholic (Leonard et al., 2000). School-age children who have grown up in families where one parent is an alcoholic have poorer social skills, peer relations, and academic performance (Sher, Walitzer, Wood, & Brent, 1991). Parental alcoholism increases a child's risk for abuse, witnessing domestic violence, and divorce, and in adolescence and young adulthood heightens risk for depression and substance abuse (Anda et al., 2002).

Overall, serious parental substance abuse creates risk because the parent's central relationship with the substance and his or her inconsistent and neglectful behavior when under the influence of drugs or alcohol creates a chaotic environment for the child: "Living with a parent with an addiction challenges the child's development of trust, attachment, autonomy, and self-esteem, and affects the child's ability to develop appropriate behavioral control and affect regulation" (Osofsky & Thompson, 2000, p. 61).

Community and Societal Risk Factors

The protective mechanism of responsive parenting is itself vulnerable to risk factors based on socioeconomic status, social disadvantage, racism, dangerous physical environments, and the generalized failure of a society to support families. Parents facing several contextual risk factors may not be able to provide adequate parenting, especially when these external stressors interact with parental and child risk factors (Ackerman, Izard, Schoff, Youngstrom, & Kogos, 1999). As children get older, they may encounter community risk factors directly, with less parental mediation than during early childhood. A child walking to school each day in a dangerous neighborhood may be exposed to frequent violence, illegal drug activity, and intimidation by gang members. If the child is aware that his parents cannot shield him from these dangers, his vulnerability to influence by antisocial peers may increase because he perceives them as more powerful than the adults who cannot protect him.

Social Policy and Risk

Compared with other industrialized nations, social policy in the United States increases risk for children, especially working-class and poor children. The United States provides far less programmatic support to children and families than do western European countries of comparable economic status. As of 2000, the United States was spending about 2.5%

of gross national product (GNP) on social assistance programs supporting families. By contrast, Sweden spent nearly 15% and France nearly 9%.
Comparing the rates of child poverty suggests the relationship between
social spending and poverty: the U.S. child poverty rate was 22.4%, while
Sweden's rate was 2.6% and France's was 7.9% (UNICEF, 2000).

Over the past 25 years, there has been a decline in the condition of
American children on a number of indicators: there have been increases
in child poverty, births to single teens, children in single-parent families,
children in homeless families, and child deaths and injuries by firearms.
Rates of child immunizations and children with medical insurance fell
during the 1980s and early 1990s, but rebounded somewhat in response
to federal child health programs established since 1993 (Children's Defense Fund, 1998).

Child poverty, an overarching risk factor, has increased dramatically. The poverty rate for children under 6 years of age is a critical indicator of risk, since the early period of development is more vulnerable to
disruption (Duncan, Brooks-Gunn, & Klebanov, 1994). The poverty rate
for children from birth to age 6 increased from the low point of 15.3% in
1969 to 22.7% in 1996. The rate dipped a bit during the second half of the
1990s but currently is increasing again (Children's Defense Fund, 1998,
2002). Nearly half of these 5 million preschool children are deeply impoverished, living in families making less than 50% of the federal poverty
level. African American and Hispanic children are more likely to be
growing up in poverty (54% and 44%, respectively); yet, poverty cuts
across all ethnic groups and is nearly as prevalent in rural as in urban
areas (McLoyd, 1998). Rural white children face the same degree of
socioemotional risk from poverty as children of color in urban areas
(Evans & English, 2002). However, since African American and Hispanic
children have higher rates of poverty than white children, they are disproportionately harmed by these societal risk factors (Conger, McLoyd,
Wallace, Sun, Simons, & Brody, 2002).

Early poverty, from birth to 6, and long-term poverty have the worst
effects. In combination, they can be devastating for children's development. The early years represent the period of greatest developmental vulnerability. *During these years U.S. children have the highest chance of being
poor* (Bradley & Corwyn, 2002). Children who lived in persistent poverty
during their early years score lower on assessments of cognitive and verbal schooling throughout their school careers, have lower academic
attainment, are more likely to repeat a grade or be placed in special education, and have higher school dropout rates. Long-term poor children
consistently have reading, math, and verbal skills deficits that are two to
three times greater than children who have been poor for a short period.
Finally, children growing up in the deepest poverty—in families whose
incomes are 50% below the federal poverty standard—have the worst

outcomes (McLoyd, 1998; Smith, Brooks-Gunn, & Klebanov, 1997; Korenman, Miller, & Sjaastad, 1995).

Once in poverty, American children are *more likely to remain in poverty* than children in any other industrialized country (UNICEF, 2000). This reality contrasts with the American ideology of opportunity and mobility. But it is consistent with social policies that limit opportunity for poor families. As of 2000, among industrialized countries, the U.S. spent the lowest percentage of GNP on social assistance programs (UNICEF, 2000). This deterioration of societal protection for children and families has been fueled by state and federal legislative and policy decisions, and by economic forces.

In the political climate of recent years, in which punitive attitudes in Congress have led to cuts in child and family support programs, the number of children affected by the devastating risk factor of poverty has been increasing (Edelman, 1997; UNICEF, 2000). However, since the *Personal Responsibility and Work Opportunity Reconciliation Act of 1996* (PRWORA, the welfare reform act) poverty has become harder to track. Although welfare reform has removed of millions of families from public assistance, it apparently has not reduced child poverty. Evidence for this comes from data on participation in the Food Stamps and School Lunch programs. To qualify for these programs, children must be at or below the federal poverty level. Even though decreases in welfare rolls range from 20 to 90% across states, participation in Food Stamps and School Lunch has been increasing, suggesting that "The economic situation for poor children in American has not improved with welfare reform but has in fact grown worse" (Lindsey & Martin, 2003, p. 169). While politicians supporting welfare reform point to success stories, only a small minority of families has escaped poverty in the transition from welfare to work. Poverty has deepened for a significant number of the most vulnerable families as welfare supports have been removed (Garfinkel, McLanahan, Tienda, & Brooks-Gunn, 2001; Winicki, 2003). Private-sector supports for families are also declining. For example, employers increasingly do not provide health insurance. Between 1987 and 2001, the percentage of children with health insurance provided by their parents' employers dropped from 64% to 51%. However, the number of children uninsured by any source has declined from about 25% to 15.5% because of congressional passage in 1997 of the State Children's Health Insurance Act (Reschovsky & Cunningham, 1998; Strunk & Reschovsky, 2002). This 15.5%, however, represents about 3.4 million children.

Poverty and Parenting

Poverty creates or intensifies many other risk factors that directly influence the child. The impact of poverty on young children is largely mediated through its impact on their parents (Conger et al., 2002). The daily stresses of chronic poverty tend to undermine a parent's sense of competence, engendering feelings of helplessness and frustration. Poor parents have little control over their lives. Economic constraints limit choices about where they will live and where their children will go to school. Poor children face destabilizing moves and school changes much more frequently than do middle-class children (McLoyd, 1998). The urban poor have no choice but to live in dangerous areas with high crime rates where their children may see violence or become victims of it.

Chronic poverty is dehumanizing and tends to damage parents' capacities for maintaining self-esteem and hope. These feelings tend to make parents become less responsive and more negative toward their children. Feelings of hopelessness, an external locus of control, and chronic economic distress are associated with higher rates of maternal depression and substance abuse, factors that further compromise parenting ability (Conger et al., 2002). Parents in chronic poverty tend to monitor their children's behavior less, with significant negative effects: "Low parental monitoring of children's peer activities has been associated with externalizing behavior problems in childhood . . . and with lower child competence in classroom peer activities" (Bolger et al., 1995, p. 1109). Parents who are poor have higher rates of single parenthood, divorce, harsh parenting, and child abuse and neglect (McLoyd, 1998).

These grim aggregate findings, however, should not be taken to mean that there are inevitable links between persistent poverty and poor outcomes for individual children. Parents who resist the stressors of poverty, provide support and adequate monitoring, and stay involved with their children's schooling provide important buffering for their children (Bolger et al., 1995). Positive attitudes in parents are linked to better adjustment by poor children: "A caregiver high in positive emotionality is likely to provide a warm, supportive, and empowering context for children's attempts to control themselves and their environment" (Ackerman et al., 1999, p. 1417). But such parents must be highly resilient themselves and must make extraordinary efforts on behalf of their children.

Other Risks Associated with Poverty

Poverty and disadvantage spawn other risk factors, including inadequate nutrition, inadequate housing and homelessness, inadequate child care, higher exposure to environmental toxins such as lead-based paint or industrial and gas/diesel pollutants, exposure to the danger of community violence, and lack of access to health care. These risks potentiate others. For example, a consequence of poor or inaccessible prenatal care is a higher rate of preterm infants born to poor families. Prematurity and neonatal health problems make the attachment process more difficult, setting the stage for the development of insecure attachments (Halpern, 1993). As children reach school age, poverty becomes associated with under-funded and therefore poorer schools (Kozol, 1991). The child who has grown up in poverty for 6 years enters school at a disadvantage because of the developmental effects of early poverty (Smith et al., 1997).

Welfare reform requires parents of infants and young children to seek full-time work. Working parents need child care, and the lack of ade-quate child care for poor families creates additional stress for parents as well as putting children at higher risk because of poor care. High-quality regulated child care is far less available in poor neighborhoods (Paulsell, Nogales, & Cohen, 2003). High-quality child care is also expensive, and therefore beyond the reach of parents working at low-wage jobs. Federal subsidies have not kept pace with the increasing costs of quality child care in the postwelfare reform years (Mezey, 2003).

Child Care: Risk or Protective Factor?

In the 1970s increasing numbers of women entered the work force, neces-sitating substitute care for their children. Between 1976 and 1998, the number of mothers who returned to work *before* their child's first birth-day rose from 31 to 59% (Brooks-Gunn, Han, & Waldfogel, 2002). Ap-proximately 70% of women with children under 3 are now working (Shonkoff & Phillips, 2000). Economic forces increasingly have made work outside the home not merely a choice but a necessity for working- and middle-class women. Since PRWORA (welfare reform) was enacted in 1996, even more women have entered the workforce, increasing the demand for child care.

While there have been debates about whether early child care is "good" for infants, the reality is that U.S. social policy provides little sup-port for early parenting, and consequently mothers, especially low-income mothers, must find substitute care for their infants in the early months of life. The Family Medical Leave Act of 1993 allows 12 weeks of job-protected unpaid leave following the birth of a child. However, only about half of U.S. workers are eligible because of the act's requirements that they work in businesses with 50 or more employees and have worked 1,250 hours during the preceding year. Many eligible low-income mothers do not use family leave because it is unpaid, and they cannot afford to take time off. A comparison of family-leave policies in Euro-pean countries provides perspective on U.S. policies: Sweden allows 64 weeks of job-protected and *paid* parental leave, and France permits 16 weeks of paid leave, followed by 3 years of job-protected unpaid leave (Kamerman, 2000; Waldfogel, 2001).

Quality in Child Care. Child care can be a protective or risk factor, depending on its quality. Quality matters—particularly for high-risk low-income children and to a somewhat lesser extent for middle-class children, whose privileged status provides protective processes that are less available to poor children (Peisner-Feinberg et al., 2001). Federal and state child care policies put low-income and working-class families at a disadvantage by failing to support a system of care that is accessible and affordable for most families with limited resources. In the United States, quality of child care is quite variable, although high-quality centers primarily serve middle-class children while low-income and working-class children in general receive lower-quality child care, whether in informal or center-based licensed care. Research and developmental theory clarify the ingredients of high-quality child care: "It is warm, supportive interactions with adults in a safe, healthy, and stimulating environment, where early education and trusting relationships combine to support individual children's physical, emotional, social, and intellectual development" (Scarr, 1998, p. 102; Shapiro & Applegate, 2002). High-quality centers also have more educated caregivers, pay higher wages, provide health insurance to staff, and have lower rates of staff turnover, which provides consistency of attachment, especially needed by infants and toddlers.

However, in national surveys of child care quality, 86% of centers were rated mediocre to poor in quality, and only 8% of infant care centers were rated as high in quality (Zigler & Hall, 2000). Lower-quality centers have fewer trained providers, pay low wages, and often do not offer health insurance benefits. The mean hourly wage in 1999 for all child care teachers was $7.42, less than one-third of the hourly wage of a public elementary school teacher (Center for the Child Care Workforce, 2001). Staff turnover is high in low-quality centers and affects young children's sense of stability and continuity.

Child Care Policy under Welfare Reform. In response to the work requirements of welfare reform, government spending on child care subsidies for low-income families doubled between 1997 and 2000. But even when funding was at its highest, 85% of eligible children *did not* receive subsidies. Currently, "due to funding limitations, only *one in every seven* children who are eligible for child care assistance under federal rules actually receives that help. Millions of low-income working families with children that need assistance do not get it because of insufficient funding for child care programs" (Parrott & Mezey, 2003). The Bush administration, aiming to shrink social expenditures and increase military spending, continues to reduce funding for child care subsidies. Many states, in response to the leveling off of federal funding in the context of a recessionary economy, have taken steps to limit access to child care subsidies (Ewen, Blank, Hart, & Schulman, 2002; Mezey, 2003).

Child Care Shortages for Vulnerable Groups. Five groups face shortages of child care spaces: infants and toddlers, children with disabilities, school-age children, children of parents who work nontraditional hours (after-noon and night shifts), and children from low-income families (Mezey, Schumacher, Greenberg, Lombardi, & Hutchins, 2002). There is a tremen-dous shortage of spaces for infants; yet, an increasing number of working mothers need infant care: 75% of infants in child care enter before age 4 months and average 28 hours a week in care (NICHD, 1997). For disad-vantaged families, early entry into care is another effect of the welfare reform act, which allows states to require mothers to return to work when their child reaches the age of 3 months (Shonkoff & Phillips, 2000). There is also a great shortage of after-school care for elementary school children, especially in impoverished areas, where risk to children is higher. Approx-imately 4 million school-age children care for themselves after school (Mezey et al., 2002).

Child Care and Risk for Disadvantaged Children. Inadequate child care resources create an additional risk for children who already face multiple risks related to low income. These children are disproportionately affected by the confluence of lack of child care slots, poor quality care, and inade-quate social policy. In general, licensed child care is less available in poor neighborhoods as compared to middle-class communities (Scarr, 1998). Experience in good child care serves as a protective factor for chil-dren, predicting increased cognitive and social competence in elementary school, particularly for those from disadvantaged families (NICHD, 2003; Peisner-Fineberg et al., 2001). Unfortunately, those children who benefit most from quality child care have the least access to it.

Racism and Minority Status

Minority status is a risk factor created from historical and structural rac-ism. Because of its historical roots, racism has been established as a value of the majority culture, now more often held covertly or even unknow-ingly than expressed overtly. In its institutional forms, including residen-tial and educational segregation and many forms of employment and economic discrimination, racism has limited opportunities for people of color, both historically and continuing into the present. In these structural forms, racism has led to economic disadvantage and disproportionately high poverty rates for African Americans and Hispanics. However, it is important to differentiate between racism and race as risk factors, because calling race a risk factor subtly shifts the source of risk to some-thing that is inherent in the individual. Race is not a cause of poverty, while racism and poverty are historically and structurally connected (McLoyd, 1998).

Racism as an attitude spans a range of beliefs, from negative stereo-typing to fears of difference to "color blindness," which denies cultural differences. Both minority and white children begin early to learn American values about race, and experimental studies have demonstrated that they already know by ages 4–6 that it is more desirable to be white (Spencer & Horowitz, 1973; Cross, 1985). Many minority children are able to resist applying negative racial or ethnic stereotypes to themselves, either because they have positive parental or other role models or because they use members of their own group as reference points for assessing themselves (Canino & Spurlock, 2000). Nevertheless, racial learning continues throughout childhood for minority and majority children not only through direct experiences with disadvantage or privilege but also through the imagery presented on television. Hirschfeld (1996) notes:

> For every episode of The Cosby Show a kid watches, he sees dozens of athletic shoe ads. These ads depict blacks as animal-like and dangerous, engaged in "violent" games of basketball played on inner-city courts and viewed through chain-link fences. When the child sees whites in these ads, they tend to be portrayed as disciplined, focused and controlled, running in parks or working out on sparkling exercise machines. What message do we expect children to take away from this? (p. 3)

Not only are ideas of white power and privilege and negative stereotypes of African Americans emphasized in such imagery, but also the images the minority child receives of himself are highly stylized and simplistic. The minority child who does not identify with the negative imagery may feel "invisible," because members of his group are not portrayed positively or with complexity (Spencer, 1990).

Some minority children may internalize negative images based on racism, although this is not a typical response (Spencer, 1985). Those who do, however—often because their parents have internalized and transmit negative racial messages—are particularly at risk for poor self-esteem and depression. In response to this risk and the general need to help children cope with racism, minority parents face added parenting stresses that white parents do not have to deal with (Hughes, 2003). African, Latino, and Asian American parents are more likely than European American parents to "make efforts to foster children's cultural pride and to teach them about their group's history and cultural practices" (Hughes, 2002, p. 16). Children who have more knowledge of their culture tend to have more positive self-concepts, better skills in solving problems, and fewer problem behaviors (Ou & McAdoo, 1993; Caughy, O'Campo, Randolph, & Nickerson, 2002). A high degree of ethnic knowledge also predicts a child's ability to understand prejudice, which provides conscious cognitive buffers against the psychological impact of exposure to racism (Quintana & Vera, 1999). African American parents are more likely than parents in other minority groups to explicitly prepare their children for experiences of bias. This represents a cultural coping mechanism by a group historically subjected to virulent racism and legal and institutional discrimination (Hughes, 2003). In a racist context, where children will face prejudice and discrimination, it is adaptive to prepare them for encounters with racism in the same sense that it is helpful to prepare a child in advance for any stressful situation such as a medical procedure.

Minority families may utilize other culturally based protective mechanisms that reduce risk. African American parents, for example, may gain support from membership in churches that have a strong communal orientation, from close ties to their extended family, and from family role flexibility such as sharing of child care by parents, grandparents, and other relatives (McAdoo, 2001). Hispanic family structure is also characterized by support from extended family networks and extraparental support of children through the system of godparents, or *compadres* (Garcia, 2001). Families from many Asian cultures embrace a strong orientation toward obligation to family, including sharing household work and communal economic contributions of individual family members (Shibusawa, 2001; Fuligni, Yip, & Tseng, 2002). These supportive mechanisms are cultural traditions. Although social support is seen as a protective factor in general, the ability to marshal support is critical for families living in poverty, because social isolation intensifies the effects of poverty. Studies of poor minority mothers found that ongoing social support increased their self-esteem, which was linked to more acceptance and warmth toward their children (McLoyd, 1998; Taylor & Roberts, 1995).

Whether exposure to racism becomes a significant risk factor depends on the balance of other risk and protective factors. Spencer (1990) has characterized minority status as "an at-risk *context* that is exacerbated by economic disadvantage" (p. 268; emphasis in original). In practice, the actual impact of racism must be assessed in the context of the individual child and her family (Williams-Gray, 2001; Webb, 2001). For some children, exposure to racism may be a clear risk because it contributes to feelings of hopelessness, negative images of the self, and depression. Other children, with the support of their parents and extended family, may regard racism as a challenge to master, in which case it does not pose the same degree of risk.

Exposure to Community Violence

In poor urban areas, children are exposed to high rates of community violence, which includes observing street fighting between gang members, seeing at close range wounded or dead victims of drive-by shootings, or becoming victims themselves. The most vulnerable children, as measured by the accumulation of other risk factors related to poverty, grow up in the most dangerous neighborhoods and have the highest rate of exposure to community violence (Buka, Stichick, Birdthistle, & Earls, 2001). As crimes involving firearms have increased in inner cities during the past 30 years, the chances of poor urban children witnessing assault and murder have increased. In areas where violence is common and chronic, many children witness *multiple* violent acts as they grow up (Selner-O'Hagan, Kindlon, Buka, Raudenbush, & Earls, 1998).

Garbarino (1995) argues that gang warfare linked to drug trafficking in these violent neighborhoods creates an atmosphere of actual violence and imminent threat akin to a war zone. In such an atmosphere, children are aware of the violence and danger of their neighborhood even though they may not have directly witnessed a murder or assault (Richters & Martinez, 1993). Neighborhoods where children are exposed to street violence also have elevated rates of family and school violence. Although it is not easy to establish directions of causality, it seems clear that many children grow up observing violence as an approach to dealing with problems or conflict (Buka et al., 2001; Lynch & Cicchetti, 1998).

Psychological Consequences of Exposure to Community Violence. Children exposed to chronic violence, whether at home or in the community, may develop symptoms of PTSD and make adaptations to trauma that interfere with development. Risk of trauma increases if the violence is intense, as in a shooting, when the child is close to the event, or when the child knows the victim or the perpetrator (Fick et al., 1997). One large-scale study found that 62% of perpetrators and 67% of victims were known to children who witnessed the violence (Richters & Martinez, 1993). When exposure to violence is repeated, or when the threat of violence remains high, the child may show a progression from symptoms of PTSD to defensive adaptations that stress toughness, emotional constriction, aggression, and uncaring behavior toward others. Children may both identify with the aggressor and the victim, developing a model of the self that requires aggressive behavior for self-protection yet also contains a fatalistic view that the child will die before adulthood. Boys are particularly likely to adopt aggression as a coping device. Although girl witnesses also use more aggression, they have PTSD symptoms and depression at very high rates as compared with males (Miller, Wasserman, Neugebauer, Gorman-Smith, & Kamboukos, 1999; Moses, 1999).

Children learn that the adults in their families and community are not able to prevent the violence from occurring. Adults trapped in poverty in violent neighborhoods may also become resigned and fatalistic, conveying to their children that violence cannot be prevented (Aisenberg & Mennen, 2000). In response to chronic trauma in the context of the failure of adult protectiveness, children may either become depressed and withdrawn or may adopt a violent stance themselves as a means of self-protection (Bell & Jenkins, 1993). Older school-age children may join gangs, model the behavior of violent older peers, and view possession of a gun as a sign of social status and safety (Garbarino, Dubrow, Kostelny, & Pardo, 1992).

Countervailing Protective Factors against Exposure to Violence. Embracing a violent lifestyle or depressive withdrawal, however, are not inevitable outcomes of living in a violent neighborhood. Consistent with general trends in resilience research, a stable, well-structured family and a safe (nonviolent) home environment significantly buffer children from the effects of violence occurring outside the home, as measured by their successful academic performance and relative freedom from behavioral symptoms. Children who receive support from competent parents and schools that promote and enforce a climate of safety appear most resilient in the face of a violent neighborhood (O'Donnell, Schwab-Stone, & Muyeed, 2002). Nevertheless, any child growing up in a violent neighborhood is at risk for victimization. In impoverished high-crime neighborhoods, protective parents, rather than drawing on support from neighbors, may attempt to insulate their children from neighborhood influences and monitor children's activities in very restrictive ways (Ceballo & McLoyd, 2002). The most adaptive parents, out of necessity, tend to overly restrict and control their children, which may interfere with normal developmental opportunities (Osofsky & Thompson, 2000).

Exposure to Media Violence

Television shows in the United States have higher levels of violent content than in any other country. The National Television Violence Study found that 60% of network TV shows (excluding public TV) regularly showed violence. Shows specifically targeting children depicted more violence than some other categories such as comedy, drama, and "reality TV" (Federman, 1997; American Academy of Pediatrics, 1995; Al-Mateen, 2002).

Children who see large amounts of media violence are at higher risk for committing violent acts in the short run, in childhood, and in the long run, as adults. The consensus of studies of children's exposure to media violence is that "the amount of TV and film violence a child is regularly watching is positively related to children's aggressiveness. Children who watch more violence on TV and in the movies behave more violently and express beliefs more accepting of aggressive behavior" (Huesmann, Moise-Titus, Podolski, & Eron, 2003, p. 203; Paik & Comstock, 1994). These effects tend to persist. A recent longitudinal study showed that both boys and girls who viewed more violence on television between the ages of 6 and 10 were at much greater risk for behaving violently as young adults (Huesmann et al., 2003). These effects were significant even after other risk factors such as harsh parenting and low-socioeconomic status (SES) were taken into account. By contrast, this study and others have shown that viewing violence as teenagers or adults does not predict violent behavior.

Young children are more influenced because their exposure occurs at a time in development when they are actively learning schemas of how the world works (Heusmann et al., 2003; Berkowitz, 1993). Media violence repeatedly presents children with behavioral scripts showing that violent acts solve problems and protect against danger. Young children tend to identify with powerful, aggressive characters, particularly when they are the "good guys" whose aggression is rewarded and glorified. These models reinforce the child's acceptance of violence as a means of responding to conflict. The stark representation of good–evil dichotomies in cartoon shows like *Batman* and films like *The Terminator* series causes young children to believe that violence is necessary and justified in the context of a dangerous world. Preschoolers are particularly likely to take in such schemas because they do not distinguish firmly between fantasy and reality and tend to believe the violent shows accurately represent the world as it is (Bushman & Huesmann, 2001). The effects of media violence can be moderated if parents clarify that the violence depicted is neither real nor an accurate representation of everyday life (Nathanson, 1999). A more powerful parental intervention, of course, is to monitor children's TV viewing and not allow them to watch violent shows.

Transactional–Developmental Variables That Increase Risk

Risk that the child's ability to cope with stress will be compromised or overwhelmed increases under the following conditions:

1. *When the child is unable to mobilize coping strategies that are adequate to cope with a stressor.* This is especially likely when the child is under 6 years of age and has not proceeded far enough in cognitive development to have established adequate appraisal strategies. The younger the child, the fewer internal adaptive coping mechanisms she will possess and the more vulnerable she will be to acute or enduring environmental stressors. Experiences of insecure attachment, maltreatment, or trauma during the first few years of life may by themselves push a child toward maladaptive developmental pathways, especially if countervailing protective processes are not present (Sroufe, 1997). Early chronic maltreatment has more severe developmental effects, for the reasons noted above and also because brain organization may be negatively affected (Perry, 2002a).

2. *When caregivers are not able or not available to reduce the child's stress.* Parenting is the critical mediator of risk. If parents are unable to buffer the child, he may be overwhelmed by environmental risk factors. Devel-

opment is a variable here as well. The effectiveness of protective factors related to internal characteristics of the child is mediated by developmental level. In general, the younger the child, the less effective such qualities as a positive attitude or above-average intelligence will be in mitigating risk and the more the child needs external protective factors that come from family support.

3. *When acute stressors interact with multiple ongoing risk factors, tipping the balance between coping and vulnerability.* For example, a child who appears resilient because of supportive parenting in spite of living in poverty in a neighborhood where violence is commonplace is traumatized by the murder of a classmate and becomes depressed and apathetic.

4. *When failures in active coping have become part of the child's expectations.* The child, through exposure to chronic stress, has learned there is nothing she can do to avoid the stress. As a result her sense of personal effectiveness decreases, and she may take the passive stance of "learned helplessness" (Lynch & Cicchetti, 1998). This is a common pattern in children who have been sexually or physically abused chronically from an early age. Such children do develop defenses to help them cope with the repeated abuse, but frequently the defenses are based on passive rather than active coping. The child begins to depend on defenses that split off emotion from experience, such as dissociation and isolation of affect (Macfie et al., 2001).

5. *When early maladaptive coping mechanisms and defenses have become rigidly established and then are mobilized in indiscriminate fashion in response to even minor stress.* For example, the young child who has been abused or has witnessed frequent domestic violence may become hypervigilant and easily aroused at any hint of aggression. Even in an inappropriate situation, as when another child speaks to him in a loud voice, he may attack the other child because his fear has become generalized. Reliance on early rigid defenses interferes with development because it limits the child's flexibility in appraising and responding to experience and prevents learning of more adaptive coping mechanisms.

6. *When the child is exposed to multiple risk factors over time and hence resilience diminishes.* The child's coping abilities are worn down and overwhelmed. Sameroff (1993) found that children whose environmental circumstances presented a high number of risk factors over time tended to do poorly. Summarizing a follow-up on children first studied at age 4, Sameroff (1993) states:

> We were disappointed to find little evidence of . . . resilient or invulnerable children. . . . At age 13 we found the same powerful relationship between environmental adversity and child behavior. Those children with the most environmental risk factors had the lowest competence ratings. . . . Whatever the child's ability for achieving high levels of competence, it was severely

undermined by the continuing paucity of environmental support. Whatever the capabilities provided to a child by individual factors, it is the environment that limits the opportunities for development. (p. 8)

CONCLUSION

It is important to conclude this extended discussion of risk factors and their potential impacts with a reminder that protective factors within the community, family, or child may be marshaled to ameliorate risk. Risk factors are not fate. Risk and protective processes are on a continuum and constantly interact. When protective processes are present across time, even in high-risk situations, children's development is guarded and resilience grows (Egeland et al., 1993; Werner, 2000).

Awareness of the presence of risk factors calls attention to the need for intervention, including preventive intervention if the effects of risk are not yet manifest. The findings of Sameroff et al. (1987, 1993) and Furstenberg and colleagues (1999) on the power of chronic and multiple risk factors suggest that the provision of protective factors should also be conceptualized from a long-term perspective. Programs aimed at decreasing risk through early intervention should not be thought of as inoculation against future risk. The protective internal characteristics of the child that are strengthened through early intervention will not stand up against multiple environmental risk factors. If early interventions work, they should be continued across the course of childhood and adolescence. Ramey and Ramey (1998) in their review of empirical research on early intervention programs have codified elements that provide the most protection for children's development:

- *Timing and longevity.* Programs that start when children are young and continue for several years have the greatest positive effects.
- *Intensity.* Intensive interventions "produce larger effects than do less intensive interventions" (p. 115). For example, a program that combines daily attendance at a good preschool with weekly home-based family sessions produces measurable benefits to disadvantaged children, while less intensive interventions make little difference. The more disadvantaged an at-risk child is, the more intensive an intervention must be.
- *Direct intervention.* Programs that intervene directly with children as well as with parents produce more change than indirect approaches such as parent training.
- *Comprehensiveness.* Interventions taking an ecological focus that includes individual and family interventions, as well as responsiveness to health, educational, and concrete needs of families, are

more effective than more circumscribed programs. The more disadvantaged and at-risk a child is, the more comprehensive intervention must be.

• *Risk/intensity relationship.* Intervention must take into account the degree of risk. While a child with few risk factors may make significant gains from a targeted, low-intensity intervention, another child with multiple risks will benefit only when intervention is both intensive and comprehensive.

• *Continuing intervention and support.* The positive effects of intervention on children in continuing high-risk situations will not be maintained unless there is continuing intervention that pays particular attention to augmenting protective processes in the child's environments.

Well-designed programs embodying the characteristics cited above can change the odds for better developmental outcomes for all children, and especially disadvantaged children. However, to be truly effective at a broader societal level, intervention programs must be continuously funded and accessible to all children who need them. Knowledge of risk and protective factors is an essential aspect of the social work practitioner's knowledge base. The next chapter illustrates the practical uses of a risk and protective factors analysis in evaluating children and their families.

APPENDIX 3.1. Summary of Risk and Protective Factors

Child Risk Factors

• Prematurity, birth anomalies
• Exposure to toxins *in utero*
• Chronic or serious illness
• Temperament: difficult or slow to warm up
• Mental retardation/low intelligence
• Childhood trauma
• Antisocial peer group

Parental/Family Risk Factors

• Insecure attachment
• Parent: insecure adult attachment pattern
• Single parenthood (with lack of support)
• Harsh parenting, maltreatment
• Family disorganization; low parental monitoring

- Social isolation, lack of support
- Domestic violence
- High parental conflict
- Separation/divorce, especially high-conflict divorce
- Parental psychopathology
- Parental substance abuse
- Parental illness
- Death of a parent or sibling
- Foster care placement

Social/Environmental Risk Factors

- Poverty
- Lack of access to medical care, health insurance, and social services
- Parental unemployment
- Homelessness
- Inadequate child care
- Exposure to racism, discrimination
- Poor schools
- Frequent change of residence and schools
- Exposure to environmental toxins
- Dangerous neighborhood
- Community violence
- Exposure to media violence

Child Protective Factors

- Good health
- Personality factors: easy temperament; positive disposition; active coping style; positive self-esteem, good social skills; internal locus of control; balance between help seeking and autonomy
- Above-average intelligence
- History of adequate development
- Hobbies and interests
- Good peer relationships

Parental/Family Protective Factors

- Secure attachment; positive and warm parent–child relationship
- Parent: secure adult attachment pattern
- Parents support child in times of stress
- Household rules and structure; parental monitoring of child

- Support/involvement of extended family, including help with caregiving
- Stable relationship between parents
- Parents model competence and good coping skills
- Family expectations of prosocial behavior
- High parental education

Social/Environmental Protective Factors

- Middle-class or above socioeconomic status
- Access to health care and social services
- Consistent parental employment
- Adequate housing
- Family religious faith and participation
- Good schools
- Supportive adults outside family who serve as role models/mentors to child

CHAPTER 4

Analysis of Risk and Protective Factors: Practice Applications

This chapter presents practice applications of the analysis of risk and protective factors. Risk and protective factors should be viewed from a developmental perspective. Infants and young children depend on external protective mechanisms—a secure attachment, protective parents, a predictable environment. As development proceeds, the child gradually becomes more capable of responding to stress using her own internal resources. For example, the school-age child can usually cope successfully with a separation from parents lasting several days, whereas a toddler, because of her cognitive limitations and the particular developmental tasks she is working on, may become symptomatic after a separation of less than a week.

HOW TO USE RISK FACTOR ANALYSIS

Risk factor analysis can be used in evaluation both predictively and retrospectively. If we identify a cluster of present risk factors, we can predict that unless some are eliminated, or protective factors are added, there may be a negative outcome for the client (Werner, 2000). Such an analysis helps us prioritize intervention goals so that we address first those issues that create the most immediate risk. We can also use an analysis of risk factors retrospectively to understand a child's current difficulties. Often we find, by asking careful questions during an evaluation, that the child's difficulties began during a period when there were several interacting risk factors. Identifying this cluster of risk factors and linking them to the current symptoms becomes our first step in understanding the child's problems. This chapter presents two cases that illustrate these two applications of an analysis of risk and protective factors.

PREDICTION OF RISK: ASSESSING CURRENT RISK AND PROTECTIVE FACTORS

The following case presentation describes a family that was thrown into crisis by the birth of a gravely ill baby. The parents' immediate adaptation to this crisis created significant stress for their older children, ages 2 and 5, and the crisis reverberated throughout the family. The case provides an illustration of how the analysis of current risk and protective factors can inform and guide evaluation and treatment.

Alan: A Case Example

Presenting Problems

Alan Emery was delivered by emergency cesarean section following a diagnosis of intrauterine fetal distress, at 2 weeks past his mother's due date. He was in extreme respiratory distress due to asphyxia caused by meconium aspiration. Meconium is fecal matter that in normal circumstances constitutes the infant's first bowel movement after birth. Alan's distress *in utero* (cause undetermined) caused his bowels to release the meconium into the amniotic fluid in the womb. Infants "breathe" the amniotic fluid as their lungs develop. Alan's lungs had taken in the meconium in the amniotic fluid, causing severe damage to them. Because of his extremely grave condition, he was rushed to a neonatal intensive care unit (NICU) at a major medical center. He was placed on a heart–lung machine for 3 days and remained in intensive care for 3 weeks before being transferred to the moderate care nursery.

Alan made a spectacular recovery with the aid of skilled medical care and cutting-edge technology. After he was out of danger, his mother, Mrs. Emery, remained very anxious and agitated, because she had been told that Alan's birth asphyxia had caused brain damage that would result in an undetermined degree of mental retardation. She asked: "How retarded will he be? Can we take care of him at home? Will he be able to go to school? Will he have to be put in an institution?" The medical staff had been concerned about Mrs. Emery throughout Alan's hospitalization because she had asked ceaseless questions about his condition but had not been able to take in the staff's necessarily tentative answers because her anxiety was so intense. Because of Mrs. Emery's increasing agitation, the NICU staff began to question her ability to care for Alan after discharge and referred the family to the Infant Mental Health Unit.

Assessment

I met with Mr. and Mrs. Emery about 4 weeks after Alan's birth, after his medical condition was stable. Even though Alan was no longer in danger, the assessment was carried out in an atmosphere of relative crisis, which waxed and waned as stress increased and subsided. Because of the crisis atmosphere, and because of emerging stressors that increased risk for the mother, infant, and other family members, it became necessary to constantly assess the balance of risk and protective factors. In order to help the reader appreciate the fluidity of a crisis situation that bred further crisis, I will first present the events as they emerged and then discuss how the analysis of risk and protective factors contributed to the intervention plan.

I was introduced to Mr. and Mrs. Emery as a social worker with the Infant Mental Health Unit at a predischarge planning meeting with the medical staff. Mr. Emery was a 46-year-old African American, while Mrs. Emery was Latina and 40 years of age. During the meeting the parents were told that tests had confirmed that Alan had sustained brain damage and severe hearing loss in both ears. The medical team also recommended a number of services and evaluations for Alan following discharge. After the meeting I talked with them in the hall. Mrs. Emery was clearly very anxious as she tried to sort through the potential meanings of brain damage and hearing loss for Alan's subsequent development. Mr. Emery was more concerned about how they would follow through on the many services that had been recommended. I offered to help them prioritize and sequence the recommendations. I also told them that I was familiar with infant development and could provide ongoing assessment of Alan's progress. They accepted these offers.

During this brief interview, I also asked about the family and learned that the Emerys had two other young children, Jimmy, age 2, and Paul, age 5. They had been staying with a family friend for nearly 3 weeks while both parents were preoccupied with Alan's condition and spending long hours at the hospital. Mrs. Emery's 15-year-old son and 19-year-old daughter from a previous marriage also lived at home. Mr. Emery told me that he was permanently disabled from working because of a serious diabetic condition. He was concerned about the cost of the follow-up services for Alan because their sole income was his Social Security disability benefits, which were currently just adequate to support the family. Mrs. Emery referred to her "nerves" and asked if I could prescribe medication. I offered to arrange for her to see a psychiatrist with our program. At this early point in the assessment I was concerned about potential risk factors associated with life-threatening illness at birth. Although my concern focused on Alan and Mrs. Emery, as individuals and as a dyad, there were other immediate family risks to consider. Risk factors that were either potential or present and contributing to stress at this point are summarized below:

Child risk factors: Alan

- Health status: residuals from heart–lung machine treatment; seizure disorder(?)
- Medical trauma as possible interference with attachment(?)
- Virtual separation from parents while in intensive care for 17 days a further interference with attachment(?)

Maternal risk factors: Mrs. Emery

- Traumatic delivery experience; traumatic reactions to child's near death(?)
- Health status: recovering from major surgery
- Psychiatric status: Intense anxiety/confusion an interference with attachment and caregiving ability(?)

Family risk factors

- Father's health status: disabling diabetic condition
- Reactions of younger children (especially 2-year-old Jimmy) to month-long separation from parents, older siblings
- Overall disruption of family routines
- Family overwhelmed by need to arrange many postdischarge services for baby
- Financial stress: marginal fixed income

Observations of Parents and Infant

Two days later I met with Mr. and Mrs. Emery as they visited Alan in the moderate care nursery. Because of the medical reports, I had prepared myself to see an unresponsive baby. I had also wondered if Mrs. Emery's anxiety would compromise her ability to respond to him. Alan, now 5 weeks old, was a large, placid-looking infant who was focusing on his mother's face as I entered the room. She was smiling and talking to him, and he watched her alertly. As she held Alan, Mrs. Emery told me how much progress he had made. He had been comatose at birth, and she had believed he "would not make it." She smiled at Alan and said in a bright, singsong tone, "Yes, you were lying so still, we thought you'd never wake up. But you did, and look at you now!"

While she held Alan, she told me the story of his birth. She had known something was wrong because the baby had stopped moving. She called her doctor, who reassured her that often there was less movement as delivery approached. But the next day she was certain that something was wrong and went to the emergency room. Immediately after she had been examined, she was taken to the operating room. She was awake during the cesarian-section surgery. She realized something was wrong with her baby when she saw the doctors frantically trying to resuscitate him. Later she would expand the story, adding that she had been convinced that Alan was dead and that the doctors were lying to her because they wanted to cover up their mistakes. However, just before Alan was rushed to the NICU, the surgeon had her touch his chest. She could feel his heart beating. Mrs. Emery commented that after being discharged following surgery she had been shocked when she saw Alan in the NICU. He was unmoving and unresponsive.

At the end of this visit, both parents voiced optimism about Alan's future. They said that if he was retarded they would make sure he got special education help. Mrs. Emery expressed apprehension about Alan's coming home, but I was struck by how much calmer and organized she seemed while holding Alan, compared to the reports of her distress and agitation. Being in physical and affective contact with her baby seemed to calm her. We arranged to meet at least one more time before Alan's discharge, which was expected in the next 5–10 days. After this interview and observation I felt more optimistic because I had a clearer picture of the family's strengths that would likely serve as protective factors. Mrs. Emery's responsive caregiving and Alan's alertness diminished my concern about the risk of poor attachment and inadequate caretaking. Some of the potential risk factors were discounted, and those that remained seemed balanced by several protective factors:

Protective factors, observed in hospital before Alan's discharge

- Mother–infant attachment is proceeding well; mother is invested in baby and comfortable caring for him.
- Baby is alert and responsive in spite of health problems.
- Relationship between parents appears cohesive: they are in agreement about the baby's needs.
- Father is invested in the baby and appropriately concerned about how to organize and manage his care.
- Availability of supportive friends (the family that cared for Jimmy and Paul) is an important backup.

In the treatment plan that was emerging in my mind, I expected to provide ongoing support for the development of attachment, monitor Alan's developmental progress, and possibly advocate for early intervention services. Our program allowed for home visits, and I expected to see the family at home once a week. I reviewed these ideas with Mr. and Mrs. Emery, and they agreed. Mrs. Emery again requested medication, and I arranged a psychiatric appointment for her for 2 days later. I also set an individual appointment with me for 3 days later. My perception of Mrs. Emery had begun to change. Although she was still anxious, her calmness when she was with Alan challenged my previous belief that she was in crisis. I was also aware that I had not yet taken the parents' histories and that I did not know what Mrs. Emery was like when she was not under severe stress. Nevertheless, the good quality of her interaction with Alan seemed reassuring.

An Emerging Crisis

However, the case was moving into a critical phase. I will describe the events of a tumultuous week. Mrs. Emery canceled her psychiatric appointment and missed her Friday meeting with me. I could not reach her by phone. In retrospect it was clear that these missed appointments were symptomatic of Mrs. Emery's intensifying anxiety and disorganization as Alan's discharge approached. I learned later that the next day, Saturday, she had been brought to the Medical Center emergency room by ambulance because of a possible heart attack. However, she had been cleared medically, given an antianxiety medication, and referred to the Adult Psychiatry Service. On Sunday Alan's physicians ordered his discharge for the following day.

The discharge decision was made on the basis of Alan's medical stabilization, the medical staff's perception that Mrs. Emery was a competent though anxious mother with good support by Mr. Emery, and their assumption that the Infant program was working with the family. I did not know that discharge was imminent, and the medical staff did not know that she had not kept her Friday appointment with me. Nor did Mrs. Emery inform Alan's doctors about her emergency room visit. When I read the emergency room summary a week later, it was also clear that Mrs. Emery did not provide the physician there with a link between her somatizing anxiety symptoms and her awareness that Alan would be discharged soon. Structural factors in a complex institution contributed to a lack of communication between professionals, and Mrs. Emery also presented a different set of concerns and different parts of her story to different professionals. *No one had the whole picture,* and in retrospect it appeared that Mrs. Emery had unconsciously disrupted professional coordination because of her deepening distress. To the list of risk factors, we now need to add some institutional ones:

Institutional risk factors
- Family relating to large, decentralized medical institution
- Inadequate or slow communication among hospital departments

Social workers who work in large institutions or coordinate clients' care across agencies must always be on the alert for structural factors that may increase risk for clients.

On Tuesday, when I learned that Alan had been discharged, I called Mrs. Emery. She said that Alan was doing well but that she was feeling terrible because she had not been able to sleep for 3 nights. She again asked me to arrange an appointment with a psychiatrist. I scheduled an appointment for the next day. At this point I did not know and she did not tell me about her emergency room visit or their referral of her to the Adult Psychiatry Service. When I was informed that Mrs. Emery had canceled her psychiatric appointment on Wednesday, I called her again. She asked me many questions with intense and pressured affect. Repeatedly she tried to establish my role: "Will you talk with me about the baby's development?" and "Isn't it the psychiatrist's job to talk to me if I want to talk about my problems?" Recognizing that she was frightened by a focus on herself, I restated our original agreement—that I would monitor Alan's development. She said, "So, you'll be the baby's therapist, and if I need someone to talk to I can see the psychiatrist." I agreed. Because of her agitated and disorganized presentation, I suggested a home visit that evening.

When I arrived, Mr. Emery greeted me and showed me that Alan was sleeping in a bassinet. He said that Alan was doing fine but that his wife was upset. Mrs. Emery appeared severely depressed and anxious. She talked in an agitated manner, and at times her thinking became tangential with some loosening of associations. She retold the story of the cesarean, focusing on how she thought the baby was dead. I said that I thought she was tremendously upset by what had happened to her and her baby and that she was worried about her baby now that he was home. She agreed and again asked for medication. Because of the psychotic features in her presentation, I suggested an evaluation by the Adult Psychiatry Service, which she agreed to.

When she was seen at the Adult Psychiatric Clinic the next day, she appeared only anxious, not psychotic. When I came for the next home visit a day later, on Friday, Mrs. Emery was clearly psychotic. She had constructed a paranoid delusional system involving being damaged by doctors. She complained that she and Alan had been guinea pigs for the hospital and that doctors had been monitoring her movements and taking pictures of her. She said that a newscaster had spoken directly to her from the TV, saying, "We know what you did." The psychosis, with its externalization of blame, persecutory delusions, and fantasies of malevolent damage, could be understood as a desperate defense against overwhelming guilt that she was responsible for her baby's damage, as well as unacceptable rage at the physician who at first did not take her concerns about the baby seriously. Given her unconscious sense of having "caused" her baby to nearly die, she was terrified of damaging him further. Her acute psychosis had been precipitated by Alan's discharge. Mr. Emery confirmed that she had never expressed delusional ideas in the past, which supported the diagnostic impression of a brief reactive psychosis precipitated by severe stress.

Reassessment: The Crisis of Mrs. Emery's Psychosis

Changes in the lives of clients often require reassessment from the perspective of the new circumstances. A case that had begun in a medical crisis had now evolved into a psychiatric crisis. Mrs. Emery had met with the Adult Clinic psychiatrist a second time, and antipsychotic medication and hospitalization had been recommended. She had refused both. She angrily told me, "That psychiatrist wanted to take me away from my baby. I told her to forget it!" (It was interesting to learn from the psychiatrist that Mrs. Emery had brought Alan to the appointment and had cared for him appropriately during the interview.) Mrs. Emery's psychosis and her refusal of treatment that focused on her as an individual forced me to reconsider the original treatment plan of supporting the family and providing ongoing assessment of Alan's development. It was uncertain that this treatment plan would be adequate, given Mrs. Emery's inner disorganization and uncertain contact with reality. Other questions had to be evaluated before deciding whether to continue with the original treatment plan or to institute a new one. The most pressing questions were whether Mrs. Emery's psychosis put Alan and her other children at risk and whether other family members would be able to moderate that risk.

The emphasis of this crisis reassessment was on *the analysis of family risk and protective factors*. While ongoing assessment in the context of intervention sometimes reveals new problems, it may also reveal new resources that were not evident in the original assessment. During the second home visit and two home visits the following week, it was evident that even though Mrs. Emery was manifestly psychotic, she was affectively in touch with Alan, responsive to his signs, and able to hold and feed him. She was also able to speak for him, telling Mr. Emery to change his diaper or her teenage son to quiet the younger children while Alan was sleeping. These warm, concerned, and appropriate responses to Alan alternated with delusional outbursts against the doctors. Even though Mrs. Emery was psychotic, Alan was not being drawn into her delusional system. On the contrary, her relationship with him seemed to be an island of reality and calm for her. Mr. Emery competently cared for Alan and kept the household going, insisting that Mrs. Emery rest. His inability to work outside the home, conventionally a risk factor, was in this case a protective factor because it allowed Mr. Emery to be consistently available to his wife and children.

At the fourth home visit, I met Mrs. Emery's 19-year-old daughter, Bettina. When I arrived she was diapering Alan. While I talked with Mrs. Emery, Bettina rocked Alan and sometimes joined in the conversation. Mrs. Emery seemed at ease with her daughter's caretaking. I had known Bettina lived at home and that she was working and attending a community college. I observed that she looked very comfortable with Alan. I commented on this, and she said she liked to take care of him. I said that it was good she was able to help her mother while she was recovering. I felt relieved that here was another competent family member who was sanctioned by Mrs. Emery as a caregiver for Alan. During this same visit I met the public health nurse who had begun visiting to monitor Alan's physical status. With Mr. and Mrs. Emery's assent, we agreed that we would each visit twice a week on alternating days to maximize professional monitoring of Alan's development and, implicitly, Mrs. Emery's status. Ongoing assessment thus revealed new protective factors that balanced the acute risk of Mrs. Emery's psychosis:

Emergent risk factors, postdischarge

- Mother's acute reactive psychosis is precipitated by baby's discharge.
- Mother's refusal of psychiatric intervention appears to escalate risk.

Protective factors, observed during home visits

- Father is competent to care for baby *and* available.
- Teenage children are part of family and able to help out.
- Baby is separated from mother's psychosis.
- Infant mental health worker (social worker) is making frequent home visits.
- Public health nurse is making home visits on other days.
- Parents have access to health care system and other supportive services.

In spite of Mrs. Emery's reactive psychosis, the presence of these additional protective factors made it possible to maintain the outlines of the original treatment plan. I was ambivalent about this decision because of the risk posed by Mrs. Emery's psychosis. The public health nurse's impressions agreed with mine that Alan was receiving adequate care and that Mrs. Emery was highly invested in him. It was very helpful to have another professional confirm my perceptions of a situation that was so anxiety-provoking. The revised intervention plan maintained the goal of monitoring Alan's developmental status but added an objective that specifically supported Mrs. Emery's recovery from psychosis. This objective was based on the observation that Mrs. Emery was not delusional in her caretaking of Alan. Rather, when she was engaged with him, she appeared neither psychotic nor anxious. She implicitly used Alan as an organizer of her experience. Hypothesizing that the trauma of Alan's near death and Mrs. Emery's irrational belief that she had damaged him had precipitated her psychosis, I believed that as Mrs. Emery saw Alan as developing and viable she would be reassured by the "real baby" and be able to give up her overwhelming guilt and rage and the psychotic defense against these feelings (Blos & Davies, 1993; Albright, 2002).

This assumption was also based on an understanding of the usual course of reactive psychosis (American Psychiatric Association, 2000; Horowitz, 1986). The features of brief reactive psychosis are psychotic symptoms such as delusions, behavioral disorganization, disorganized speech, and hallucinations. In nearly all cases there is a major stressor that precipitates the psychotic episode. By definition, it is time-limited, lasting from a day up to a month. The psychotic symptoms diminish as the stress decreases, and gradually the person returns to his or her previous level of functioning. Brief reactive psychosis is not related to schizophrenia. It is more common in people with personality disorders (American Psychiatric Association, 2000). Horowitz (1986) sees reactive psychosis on a continuum with other stress response disorders as an extreme expression of posttraumatic stress disorder. An additional—and crucial—consideration in this case was that Mrs. Emery had intensive and coordinated support from many sources, most prominently her husband, but also her adolescent children, the public health nurse, and myself (Ramey & Ramey, 1998).

A Realistic View of the Baby Decreases Stress

Within a month following Alan's discharge, Mrs. Emery showed only occasional flashes of psychotic symptoms. As she invested more and more in Alan, she became increasingly oriented to reality. Our collaborative work during this period focused on a weekly assessment of Alan's development. At each home visit, we watched Alan together. Mrs. Emery would tell me her observations of Alan's behavior and raise questions about its meanings. She was convinced that he responded to sounds by turning his head, which led her to question the diagnosis of severe hearing loss. I suggested that she explore this question with Alan's pediatrician. It was obvious to both of us, however, that Alan was developing within normal limits affectively and socially. At 2 months, he was smiling, responding with pleasure when he was cuddled, and crying when he was uncomfortable. To Mrs. Emery, who had already cared for four babies, these were heartening signs that Alan, in spite of his traumatic early history, was a normal baby in many ways. Gradually, we were putting together a coherent picture of Alan that included his strengths and limitations. Increasingly, I felt that this accurate view of the real baby in front of her was replacing the terrifying first image of Alan as unmoving and lifeless. As this occurred, her psychosis disappeared.

Who Is at Risk?: A Family Perspective

Parallel with this assessment and intervention on Alan's behalf, another story of family stress was unfolding: Jimmy's and Paul's reactions to the separation from both parents and to Mrs. Emery's reactive psychosis. Their behavior made clear that it was essential to extend the assessment of risk beyond the identified client. Each child expressed distress in behavior typical of his age.

Jimmy, at 25 months, was extremely needy following the month-long separation from his mother. He tried to follow her everywhere, made constant demands for snacks, and had tantrums if he was refused anything. Such behavior represents normal responses of a toddler to stress. However, his mother, given her intense preoccupation with Alan, could not tolerate having another child with difficulties. Instead of being able to read Jimmy's behavior as the anxious reactions of a young child whose attachment has been disrupted, she saw his actions as "bad" and "mean." The unhappy combination of Jimmy's 2-year-old oppositionalism and his severe anxiety regarding attachment was leading to behavior that brought punitive responses from his parents. It also appeared that Jimmy's behavior represented for Mrs. Emery an acting-out of the "craziness" she was trying so hard to suppress in herself.

Paul was dealing with his own separation distress by trying to win his parents' approval by being the good boy. This too was consistent with his developmental level. At age 5 he was in the process of internalizing a conscience and was thus eager to suppress negative or hostile impulses in himself. He was using Jimmy as a scapegoat, displacing his own angry feelings onto Jimmy and at times goading him into misbehavior. Then, when Jimmy misbehaved, Paul would seek his mother's attention by telling on Jimmy. In a particularly poignant example of this dynamic, Jimmy went to his mother's room and smeared his face with Mrs. Emery's cosmetics, and Paul rushed to tell his mother. Mrs. Emery punished Jimmy. She was still caught up in the blunted and concrete thinking of an individual recovering from psychosis and was unable to see that Jimmy's behavior might represent an attempt to get close to her by putting on the cosmetics he associated with her smell and touch.

Jimmy's and Paul's problems were at first difficult to incorporate into the treatment plan because Mrs. Emery was so exclusively concerned about Alan. Further, given her guilt-ridden psychosis and anxiety, it was not possible to link Jimmy's behavior to the separation or to suggest she change her reactions toward him. In the short run, I addressed their issues by suggesting to Mr. Emery that he give them more attention, and I also employed emergency "sidewalk counseling." I would talk to the boys outside and put into words the upset and worry they had experienced during the separation and their confusion about how different their mother had become since returning home. After 2 months of home visits, when Alan was about 4 months of age and Mrs. Emery had begun to feel more confident about his development, she was able to turn to Jimmy and Paul and tell them she understood their upset. With her returning capacity for empathy, she was more able to respond warmly to them as she had before the crisis of Alan's illness.

The analysis of risk should be applied to all family members, not just the identified client (Blos & Davies, 1993; Lynch & Cicchetti, 1998). The Emery case demonstrates how accumulating risk factors can put other family members at risk. Clearly, Mrs. Emery's separation from Jimmy and her angry punitiveness toward him were putting his development at risk. The risk was intensified by his developmental status as a toddler. While Paul was less obviously at risk, his excessive tattling on Jimmy suggested that he was also struggling with reactions to the separation and loss of his mother's emotional responsiveness.

Lessons from the Analysis of Risk and Protective Factors

Especially in emergent crises it is important to do a careful analysis of risk and protective factors and try to figure out how to augment the protective factors as a means of reducing the risk factors. For the purposes of intervention planning, it is necessary to distinguish between immediate and potential long-term risk factors. For example, preliminary assessments suggested that Alan would be mentally retarded. However, that risk factor was not of immediate importance. By contrast, Mrs. Emery's intense anxiety was of more immediate concern. Further, new and unexpected risk factors emerged when Alan's discharge increased the stress on the family. Ongoing assessment of the balance of risk and protective factors became critical when Mrs. Emery's psychosis emerged, given its potential to compromise her ability to care for Alan. Was Alan at risk for neglect? For abuse? Would a Protective Services report need to be filed? Should Mrs. Emery be hospitalized? Since she refused hospitalization, should she be committed? The answers to these questions had a bearing not just on treatment goals but on *serious case management decisions* that had the potential to change this family's life.

When she was psychotic, Mrs. Emery established a clear split between, on the one hand, the physicians she delusionally believed had damaged Alan and, on the other, those helpers, including myself, the public health nurse, and Alan's pediatrician, whom she saw as helping her with her baby. Mrs. Emery implicitly realized that I accepted her requirement that I focus on the baby, not her, and that I take a positive approach that avoided any hints of blame that would reverberate with the overwhelming self-blame the psychosis was defending against. I was very reluctant to raise any issue that she would perceive as criticism. Essentially, I felt that if Protective Services and/or the legal system became involved, the Emerys would shift from being voluntary to involuntary clients and that their view of me would shift from helper to harmer. I believed that Mrs. Emery, given her delusional state, would only be able to see a Protective Services report as cruel and punitive toward her, and so my alliance with her would be destroyed. I also believed that such an "insult" would help perpetuate her psychosis because she would see it as another example of persecution by a professional. Yet, if abuse or neglect is suspected, social workers are required by law to report it. The ability to do home visits and the careful analysis of risk and protective factors enabled me to see the particular strengths of this family and the particular quality of Mrs. Emery's psychosis. This analysis yielded the conclusion that Alan was not at risk for abuse or neglect, in spite of being exposed to the typically high-risk situation of a parental psychosis.

RETROSPECTIVE ANALYSIS OF RISK AND PROTECTIVE FACTORS

The retrospective analysis of past impacts of risk factors must be based on a detailed knowledge of development. In evaluating an older child, the practitioner tries to learn what stressors the child has been exposed to throughout her development and what protective mechanisms may have moderated those stressors. Often such an analysis illuminates connections between the child's current symptoms and past risk factors, leading to an understanding of how the child adapted to past stressors and how those adaptations carry over into her current behavior.

Assessment of External and Internal Adaptations to Risk

Children may adapt to harsh parenting, abuse, or witnessing domestic violence in early childhood by developing behavior problems, which may show up as defiance of adults and aggression toward peers. These children are likely to come to our attention when they reach school age because their behavior is so problematic. However, in assessing the potential impacts of early risk factors, it is important also to look at developmental progress, adaptation, and current symptoms in terms of the child's internal life. Some resiliency literature inappropriately tends to equate behavioral adaptation with mental health (Luthar, Cicchetti, & Becker, 2000). But a school-age child may appear to be functioning well superficially, in that he does his work and does not get into trouble, yet may be beset with anxiety that interferes with peer relationships and the development of autonomy. Indeed, although disruptive behavior problems are more likely to lead to a referral of a child, anxiety disorders are the most common type of childhood psychiatric problem (Albano, Chorpita, & Barlow, 2003). Children may be functioning adaptively, judged by behavioral measures, yet score high on measures of internalizing symptoms such as anxiety and depression (Luthar & Zigler, 1991). Resilience is often a mixed picture—a child is resilient in some areas but vulnerable or rigidly defended in others. Resilience developed in response to severe stress and risk conditions often has costs (Luthar et al., 2000).

Assessing the Evolution of Early Risk Factors

In retrospective analysis of the impact of stressors on young children, it is particularly important to try to understand the quality of attachment during the period of risk and to determine whether the attachment has been a significant protective factor over time. During the first 2 years of life coping is primarily a transactional process, with the infant signaling distress and the caregiver responding with soothing or stimulation, which restores the infant's affective equilibrium. Only gradually does the child develop effective internalized coping mechanisms. During the preschool years, the child's ability to regulate affect and behavior and to organize experience cognitively continues to depend in a large degree on parental responsiveness and on transactional patterns of affect and behavior regulation. Toddlers and preschoolers, because of normative limitations in level of cognitive development, are prone to interpret experience in concrete, egocentric, and magical ways that confuse cause and effect and fail to distinguish between thought and action. These cognitive limitations, as well as immature internalized mechanisms for dealing with stress, leave the young child vulnerable to stressful or traumatic experiences. The younger the child, the more likely that she will become behaviorally disorganized and traumatized when stress is extreme because she lacks skills for mastering stress through cognition or action.

Parents play a critical role in supporting and developing the young child's capacity for affect regulation by providing comfort, by modeling coping strategies, and by explaining and clarifying their experiences, particularly those that are stressful for the child. If the parent is unable to help the young child modulate his reactions to serious stress, the child has the frightening internal experience of having to confront the anxiety-producing stressor alone. In this emergency, the young child is likely to develop an array of defenses that may include dissociation and other forms of affective inhibition, as well as tendencies toward being controlling and relying on fantasies of omnipotence and more action-oriented defenses such as acting out, restlessness, and identification with the aggressor (Pynoos et al., 1996). These defenses are reinforced by the child's affective reactivity to current stimuli reminiscent of the stressful situation and, for some children, conscious ongoing fantasies that the stressful or traumatic events will be repeated. This interplay of fantasy and defense then may be carried along through time, shaping the child's emotional life and orientation to the world. However, what adults usually see, and often misread, are the behavioral manifestations of the child's defenses. They are less likely to be aware of the child's fantasies and fear of repetition of stressful or traumatic events (Scherringa & Gaensbauer, 2000).

When the parent is unable to help the child modulate her reactions to stress, a problem that began in a linear process of cause and effect is often transformed into an transactional problem that is best thought of as bidirectional and circular. The child's symptoms are unfortunately reinforced and maintained by parental responses. For example, in the previous clinical illustration, Jimmy Emery's attachment with both parents was disrupted by the month-long separation following his brother's birth. Jimmy reacted with anger and despair. When he came home he expressed these feelings in the nonverbal behavior typical of toddlers. He was defiant, insistent on getting his way, and apparently intentionally destructive, as when he made a mess of his mother's cosmetics. His mother, especially during her brief psychosis, responded with frustration and anger, punishing him for actions she was only able to read as misbehavior. Her reactions increased his sense of her emotional distance and led to increased anger and misbehavior. The adaptive task for Jimmy and his mother was to find a way to reestablish a secure attachment before these symptom-based transactions evolved into a characteristic style of interaction between them. Fortunately, the resolution of her psychosis and the lessening of her anxiety about the baby allowed her to see Jimmy more sympathetically and to respond to him in more nurturant ways, which, also in circular fashion, helped him feel more connected to her and led to less symptomatic behavior. In cases where symptoms have persisted for a long time, it is necessary to identify in the risk factor analysis transactional patterns that perpetuate the symptoms.

Alex: A Case Example

Presenting Problems and Assessment

Alex Carty was an 8-year-old European American boy whose presenting problems included aggression toward his mother and sometimes toward peers at school, restlessness and disruptiveness in class, and difficulty concentrating on schoolwork. Shortly before referral he had hit a girl in the head with a rock and injured her. The school social worker described him as "impulsive, aggressive, and possibly on his way to a conduct dis- order." Both his mother and teacher saw him as an anxious, "jumpy" child who always seemed to be on alert. His parents had divorced 3 years previously. Alex's father had been abusive to his mother and to Alex. Alex had witnessed many physical fights and arguments between his parents. Beginning at age 2, he also became the object of his father's impulsive verbal and physical attacks. His mother, who had been victim- ized herself, had been unable to protect Alex. The attachment relationship could not mediate the experience for Alex because his mother was depressed, overwhelmed, and traumatized herself. The parental separa- tion occurred when Alex was nearly 5. His father left the state and cut off contact, so Alex had not seen his father for more than 3 years. At the time of the evaluation, Ms. Carty alternated between angrily rejecting Alex for his aggressive behavior toward her and children at school and feeling guilty that she had not stopped his father from hurting him. Her view of him was similarly inconsistent, alternating between seeing him as being very much like his father versus thinking of him as a vulnerable child who had been abused. In the retrospective examination of risk and pro- tective factors, several issues seemed salient:

Risk factors: Ages 2–4

- Frequent witnessing of father's physical attacks and emotional cruelty toward his mother
- Frequent verbal abuse by father
- Several incidents of physical abuse by father
- Mother's traumatization and depression interrupted interactive coping that might have mitigated Alex's stress
- Identification with father as an aggressive male model, followed by loss of father
- Alex's cognitive immaturity and lack of internal coping mecha- nisms at time of abuse

Protective factors: Past

- Responsive parenting by mother, first 2 years(?)
- Cessation of violence and abuse due to parental divorce

The transactional patterns between Alex and his mother that had devel- oped in response to their difficult history were helping maintain Alex's symptoms. At the same time, Mrs. Carty's present concern about Alex suggested that transactional protective mechanisms could be utilized to help resolve Alex's difficulties:

Risk factors: Current

• Mother negatively identifies Alex with his father and is frequently critical of him.
• Mother does not set effective limits on Alex's aggression toward herself, which reinforces his use of aggression as a coping mechanism.

Protective factors: Current

• Mother's current concern about Alex is indicated by her dissatisfaction over her negative attitudes toward him.
• Involvement of both Alex and Mrs. Carty in treatment.

Alex's presenting symptoms of aggression, impulsivity, anxiety, and hyperalertness were consistent with research on the outcomes of early physical abuse and witnessing violence (Dodge et al., 1994; Lehmann, 2000). It seemed likely that his symptoms represented posttraumatic dynamics associated with early experiences of witnessing violence and being abused. As treatment proceeded and increasing evidence of PTSD accumulated, this hypothesis was confirmed. Significantly, the interpretation of Alex's current symptoms as rooted in past trauma helped Ms. Carty see Alex more empathically and provided her with a rationale for working to change her parenting style by establishing firmer limits, which provided Alex with a greater sense of safety.

Comment on Diagnosis

During the assessment, Alex did not meet the full DSM-IV criteria (American Psychiatric Association, 2000) for PTSD, although several symptoms of the disorder were present and were likely related to trauma. As the therapeutic relationship developed, Alex made clear links via play and words between his current symptoms and his traumatic abuse. But we should note that his symptoms could be conceptualized in other ways. If we looked at his current symptoms without reference to the history and did not give sufficient weight to the anxiety in his presentation, the school social worker's suggestion that he was on his way to a conduct disorder might seem plausible. From the perspective of knowing that Alex had been abused and had witnessed a great deal of violence, the symptoms of impulsive aggression and fighting more likely represented trauma-based defenses. But what had started as desperate coping devices expressed via the behavioral repertoire available to a 2-year-old were now disconnected from their experiential sources. They had become generalized ways of relating to the world, and in the eyes of others had become pure behavior, or just the way Alex was. The long time between the trauma and the present, and the long time during which Alex's symptoms seemed to have a life of their own, had thoroughly masked the connections between trauma and later symptoms. The assessment of past risk factors helped me stay alert for posttraumatic play and other indicators of memories of abuse as treatment unfolded.

Intervention: The Exploration of Trauma

The account of my work with Alex will be selective, focusing on how the hypotheses regarding early trauma as a risk factor were confirmed by Alex's play material. I will briefly summarize the main themes of our work and then describe in detail a dramatic session in which the connections between the father's past abuse and Alex's current thoughts and behavior could be addressed directly.

I saw Alex in a nondirective play therapy that at first emphasized the development of our relationship. Given his abuse by his father, I was concerned that he would be anxious about working with a male therapist. However, it soon became clear that he was more ambivalent than fearful of me, as the themes of wishes for a male to identify with and mistrust of males emerged in his play. Though it was clear he was very interested in me, in his play with soldiers he repeatedly defeated my army men while saying that his were invulnerable. A prominent theme in this play was trickery. For example, he told me that one of his tanks had been abandoned and that my soldiers could take it over. He gave me instructions about what my soldier was supposed to do, saying, "You go inside the tank. You're looking around, but it's too dark to see. You light a match. You say, 'Hey, what's all that liquid?' It's gasoline! BOOM!" Variations on this theme of trickery and complete dominance continued across many sessions, taking on the quality of posttraumatic play with its repetitive, unvarying, and driven quality. Alex's mother had told me that his father had sometimes been kind and engaged with Alex and other times became abusive abruptly. I understood his play as a reversal of his experience: he became the sadistic trickster, and I became the confused victim. He had coped with ongoing fears of being hurt by identifying with the aggressor. He had also responded to the anxiety associated with being abused by adopting a defense or coping mechanism organized around a fantasy of being in omnipotent control. Alex's play presented both the fears (his play was full of violence) and the defense (he was in total control, his soldiers never lost). This coping mechanism was helpful to him as a fearful and vulnerable 3- and 4-year-old. However, ongoing fearfulness and reliance on omnipotent fantasy as a defense interferes with the developmental tasks of the school-age child and with the growth of more adaptive coping mechanisms such as reasoning about problems.

I commented on Alex's play by saying that kids did not like being tricked and hurt. In response to my empathy about his fears, Alex became more trusting of me, which allowed him to use our sessions to work through some internal dilemmas that had seemed unsolvable at an earlier developmental stage. The therapeutic relationship in work with children has many of the characteristics of an attachment relationship, including the function of transactional affect regulation. Specifically, the child comes to rely on the therapist to provide empathy and a background of security as he represents dangerous, frightening situations in play. Affects and fantasies that would overwhelm the child if they were discussed directly can be explored in displacement, via play and indirect interpretations, in the safety of the therapeutic relationship.

A Detailed Account of a Play Therapy Session

I will present the process of an hour in which Alex clarified what his father's abuse had meant to him and how it had shaped his current concerns and behavior. This session followed many hours of relationship building and many hours of symbolic play representing traumatic themes. Alex built a long car out of several green Lego squares. He said, "Let's drive it," and we carefully lowered it to the floor. As he pushed it, it broke it in two and he said, "Now you've got one too." We drove our cars a bit and he said, "You know we're in space. We're on the planet Pluto. Is Pluto close to the sun?" I said, "No, it's the farthest in our solar system." He put an orange foam ball on top of the file cabinet and said, "That's the sun." He instructed me to drive my car under a chair, which he called a cave, and then told me to drive it out. He became a giant Plutonian monster tromping toward my car, and I quickly scooted it back into the cave. Then he told me to be the monster. I moved with giant steps toward his car, but he said, "You can't see. My car's got reflectors, and the sun's blinding you." Then he became the monster again and stepped on my car and smashed it. I said, "It doesn't matter if you're driving your car or being the giant, you're the one who's got the power and you're the one who wins! This play makes me think maybe there was a time when you were little when you didn't have any power and that scared you a lot. Maybe somebody did something that made you feel that way."

Alex said, "Yeah, my dad."

"What happened?"

"When I was 3 years old I was wrestling with my dad and I scratched him and bit him, and he just picked me up and threw me in my room." (He goes through the motions of picking someone up by the back of the neck and flinging him through the air.) "I just hit the wall. Do you know I got a dead tooth?" (He opens his mouth to show me.)

"I can't see which one it is. How did it happen?"

"My dad. I hit the wall with my face, and now my tooth is dead."

"Is this something your mom told you or something you remember?"

"I remember it."

"Do you still worry about your dad sometimes?"

"Wouldn't you worry if you thought he was going to come and take the kids?"

"Where did you get the idea that your dad might do that?"

"I heard him tell my mom. He said if she ever divorced him he'd come and take the kids."

"Now I can understand why you like to be in control and have all the power—because you really worry what might happen if your dad would come and you couldn't stop him from taking you."

Alex was looking worried and agitated. He said, "I know I'd still recognize him." Then he looked uncertain. I said, "Maybe you're worried you wouldn't recognize him."

"Even if he wore a mask, I'd know him as soon as he spoke. I'd say, 'I know it's you.' I know what I'd do then, I'd run down the hall by the office.. ."

"Oh, you're imagining he'd come to school."

"Yeah. I couldn't stay in the classroom because there aren't any doors that lock. I'd get in the bathroom by the office because it's got a deadbolt and once I got the door locked, I'd say, 'Ha, ha, you can't get me.' "

Discussion

Alex's fully imagined fantasy of his father's coming to kidnap him was one he had lived with alone. The fantasy had some adaptive elements, in that he had developed a careful plan for getting away. Yet, the fantasy was also stuck in a 3-year-old's perspective. In the fantasy, as in his subjective experience of the abuse episodes, he imagines himself alone with his father. There is no one to help him, and he must find a way to take control of the situation on his own. His solution has an omnipotent quality—he heroically saves himself. This hidden fantasy is a vivid example of the "fate of the stressor" once it is internalized as a fearful expectation. Alex's aggression toward other kids at school suggested that he had generalized this fear to situations unrelated to the original trauma. His reliance on identification with the aggressor, a coping mechanism held over from an earlier developmental period, was interfering with current developmental tasks of moving into the world of peers and establishing higher-level coping devices.

My interventions in subsequent sessions focused first on specifying the omnipotent coping device as represented in play and describing how it had originated in response to his father's violence. I said, "I understand why your guys always have to win. In your inside feelings, it's very scary if they get beaten. If they would get hurt, even in pretend, I think it would remind you of how you felt when your dad hurt you when you were 3." Then I helped him think through more adaptive coping devices. For example, I introduced a developmental perspective on his fantasy of being kidnapped at school, saying, "When you were 3, you didn't know how to get help. Maybe you didn't even know some of the words to get help yet. And your mom couldn't help you because she was so upset herself, so I can understand that you felt like you had to do everything yourself. But now you're older and you know a lot more about getting help." I suggested some ideas and strategies he had not imagined, saying, "If you saw your dad at school, you could tell your teacher or you could tell the principal. They would try and stop him. If necessary they would call the police to come and protect you. You and I can talk your worries over with your mom, and she can talk to the principal to let him know not to let anyone take you from school." One aim of these interventions was to help Alex see, from the perspective of his more advanced developmental level, that he had more resources to deal with potentially traumatic situations than he had at age 3. A second aim was to suggest and help him apply a concrete, cognitive perspective on solving the problem that worried him. A third aim was to modify his internal coping mechanisms so that he relied less on omnipotent fantasy and more on rational, intellectualized ways of regulating anxiety that were more consistent with his current level of development.

In summary, the identification of early risk factors, whose potential impact is assessed in terms of the child's developmental level when they occurred, helps the practitioner generate hypotheses about the sources of the child's current symptoms. In Alex's case, the linkages between past trauma and current symptoms, defenses, and conscious fantasies were vividly revealed as he learned to trust the therapeutic relationship. For Alex, trauma was not yet a past experience relegated to memory but a daily source of fear. One of the features of PTSD is intrusive memories of the event. It appeared that Alex was thinking frequently of his father's abuse and that he had carried the memory forward in time, transforming it into a fear that his father would hurt him in the future. From the perspective of his fears, his symptomatic behavior, inappropriate and generalized as it was, made sense. The analysis of past risk factors allowed me to understand how early trauma influenced this child's current behavior.

EXERCISE

Using the form below, analyze the balance of risk and protective factors for one or more of your clients. Include past and current factors.

Assessment of Risk and Protective Factors

Child risk factors   Child protective factors

_____   _____

_____   _____

_____   _____

Family risk factors   Family protective factors

_____   _____

_____   _____

_____   _____

Social/environmental risk factors   Social/environmental protective factors

_____   _____

_____   _____

_____   _____

PART II

The Course of Child Development

Introduction to Part II:
A Developmental Lens on Childhood

In Part II, Chapters 5–12 present an overview of child development for use in mental health practice. When we meet a child, we are confronted with the need to form an objective view of her development. We must assess how well she is responding to current challenges of development. We also need to develop an empathic understanding of the child's current situation and past experience. We must appreciate her external experience—environmental circumstances, caregiving, significant events—as well as her internal responses—how she reacted to her experience, how she understood it, what coping strategies and views of herself she formed in response to the experience—all in the larger contexts of her family, community, and culture.

BARRIERS TO UNDERSTANDING
THE CHILD'S PERSPECTIVE

To the beginning practitioner, children's ways of thinking and responding to the world can seem mysterious. It feels harder to reach an empathic understanding of a child's experience than an adult's. We can more readily understand adults because they communicate and think in ways similar to our own. Adults express themselves primarily in words, whereas children tend to express themselves through behavior and play characteristic of their particular level of development. Most adults have at least some capacity for logical thinking, reflection on their experience, and integrative modes of thinking, such as being able to move back and forth between the abstract and the concrete, the general and the specific, the past and the present. In the course of normal development, these cognitive abilities are not well established until adolescence. Children think differently from adults, and the younger the child, the more cognitive divergence we see.

Children live in the present and tend not to make links between past and present experiences. They have little interest in reflecting on their experience. They tend to think in very concrete and specific terms. It is also more difficult for adults to empathize with the child's experience of the world because they have evolved beyond the more primitive thinking characteristic of young children, making it difficult for them to understand the young child's view of reality. Younger children, for example, often bend their perceptions to fit their wishes.

> I was playing in the backyard with my 2½-year-old grandson when big thunder clouds began to roll in. I said, "Hayden, it's going to rain." He said, "No, it's not going to rain!" I said, "But I can see big dark clouds coming, and I can hear thunder booming in the distance, so it probably will rain." Hayden remained adamant, "Nope, it won't. Let's play." Hayden was quite capable at 2½ of observing the signs of a coming thunderstorm; however, in this instance he wanted to keep playing, and that wish overrode both prior knowledge and current perception. My first "adult thought" response was to try to convince him using logic, but then I said, "I bet you don't want it to rain because we're having fun."

Another barrier to empathy is the typical adult reaction to the ways children sometimes express their distress. Children's symptomatic behavior—aggression, oppositionalism, throwing tantrums, refusal to follow rules, behaving "irrationally" in myriad ways—can be perplexing and disturbing to adults. This can lead to attempts to simply get rid of the behavior instead of trying to understand what it expresses. The adult's understandable impulse to control the child short-circuits empathy. A related problem is the difficulty in conceptualizing the symptomatic behavior of children. Often the reasons for children's symptomatic behavior are obscure. Diagnosis of children seems harder than adult diagnosis because children often do not readily fit into available diagnostic categories; instead, they may present with a variety of symptoms—behavior disturbances, anxiety, social withdrawal—that are consistent with several diagnoses. Further, it is often hard to differentiate children's difficulties from the transactional context of family interactions. In adults, symptomatic behavior can often be understood in the context of regularities in personality. That is, the adult's symptoms as well as strengths may seem more consistent and predictable because they reflect an established personality. The same cannot be said of children, who to a much greater degree are changing as development proceeds and are more reactive to changes in their family circumstances.

The best way to overcome the obstacles to understanding children is to gain a working knowledge of development.

DYNAMICS OF DEVELOPMENTAL CHANGE

Development is not simply additive, but comes in "packages" (Sroufe, 1989). Emerging capacities transform capacities that developed earlier, so that the child, across multiple domains of development, appears to be a different kind of person. For example, as changes in the school-age child's cognitive abilities create firm distinctions between fantasy and reality, the role of fantasy undergoes a reorganization. The school-age child still utilizes a great deal of fantasy, but unlike a 4-year-old he has clearer ideas about what is pretend and what is real, and he is less inclined to impose fantasy onto reality. This more accurate reality orientation, in turn, influences perception, views of self, social behavior, and play. This new organization of the self in middle childhood can be used as a yardstick to differentiate a 9-year-old functioning age-appropriately from another 9-year-old who is still relying on a fantasy approach to reality, which in turn prevents him from integrating and using his new cognitive capacities in age-expected ways. The more complex organization of the child's abilities means that a school-age child is not simply a more advanced preschooler but fundamentally thinks, communicates, behaves, and sees the world *differently* from a preschooler (White, 1996; Case, 1998).

INTERACTIONS BETWEEN MATURATION
AND ENVIRONMENT

At the same time, new environmental demands, if not grossly mistimed in relation to the child's existing capacities, stimulate and shape development (Kagan, 1984). For example, children entering elementary school face major adaptive tasks determined by their new environment. They must learn to sit still, to work quietly, to listen for and follow directions, and to concentrate on structured academic tasks. They must learn to inhibit impulses to play or impose fantasy on their current experience, because those impulses, so typical of the preschool child, are not adaptive in a second-grade classroom (Rimm-Kaufman & Pianta, 2000). Finally, emerging development may be enhanced or slowed by concurrent events in the family's life. The birth of a sibling may create enough stress to temporarily compromise a 3-year-old child's emerging sense of independence from his mother and his growing interest in play with peers. But the direction of change in response to environmental stress is not always predictable. "Resilient" children have been described as responding to stress by becoming more effective. For example, a 10-year-old boy responded to his parents' separation by becoming more conscientious and competent in school.

THINKING DEVELOPMENTALLY IN ASSESSMENT AND INTERVENTION

To assess children accurately the practitioner must be aware of steps and timing in the evolution of different lines or domains of development, transformations that distinguish one developmental period from another, tasks the environment poses at each stage, and circumstantial challenges that may affect the course of development (A. Freud, 1963).

In each stage of development, new capacities emerge that can be drawn upon to help children. The developmentally sophisticated practitioner knows how to use the "tailwinds of development" to push forward the aims of treatment. For example, the young school-age child, because of her increasing internalization of right and wrong, ability to understand sequences and cause and effect, and wishes for tangible signs of accomplishment, can join with her parents and clinician in devising a behavioral plan that makes connections between compliant behavior and positive reinforcers. An 8-year-old can conceptualize the idea that if she gets ready for school on time each morning, she will gain credits that add up to a reward at the end of the week. Becoming involved in the planning helps the child invest in the plan and increases her motivation for change. On the other hand, capacities not yet present in the child cannot be used to advantage in intervention. A 3-year-old is much less able to participate in behavioral treatment planning, because her ability to understand cause and effect is still quite limited.

ORGANIZATION OF DEVELOPMENTAL CHAPTERS

In each of the chapters on development (Chapters 5, 7, 9, and 11) I present summaries of the major adaptive tasks for each phase and details of progress in the following eight developmental domains:

- Physical development
- Relational and social development
- Cognitive development
- Language and communication
- Expressive development, including play and fantasy
- Regulation of affect and behavior, including defense and coping strategies

- Moral development
- Sense of self, self-organization, and relation to reality

Each developmental chapter will be followed by a practice chapter illustrating applications of developmental knowledge to the realities of practice. The practice chapters (6, 8, 10, and 12) briefly describe how level of development influences a child's behavior, play, and capacity to relate, and discuss appropriate assessment and intervention approaches for each period of development. Each practice chapter presents one or more detailed case narratives, which illustrate how a developmental perspective can be utilized for each stage.

CHAPTER 5

Infant Development

This chapter examines the infant's developmental tasks and the interactions that support them within the attachment relationship, describing what the infant brings to these tasks and how parents and other caregivers facilitate the infant's adaptation. It also presents an account of the infant's gradual development of a sense of self and how this is promoted through the relationship with the caregivers. Cognitive, affective, and social development are woven together and are facilitated by the parent's interactions with the infant. The rapid rate of development and how it unfolds within the caregiving matrix will be highlighted. In contrast to subsequent developmental chapters, this chapter presents an integrated narrative of infant development as the outcome of transactions between maturation and caregiving. Later chapters will focus more on domains of individual development and somewhat less on caregiving, since in the phases following infancy the child increasingly becomes more of an autonomous and separate self.

THE INTERACTION BETWEEN MATURATION AND CAREGIVING

Infant development is inseparable from the progression of the infant's relationship with caregivers. Contemporary accounts of infancy emphasize the role of parents and other caregivers in supporting the infant's gradual development of competence and a distinct sense of self (Crockenberg & Leerkes, 2000). The infant needs adult partners who can help her negotiate the developmental tasks and opportunities that maturation opens up. Infants have built-in capacities that allow them to organize and find patterns in their experience, while the caregiving and interactional activities shape what their experience will be. The experiences caregivers present to the baby reflect the values and emphases of the parents' particular culture (Lewis, 2000; Small, 1998). As described in Chapter 1, attachment relationships provide the context for interactions that promote development. For this reason, *the quality of attachment is a crucial variable.*

BRAIN DEVELOPMENT:
THE IMPORTANCE OF EARLY EXPERIENCE

As discussed in Chapter 2, brain development is most rapid during the first 2 years of life. During the last 2 months of gestation and throughout the first year after birth, the brain grows rapidly through the production of synapses and dendrites. The dense branching and outreach of dendritic fibers links billions of individual neurons and, on a broader scale, the different regions of the brain (Johnson, 1997). This integration of the circuitry of the brain, along with myelination of nerve pathways, makes possible the development of sensory, perceptual, emotional, regulatory, motor, and cognitive functions (Nelson, 2000b). After birth, brain growth and the particular ways brain functions are organized are subject to the influence of the infant's environment. Experience influences which neural pathways will be strengthened, which will remain available, and which will atrophy. Appropriate caregiving and stimulation enhance brain development, whereas understimulation and poor or traumatizing caregiving retard or shape brain functioning in maladaptive ways. From the perspective of brain growth and its effects on subsequent development, the transactions between infants and caregivers take on critical importance.

METAPHORS OF INFANT–PARENT TRANSACTIONS

Kenneth Kaye (1982) proposes a useful metaphor to describe how the parent facilitates infant's developmental progression; he suggests that the infant is like "an apprentice in the shop of a master craftsman. The apprentice learns the trade because the master provides protected opportunities to practice selected subtasks, monitors the growth of the apprentice's skills, and gradually presents more difficult tasks" (p. 55). Kaye notes that "An adult can take over the planning of a skilled action and have the infant perform those subskills of which he is capable" (p. 65). An infant–parent game like patty-cake provides a typical example of an infant participating partially in a scenario planned by a parent. As early as 7–8 months, infants can imitate gestures and can learn to clap at the appropriate times as a parent recites "Patty-cake, patty-cake, baker's man . . . "

> At 8 months, Andrea became an apprentice as her grandmother sang the gospel song "This Little Light of Mine (I'm Gonna Let It Shine)." Her

grandmother demonstrated a gesture, holding one finger up and waving it back and forth, when she sang the chorus, "Let it shine, let it shine, let it shine!" Andrea raptly watched her grandmother's finger waving and always smiled when she heard that part of the song. Soon Andrea was waving her finger when she heard the chorus. She could not sing yet, but she could join in the song because her grandmother had taught her a way to participate that was within her reach.

This example also clarifies the emotional component of the master–apprentice relationship between caregivers and babies. The excited and happy engagement between Andrea and her grandmother supports the intrinsic motivation to develop new skills (Siegel, 1999).

A second useful, and complementary, metaphor for the caregiver's function in promoting development is "scaffolding" (Bruner, 1985). In its dictionary definition, a scaffold is a temporary framework that supports workers and materials while a building is being erected. As applied to development, the parent provides support—a "scaffold"—for the infant's cognitive, emotional, and motor development until the infant has accomplished a particular developmental skill and can use it autonomously (Rogoff, 1998). An early and quite literal example of scaffolding is that in the first few months the caregiver compensates for the infant's inability to reliably control his head movements. A young infant's neck muscles are not strong enough to prevent his chin from slumping to his chest, which limits his ability to scan the environment visually. However, if a caregiver provides support for the baby's head by holding him at the proper angle, he can look out at the world and see what is going on, opening up a wider visual horizon.

A later example of scaffolding, common in interactions between parents and 6- to 7-month-olds, is that the infant repeatedly drops a toy and the parent picks it up and hands it back to her each time. This infant is experimenting with control of her hands, control of an object, with a rudimentary concept of disappearance and reappearance, as well as engaging in a fun game with her parent. But if the parent does not support the infant's actions by retrieving the toy each time, she cannot exercise her abilities. Scaffolding makes possible actions the baby could not do on her own. Parental scaffolding clearly continues throughout childhood, but it is most evident during the first 3 years.

CAREGIVERS' ADAPTATIONS
TO DEVELOPMENTAL CHANGE

Stern (1995b) states, "The infant and his parent are in the throes of the greatest and fastest human change process known: early normal development" (p. 3). The speed of the infant's development requires frequent changes in parenting behavior. A task of parenting is to know when to raise the scaffold in response to the infant's changing abilities. Sander (1975) describes the developmental process as requiring frequent adaptation by the parent:

> With one component, the infant, rapidly growing and consequently rapidly changing, new qualities and quantities of infant behavior are constantly introduced into the content of interaction. The regulation of infant functions, based on behaviors that have become harmoniously coordinated between mother and infant, will become perturbed with the advent of each new, and usually more specifically focused and intentionally initiated, activity of the growing infant. Thus adaptation or mutual modification on a new level is required. (p. 135)

The overall direction of these adaptations is toward the infant's "progressive assumption of control of situations as part of the widening of his scope of self-regulation vis-à-vis the environment" (Sander, 1975, p. 135) and toward the parent's gradual relinquishing of control.

In this model, periods of comfortable and coordinated interaction, during which the parent has adapted to the infant's developmental status, alternate with periods of "perturbation," when the parent must change his or her behavior in response to new developments in the infant. A good example occurs between 7 and 9 months, when the infant begins to crawl. This is a momentous change for the baby because now she can cover ground on her own. She does not need the parent to carry her from place to place. She has much greater control over her movements and can explore her immediate world more easily. Because the crawling baby is more autonomous, the parents must adapt by "baby-proofing" the house. A speedily crawling infant can get into all sorts of trouble. Parents have to redesign the environment to keep the baby safe. At the same time, parents must adjust to new attachment demands of a mobile baby who can come to them when she wants contact.

THE NEONATAL PERIOD: BIRTH–4 WEEKS

Infancy research has changed the once-dominant view that infants have few abilities at birth, and now we recognize that infants do not have to learn to perceive the world. Instead, "perception is prestructured" and learning processes "build upon these predesigned or emergent structures" (Stern, 1977, p. 57). Infants are born with a number of abilities that become the bases of future development. In full-term infants these abilities are either present at birth or become evident during the neonatal period, the first 4 weeks of life. The senses of sight, hearing, smell, touch, sensitivity to pain and responsiveness to changes in the position of the body are all present at birth (Bertenthal & Clifton, 1998). By age 1, most of these capacities have reached a level similar to an adult's. Newborns can see close objects 8–10 inches away with fair acuity, similar to the effect of a soft-focus photograph. They are better at seeing strong contrasts rather than subtle gradations of color and light. They can visually track slow-moving objects. During the first 6 months, an infant's visual acuity increases greatly, then gradually improves to 20/20 by age 4 (Kellman & Banks, 1998). Newborn infants show a preference for looking at the human face over other objects. They can hear well, though their hearing will not reach adult level until about age 2 (Werner & VandenBos, 1993). They respond particularly to the sound range and intonation patterns of the human voice, with a clear preference for female voice tones, and even a specific preference for their mother's voice (Snow & McGaha, 2003). They can orient to sights and sounds, remain alert for short periods, modulate affective and physiological states (such as turning away, withdrawing in the face of overstimulation), and use the comforting of a caregiver to decrease arousal (Brazelton, 1990).

During the first year of life the infant's capacity to discriminate between sounds, colors, objects, characteristics of persons, and other differences develops rapidly. From birth onward, and with increasing acuity, infants notice differences and similarities and remember them. This early ability to discriminate at the level of the senses later becomes the basis of categorical thinking and generalization (Haith & Benson, 1998). An example of very early recognition and discrimination of smells came from MacFarlane's (1975) classic study of nursing newborns. By 3 days of age they had already learned the smell of their mother's milk. Nursing pads soaked with their mother's milk and milk from another woman were placed on either side of the baby's head; invariably, she turned toward the pad with her mother's milk on it.

One of the most surprising human abilities that is innate and observable in earliest infancy is cross-modal perception, which involves the ability to translate and generalize from one perceptual mode to another and integrate the information gained from each. For example, if I put my hand into a bag filled with stones of different shapes and sizes and choose one without seeing it, I can later see the stone without touching it and know it was the one I chose. Experimental studies have shown that newborns can make such cross-modal transfers of information. Three-week-old infants with their eyes covered were given differently shaped pacifiers. After they had sucked on them, they were shown the two different pacifiers. The infants looked much more at the pacifier they had sucked on, indicating they recognized the object across sensory modalities (Meltzoff & Borton, 1979). Integration of the senses is not something that is learned but rather is innate. The capacity to integrate information gained from different sensory modalities increases through the preschool years and becomes one of the perceptual foundations for learning. Children who lack integration in their sensory systems have more difficulties in attentional capacity, language, and visual-spatial skills (DeGangi, 2000).

Neonates also have a number of physical reflexes. Some reflexes, including rooting toward and sucking at the breast and grasping with their hands, become the basis for early social interactions with caregivers. Newborns also show pleasure through smiling and calm alertness, on the one hand, and distress through fussiness or crying, on the other, "teaching" their caregivers what they like and do not like. The parent's observation of what pleases or distresses the newborn leads to efforts to extend pleasurable states or to end distress. Through this, the infant begins to understand contingent responding and to develop expectations of how caregivers will respond to his signals. The infant with a responsive parent learns very early that when he cries he will be picked up.

The newborn's "innate" capacities have genetic components but have also been shaped by prenatal influences and by the birth experience. Brazelton (1996) points out that "prenatal experiences have been incorporated into the developing brain and have been fueling the development of this brain. We now know that nutrition, infection, drugs and psychological experiences of the mother are indeed transmitted to her fetus and affect both the current behavior and developmental potential of the child" (p. 131). The idea that the mother's psychological state can impact the fetus *in utero* may seem surprising; however, a number of studies have linked high levels of anxiety and stress in pregnant women with low birth weight and prematurity, as well as higher levels of fetal activity and higher levels of irritability after birth (Paarlberg, Vingerhoets, Passchier, Dekker, & van Giegn, 1995). Infants whose births have been physically difficult or who have been affected by anesthesia during delivery or medical procedures after birth often are less responsive and alert during the days following birth. They need time to recover (Friedman & Polifka, 1996).

In the first week after birth, infants begin to show the capacity for "state modulation," exemplified, on the one hand, by the ability to remain alert and attentive and, on the other, by the ability to shut out or habituate to stimuli in order to remain asleep (Brazelton, 1990). For example, one episode of the Neonatal Behavioral Assessment procedure involves shining a light 10 times above the eyelids of a sleeping newborn. The baby reacts to the light at first by jerking her body; however, by the fourth time the light is shone, she does not move and remains asleep, indicating that she has quickly habituated to a familiar stimulus (Brazelton, 1992). The ability to habituate supports the development of self-regulation. She does not have to react to familiar things and situations, which lessens the frequency of arousal and allows her to remain more calm and alert during the brief periods when she is awake.

Times of calm looking out at her surroundings last for brief periods and total 2–3 hours of each day for the newborn, but time spent in this state increases gradually over the first 6 weeks (Thoman, 1990). The baby's growing ability to maintain this state supports her orientation to the external world, which in turn allows her to begin to take in information. The clearest evidence for very early learning ability comes from studies demonstrating that newborns can discriminate their mother's voice from a stranger's after only 3 days of contact with the mother (DeCasper & Fifer, 1980). Infants also quickly learn to notice novel stimuli and to discriminate between the novel and the familiar. Habituation to the familiar—recognizing and giving less attention to stimuli they already know about—increases rapidly during the first year. Maturation of the sensory areas of the cerebral cortex promotes more rapid habituation by increasing the speed at which the brain processes information (Richards, 1997).

During the neonatal period infants vary in their abilities to regulate internal states, to habituate to stimuli, and to maintain states of alertness. In the early weeks, newborns either cry or are in a distressed state close to crying about 2–3 hours a day. Parents frequently can relieve the distress signaled by fussing or crying by comforting or feeding the baby. During the neonatal period caregivers gradually differentiate types of crying reflecting tiredness, hunger, anger, or pain, and learn to provide appropriate responses (St. James-Roberts & Plewis, 1996). At the ends of the regulatory continuum, however, some infants may be lethargic and withdrawn, whereas others are hypersensitive, crying frequently, and unable to calm themselves. Hypersensitive infants have more trouble developing smooth patterns of self-regulation (Barton & Robins, 2000). They are more reactive and less able to habituate, which means they are more frequently responding to external stressors by becoming physiologically aroused. Consequently, they startle more easily and cry more. The frequent crying of hypersensitive infants reflects not only distress but also an attempt to block out intruding stimuli. However, crying is an "expensive" defense because it keeps the infant in a state of distressed arousal and can have an impact on the early relationship with parents (Maldanado-Duran & Sauceda-Garcia, 1996). *In the early weeks, therefore, parents and infants face a task of mutual adaptation initiated by the parents.* Parents must learn to "stimulate lethargic babies and contain overreactive infants" (Brazelton, Nugent, & Lester, 1987, p. 800).

AGE 1–3 MONTHS

During the first 2–3 months of life, the infant has two basic developmental tasks: (1) to develop a basic capacity for self-regulation and (2) to become oriented to the external world, particularly the human world represented by caregivers (Greenspan & Greenspan, 1985). Between 1 and 3 months, the baby is becoming more alert and more settled. Compared to the neonatal period, when he slept most of the time, he is awake for longer periods and is getting more interested in his environment. He is also learning how to regulate internal states.

Self-Regulation and Mutual Regulation

"Regulation" refers to processes that maintain feelings of well-being, control the amount of stimulation coming in, and modulate the degree of arousal. During infancy, caregivers provide an external structure of regulation by responding appropriately to the infant. Slowly, the infant expands her strategies for self-regulation. Self-regulation and mutual regulation proceed together in infancy. It is difficult to separate the two, because the parent's responses to the baby's distress provide the scaffolding that enables the baby to work on calming herself. During the first 3 months, regulation has two components: regulation of body rhythms and regulation of arousal.

Regulation of Body Rhythms

Infants at birth do not have regular patterns of sleep, eating, and elimination. Gradually, with the parent's help, they develop regular patterns, which gives a beginning sense of predictability to their experience. For example, a newborn sleeps about 16 hours a day, with the same proportion of sleep and wakefulness during the day and night. By about 6 weeks, the circadian rhythms are becoming established, and the infant is sleeping primarily at night, with well-defined nap periods during the day (Sadeh, Dark, & Vohr, 1996). Although this is primarily a biologically and maturationally based change, it is encouraged by the parents' own sleep and wake cycles. Young infants sleep for short periods of a few hours and often wake up briefly at night. They often wake sufficiently to need the parents' help to go back to sleep. Gradually, they develop self-soothing techniques. However, a recent study showed that 50% of 1-year-olds who woke at night needed comforting from parents to go back to sleep (Goodlin-Jones, Burnham, Gaylor, & Anders, 2001). "Sleeping through the night," a milestone parents wish for, has a gradual evolution.

Concurrent with the development of relatively regular sleep patterns, the infant, with the parents' encouragement, begins to eat primarily during the day. By responding to the infant's signs of hunger and at the same time establishing a general schedule of feeding times, the parent helps shape the infant's experience of hunger, feeding, and satiation into a regular pattern. By 3–4 weeks, following a period of weight loss while feeding patterns were being established, the infant has regained his birth weight, which helps parents feel they are succeeding. As caregivers respond to the baby's needs as well as shape his experience in accordance with their own needs and routines, the baby feels a sense of regularity and predictability.

As the baby's rhythms of sleep and wakefulness, feeding and elimination, become more regular, she feels more predictable to the parents. Parents describe that infants become more "settled" in this way between 1 and 2 months. The parents' perception that the baby is more settled is also based on the fact that the parents have spent enough time caring for the baby to get to know her characteristics and behavioral patterns (Leach, 1978). For example, they have learned to distinguish between types of crying due to hunger, discomfort or pain, alarm, and fretfulness related to tiredness or lack of regulation (Thompson, 1998). As parents learn their baby's cues, they begin to feel more competent (Porter & Hsu, 2003). Parents of 1- to 2-month-olds begin to say they "know" their baby and start to ascribe personality characteristics to her.

Regulation of Arousal and Emotion

The second component of self-regulation is called *regulation of arousal and emotion*. At first this is primarily a mutual process, with the infant signaling discomfort and the caregiver moving in to reduce the baby's distress and arousal. During the early months infants depend on parents to feed them when they are hungry and pick them up when they are distressed. If the caregiver is responsive and predictable, the baby develops expectations that he will be fed or comforted within a certain time frame. Out of this awareness, the infant develops a beginning ability to wait. His parent's responsiveness helps him manage his anxiety and distress, because he learns that his needs will be met (Siegel, 1999). Good experiences with mutual regulation lay the groundwork for self-regulation and in the long run promote autonomous coping and resiliency (Crockenberg & Leerkes, 2000).

The young infant is also learning to regulate arousal by depending on the self. By 3–6 weeks, when she is coordinated enough to reliably get her hand to her mouth, she discovers that if she sucks on her hand or thumb, she feels calmer. She discovers that she can calm herself by looking at her parent's face or by watching the mobile above the crib. Another means of self-regulation under the infant's control is called gaze aversion. If a parent is behaving in a manner that is too stimulating, the infant looks away. The infant shifts her attention away when she is becoming aroused to the point of distress (Stern, 1974).

The increasing maturation of the central nervous system during the first month of life also contributes to the capacity for self-regulation by making the infant's reactions to stimuli more predictable and organized. He can delay reactions to hunger. He is less fussy and reactive, which means his states of calm alertness last longer. When he is awake his attention span is greater and his awareness focuses more on observing and exploring people and objects (Emde, 1989). While maturation of the nervous system helps smooth out the full-term 1-month-old's degree of reactivity, a baby born prematurely will take longer to appear more settled and capable of regulating arousal. The premature infant's central nervous system development is "behind" by the number of weeks of prematurity. Illness, intrusive medical procedures, and a period of time in the neonatal intensive care unit (NICU) are frequently associated with prematurity and also contribute to slower early development. Consequently, it is normal for a premature infant to be more easily overstimulated, more reactive, and unsettled for a longer period (Minde, 2000).

In spite of gradually emerging mechanisms for self-regulation, it is necessary to stress that in infancy (and in early childhood as well) the baby's ability to self-regulate is neither sophisticated nor effective in the face of significant distress. The infant depends on the parent to see her distress and to take measures to reduce it (Buss & Goldsmith, 1998).

Temperament and Self-Regulation

As the infant becomes more regulated and more social, the amount of fussy crying and "colicky" discomfort diminishes. Newborns tend to cry easily and to have a low threshold for distress; in normal infants by 3–4 months, however, crying has become much less frequent because of improved self-regulation. However, some infants remain fussier, harder to comfort, and more irritable. These babies have been described popularly as suffering from colic, which involves frequent and prolonged crying, seemingly in response to pain, though in fact the etiology of colic has not been established. Recent research has suggested that colicky babies have lower thresholds for arousal, more disturbed sleep, and delays in establishing circadian rhythms (White, Gunnar, Larson, Donsella, & Barr, 2000). The phenomenon of colic overlaps with the "difficult" temperament style (Rothbart & Bates, 1998). While difficult temperament in infancy has not been found to be a stable characteristic across childhood (Bates, Wachs, & Emde, 1994), it can persist if caregivers are unable to help calm and contain the baby or if their responses actually reinforce the baby's lack of regulation. Fussy, irritable behavior that persists after the first 2–3 months due to temperamental factors (or due to prematurity, illness, or prenatal drug exposure) creates an adaptive hurdle for the infant and her parents.

Parental Responses to "Difficult" Infants

Many parents with "difficult" infants find ways to reduce their irritability. Some find that containing techniques, such as holding the baby a great deal or swaddling him tightly in blankets, reduces irritability and increases security. Others discover that their "difficult" infant is hypersensitive to stimuli and in response take steps to reduce new stimuli or slow the pace of events in the infant's environment. Or they interact with him using only one sensory modality at a time; instead of overstimulating him by talking to him and jiggling him simultaneously, they talk to him while holding him still (Brazelton, 1992). These are examples of the concept of "goodness of fit" in the sense that the parent responds adaptively to the infant's difficultness (Bates et al., 1994).

Some parents with difficult infants, on the other hand, respond with frustration, irritation, or anxiety to the infant's constant fussiness and disregulation. They experience their baby as impossible to console and may blame themselves or the baby. These parents may not respond adaptively, and instead express anger, handle the baby roughly or abruptly, or emotionally withdraw and leave the baby to "cry it out." In such cases, the parent's behavior reinforces the infant's temperamental tendencies toward irritability, hypersensitivity, and disregulation. A cycle of mutually negative feedback can be established, which in turn interferes with secure attachment (Crockenberg & Leerkes, 2000).

Orientation to the World: Beginnings of Interaction

During periods of calm, we also see the baby becoming increasingly attuned to the external world and particularly to her mother or primary caregiver. In the first 2 months the baby's sensory modalities become more organized and acute. As early as 2–3 weeks we can observe an infant staring intently at her mother's face or looking at her fist or listening to voices. Over the next month she begins to expect certain events will occur when she feels certain things. For example, when she is hungry she expects to be fed. She has taken in and remembers the rhythms and routines her caregivers have organized for her. The 2-month-old orients to sight and sounds and also becomes more interested in objects. She can visually track objects that are moving. Her body registers excitement when she sees a bright-colored toy, and she will try to grasp it, though usually without success, since the aim of her reach is not yet accurate because she cannot yet coordinate motor movements with visual perception (Von Hofsten, 1992).

By 6–8 weeks infants show a preference for face-to-face interactions and are very responsive to their caregivers' facial expressions, movements, and voice tones (Reed, 1995). They study their caregivers' faces and begin to establish eye-to-eye contact and to smile at about 4–6 weeks. Their faces begin to express a range of emotions, and by 3 months they can recognize and respond to the emotions of their caregivers (Siegel, 2001). They can share affects and already are aware of violations of affective expectations. For example, in an experimental procedure, if a parent shifts from interacting with a 3-month-old infant to a "still face"—a silent, blank expression—the baby will become worried, distressed, and more active. She attempts to cope with the temporary "loss" of her mother by making active bids for her attention, by smiling, vocalizing, or moving her arms and legs, trying to "get the mother to come back to life" (Stern, 1995b, p. 102). This experiment clarifies that 2- to 3-month-olds discriminate between different types of emotions, have begun to internalize expectations about the affective components of their relationships with parents, and are very sensitive to interruptions in the flow of affective exchange (Tronick, Als, Adamson, Wise, & Brazelton, 1978). While the still-face experiment imposes only a brief disruption of affective exchange, it points to the more difficult situation of infants whose caregivers are inconsistent in their emotional responsiveness. Parents who are depressed, subject to radical swings of mood, or preoccupied and anxious due to stress may present an affectively disturbing image to the infant, leaving her without a model for sharing and organizing affects. This sets the stage for the development of ambivalent attachment. Inconsistent emotional response by a parent also may leave the infant to cope with distress and arousal on her own too frequently, with negative effects on future self-regulation (Siegel, 1999).

The Development of Interaction Patterns

In normal interactions between parents and 3-month-old infants, the behavior of caregivers tends to mimic the give-and-take of conversation. The baby makes a gurgling sound, and the parent responds with a happy "Oh, you're trying so hard to talk, aren't you?" The baby smiles in response, and the parent smiles back and says, "You keep makin' those big noises and pretty soon you will talk!" The parent structures the interaction into the turn taking that characterizes conversation by waiting for the baby's responses and then commenting on them. The parent carries the load in these early interchanges by initiating speech, imitating the baby's facial expressions, and affectively underlining the baby's affects (Stern, 1985). But the baby is learning about the structure and the pleasures of human interaction, and in a few months will be initiating "conversations" and taking an active role in perpetuating them (Marvin & Britner, 1999).

By 3 months infants are regularly smiling and cooing during face-to-face interactions. In response to the infant's interest, caregivers begin to talk to him more. Observational studies across cultures show that parents' "infant-directed speech," or "parentese," has some universal features, including a gentle, high-pitched tone, slower cadence, and short, repeated utterances that sound exaggerated (Kaye & Fogel, 1980; Reed,

1995). Infants respond by laughing and cooing and making other sounds. Infants and parents begin to "talk" to each other, with the parent using simple phrases and the infant making cooing sounds. These vocalizations are not random but rather represent the infant's first clearly communicative behavior. Laughing is a response to feelings of pleasure in an interaction. Cooing has a communicative intent, as is known by any parent whose 3-month-old infant has stared into his or her eyes while cooing repeatedly. It is clear that the attachment relationship is beginning to develop.

AGE 3–6 MONTHS

The continuing development of attention, perception, sensory acuity, and memory between 2 and 3 months, along with repeated experiences with caregivers, allows the infant to make clear distinctions between caregivers. This makes possible and leads to the development of attachment. That is, the baby learns to recognize his mother—her face, voice, odor, gestures, touch, characteristic affective tone, how she handles him, and even what kinds of interactions she prefers. Already at this age the baby knows his mother (assuming that she is the primary caregiver) and prefers her to others, although he will also have a strong preference for others, such as his father, grandparent, or child care provider, who regularly care for him.

Attachment

There are several hallmarks of the infant's behavior during the attachment phase, many of which demonstrate that infants make preferential attachments to the particular people who are their primary caregivers:

- An increase in social smiling occurs, with special smiles for parents.
- The infant shows a strong interest in face-to-face, eye-to-eye contact with caregivers.
- The infant increasingly attempts to engage the parent through looking, smiling, cooing, babbling, and motor activity.
- Primary caregivers now can comfort the baby by means other than holding: with voice, looks, or the presentation of a toy.
- The infant responds differently and preferentially to her mother, father, and others, reserving the brightest smiles for her primary caregiver, or beginning to show distress if, for example, her mother hands her to a babysitter. Infants who are in day care often reflect their preferential attachment by "storing up" reactions to the absence of the parent and

then going through a fussy and sometimes passionate crying episode when their parents pick them up (Brazelton, 1992).

• The infant demonstrates that she has developed different expectations of different people. For example, she may attempt to engage her mother or father in play but not her grandmother; though she enjoys playing with her father, she may prefer comforting from her mother.

As attachment develops, the particular characteristics of the caregivers begin to shape the infant's view of himself and relationships. The infant learns the parent's expectations, preferences, facial expressions, and affective tone and mirrors them. If the infant has multiple caretakers, by 6 months he will register his awareness of their differences by interacting with them in different ways (Stern, 1995a).

Play

The development of relationships, cognitive abilities, and the infant's growing interest in the external world can be clearly seen by observing babies while they are playing. As the infant becomes more coordinated and able to see at a distance as well as close up, there is a general spurt in her interest in the external world. She wants to look at everything and explore everything with her fingers and mouth. She is particularly attracted to her caregivers and to new objects in her environment. She can be observed scanning her surroundings and listening to sounds intently. Between 3 and 6 months, the infant's interest in the world and in her caregivers leads to the development of play. Play in infancy is primarily exploratory and interactive. Although infants show pleasure in play and actively seek stimulation, at first they do not initiate play interactions. In the early period of play development, the parent takes the lead in play, socializing the infant in the "baby games," such as peek-a-boo, that are traditional in the parents' culture. Parents facilitate the infant's interest in play interactions through exaggeration. They speak, gesture, and make facial expressions that are much more dramatic than they would use with an older child or an adult. Stern (1974) suggests that the parent's more dramatic animation helps the infant reach "an optimal level of arousal" to engage in play interactions (p. 410). He suggests that there is an optimal range of stimulation for helping the infant to become engaged and continue to play. Understimulated infants are not drawn into sustained interactive play; overstimulated infants turn away or withdraw, short-circuiting engagement. Parents usually are able to discover the optimal level of stimulation for their particular baby unless factors like parental emotional disturbance, psychosocial stressors, or serious deficits in the infant interfere.

Types of Infant Play

Several forms of play predominate during the first year, including the following:

Vocal Play. Infants enjoy listening to themselves. By 4 months, they have a repertoire of sounds, including grunts, squeals, trills, and vowel sounds such as "ah," "ooh," and "oh." Babies can be overheard "talking" in their cribs. This playful vocalizing has a self-sufficient quality. The baby is not trying to communicate but rather is experimenting with and enjoying the sounds he can make. At about 6 months, this vocalizing becomes babbling, which combines consonant and vowel sounds ("ba-ba," "um-um") and reproduces inflection tones and speech rhythms he has heard from his caregivers (Locke, 1993).

Exploratory Play with Objects. Infants explore objects with their eyes, hands, and mouth. They are interested in shape, color, and texture as well as in the movements and sounds objects make. Jean Piaget (1962) labeled this type of play "sensorimotor play," describing it as the infant's way of learning about the properties of objects by looking at, touching, and manipulating them. While exploratory play does serve this cognitive function, it also provides the baby with feelings of pleasure, which is a central element of all forms of play. Parents facilitate exploratory play.

> For example, a father shakes a rattle to attract his 4-month-old daughter's attention to it. She looks at it with interest and reaches for it. He brings it close enough to her hand for her to grasp it. As she looks at it and then brings it to her mouth, he says, "How does it taste? Like plastic, I bet!" Then, if she has not yet made it rattle herself, he shakes her hand to demonstrate its sound. She looks strongly interested, pauses as if she is figuring out what to do, and then begins to bang the rattle. Her father says, "You did it!" When the infant's interest wanes, she drops the rattle. The father notices that she has disengaged and hands her something new, and the play continues a bit longer. Although this play focuses on the rattle, it has a strong interactive quality and sense of shared pleasure. The interaction also has a strong element of scaffolding. The parent, out of his knowledge of his baby, sets up a situation and process through which the infant enjoys the toy and learns about it. His observation of her disinterest causes him to give her a new object. This too is based on his knowledge of her—that, as is typical of 3- to 6-month-old infants, she hungers for novelty and often becomes bored by familiar toys.

Interactive Play. Between 4 and 5 months, the infant begins to initiate interactions on his own, often by vocalizing or smiling at the parent. It is now clear that the attachment relationship is being used for something else besides getting comforted and feeling secure. It is being used by the baby as a vehicle for communication and for developing a sense that he can be a force in the world. The baby joins in interactions and works to keep them going. The exchanges between parent and baby begin to last longer and to become increasingly complicated. At this point, the baby is remembering the kinds of interactions that are pleasurable and tries to get the parent to repeat them. Behaviorally, the infant is expressing what the toddler or pre-schooler will later say in words: "That was fun, let's do it again—over and over."

The baby is also more aware of the environment, scanning it visually and reaching out for objects. Parents, by watching what interests the baby, are now following the baby's lead. For example, a parent becomes aware that the infant is looking at a toy and then brings it within the baby's reach. Or, after the baby has learned from repetitions of this experience that looking and reaching are signals of wishes, she reaches for the toy with the expectation that her father will bring it close enough for her to grasp. At the same time, especially during the 5th month, the baby is becoming more competent in using her hands as well as her eyes and hands in coordination. She can shake a rattle that has been placed in her hand, shift it from one hand to the other, and reach for objects with good aim. The baby's increasing effectiveness in signaling, in taking the initiative, and in grasping, holding, and manipulating objects, all of which is "scaffolded" by the parent's actions, leads to a sense of "competence and voluntary control over . . . her environment" (Brazelton & Yogman, 1986, p. 7).

Baby Games. Parents also play ritualized, repetitive games with their infants. The mother teaches the baby a game, sometimes of her own spontaneous creation, and more often one traditional in her culture. In American culture, for example, parents often play peek-a-boo, "I'm gonna get ya," and "tickle" games with their babies. These games operate on the principle of repeat and vary.

> For example, a mother changes her 5-month-old's diaper and then lightly tickles her stomach. The baby becomes excited. The mother pauses, to allow the suspense to build, then says, "I'm gonna get ya," and tickles the baby more forcefully. The baby laughs. The mother pauses and looks at the baby. The baby, anticipating the next tickle, kicks her legs and begins to squeal. The mother says again, with more drama, "Ah-m-m-m gon-na get ya!" The baby shrieks and laughs. But after the next tickle, the baby not only laughs, somewhat hysterically, but also looks away. Then the mother, sensing that the baby is at the edge of being overaroused, lowers the intensity of her behavior or perhaps shifts to another game, so that the infant's arousal decreases to a comfortable level.

This is a good example of mutual regulation, in which both partners attend to one another's behavior and affects in order to keep an exchange going at a pleasurable level. The mother is gearing her actions and monitoring the baby's responses with the implicit goal of keeping the level of stimulation within an optimal range. The infant signals, through her responses, when the parent's play behavior is at the right level of stimulation as well as when it is too much or not enough. The parent uses this feedback to either maintain or modify her play behavior (Uzgiris & Raeff, 1995).

Winnicott (1971) suggested that if the parent adjusts her behavior by following the baby's cues the baby experiences the pleasure and excitement of feeling in control of the play. In peek-a-boo, for example, the mother controls her disappearance and appearance, but the infant feels that he is making things happen. And, in the sense that his responses encourage his parent to disappear and appear over and over, he is in control. By 8–9 months, the baby actually will control the game by covering his own face. Before 6 months, parents almost always initiate games, but by 8 months infants can clearly signal that they want to play a game. An 8-month-old, for example, will clap his hands to show his parent that he wants to play patty-cake.

Baby games contain humor, suspense, and excitement, which both players share. Infants will not play with any adult, however. They experience a range of positive affects and humor when they are playing with people they know and trust (Trevarthen, Murray, & Hubley, 1981). This is an essential idea, since the parent's behavior in baby games—tickling, poking, presenting toys and taking them away, hiding from the baby—has strong elements of teasing. The crucial difference between hostile teasing and baby games occurring in the context of a secure attachment is that the parent does not push the infant's arousal to the point where anxiety and helplessness supplant pleasurable excitement. The parent gives in—by showing himself in peek-a-boo—before the baby feels helpless, and the baby has the exhilarating feeling of making the parent come out of hiding.

Baby Games as Indicators of Difficulty

Parent–infant games can also reveal parental difficulties that may put the infant at risk. Fraiberg's (1974) clinical studies show that the observation of baby games may provide a sensitive index of how the parent–infant relationship is developing. Fraiberg describes teasing that gives a parent pleasure even as the baby becomes distressed and disorganized—for example, repeatedly pulling a bottle from a baby's mouth during a feeding, or "rough-house" play at the border of abuse that becomes frightening or painful to the infant.

In an example I observed, a mother put a ball in her 7-month-old son's hand and swung his arm hard in a throwing motion and said, "Throw the ball at daddy." The baby laughed at first, but as his mother kept manipulating his arm he became somber and looked frightened. Then he began to whimper. She was oblivious to this because she appeared caught up in expressing hostility toward her partner. This was registered by her aggressive facial expression as well as her behavior. As the "game" continued, the mother kept repeating, "Throw it at Daddy! Boom!" The ball had turned into a bomb! She was using her infant, in the context of playing a game, to act out anger.

This example presents common features of disturbed baby games: the parent's insensitivity to the baby's needs and feelings, the baby's becoming overaroused to the point of distress, and the parent's exploitation of the baby to satisfy or act out his or her own needs. Baby games with these qualities, in contrast to mutually pleasurable games, suggest risk for the infant and point to the need for a careful evaluation of the parent's difficulties.

A NORMAL INFANT AND A COMPETENT PARENT: A CASE EXAMPLE

The following observation of an infant and parent interacting with a toy illustrates some themes of the account of infant development so far. This description highlights the following:

- The developing competencies of the infant
- The infant's intense involvement with the external world
- A smoothly functioning infant–parent partnership in action
- Sharing of pleasurable affects that characterizes play during the attachment period
- Parental scaffolding of the infant's experience

Four-month-old Rashid and his 19-year-old mother are participating in a developmental guidance program at a teen health center. In this program, a social worker engages the parent in discussions of infant development and parenting through the viewing of videotaped play sessions with her baby. The intervention attempts to support existing strengths and to increase the parent's ability to observe and understand her baby (Share, Givens, Davies, Eley, & Chesler, 1992; McDonough, 2000).

Ms. Jamison is an African American single mother. She and Rashid live with her mother and father and siblings. She receives solid emotional and concrete support from her family. Rashid is cared for primarily by his mother but also has warm attachments with his grandmother and his mother's sister. Rashid appears to be developing well, and his mother is warmly engaged with him. As she talks to the social worker who is videotaping them, Ms. Jamison speaks easily about Rashid, raising questions about him and conveying that she knows him well.

The worker suggests that Rashid might be interested in some of the toys. His mother gently places Rashid on his back on a blanket on the floor, then puts a "gym" with *Sesame Street* characters suspended from a bar above him. She positions it above his chest so that he can both see and reach the figures. She says "Look at them" and swings them gently. Rashid is already looking raptly. As he takes in the brightly colored, slowly swinging figures, his legs and arms begin to move rhythmically in excitement. His mother laughs at his excitement, and he turns toward her, catches her eye, and smiles. She says, "You like it! You want them!" Rashid smiles and kicks his legs. Then he calms momentarily as he stares at the figures. Rashid continues to alternate between attending to the toy and responding to his mother's voice with smiles. His mother points to the different characters, saying, "Here's Bert, here's Ernie, here's Big Bird." After she does this, Rashid vocalizes and touches the figures with his feet. He reaches for them with his hands but is not able to grasp them. His mother suddenly realizes that she has placed the gym so that the characters face away from Rashid. She turns it around and, speaking for Rashid, says, "I can't see their faces, mom. There you go. Now I see 'em." She discovers that Big Bird makes a squeaking sound, and she squeezes it while Rashid watches. Rashid reaches for it but is not yet coordinated enough to grasp it. She says, "I'll squeeze it for you," and he kicks his legs in excitement. After a minute Rashid's attention wanes, and his mother says, "OK, you're getting tired of this—you're just looking at your shoes now." She props him up to a sitting position, so he can see the toy from a different perspective. He looks for several seconds, then shifts his gaze away from the toy. She says, "OK," and picks him up, and he smiles at her.

From this brief observation, which lasts only 5 minutes, we can identify two fundamental forces that interact to shape infant development. The first is Rashid's motivation to take in and master his environment. Rashid shows interest in the world that is characteristic of his age. He uses his already well-developed attentional skills in a sustained engagement with a new and interesting toy. Even though he does not yet have the physical skills to accurately reach out and grasp the toy, he is highly motivated to do so, and he keeps trying despite his lack of success. He "grasps" the figures with his eyes, however, and registers pleasure by smiling, gurgling, and kicking his legs. He shares his excitement and interest with his mother. Overall, he takes an active role in shaping his own experience. While this view of the infant as active may seem a truism, it serves to correct an older view of the infant as a passive recipient of what the environment presents (Emde, 1996). This view of the infant as actively initiating behavior and striving to become more competent becomes even clearer during the second half of the first year, when, for example, the infant will crawl energetically to reach a toy at the other end of a room.

The second shaping force illustrated in this vignette is how adult behavior provides structure and direction to the infant's experience. Rashid's mother does many things that facilitate his experience with the toy. She helps focus his attention by pointing to the figures and swinging them. She affirms his pleasure in looking at them by commenting in warm tones and by smiling back when he smiles at her. She reinforces his interest in the toy by mirroring it and focusing her attention on the toy at the same time he does. She is able to take his perspective when she realizes that the figures are not facing him; she acts on this perception by turning the toy around, which changes and extends his experience of it. She explores the toy herself and discovers that it makes a noise; she shows this to Rashid and squeezes it several times, realizing that he is interested. Observing him reach toward it, she imagines he would like to make the noise himself and squeezes it for him. Finally, she is attentive to his decrease in attention and gives him a chance to look at the figures from a new angle. This temporarily increases his attention. When his interest wanes, she realizes it and picks him up.

This is an ordinary example of a parent interacting with an infant in response to his interest in an object, but when the actions of the parent are listed *it becomes clear how much she facilitates and shapes the infant's experience.* The parent knows more, sees things in a broader perspective, and is more organized than the infant. She uses her skills in perspective taking, her ability to recognize Rashid's affective and motoric signals of interest (and waning interest), and her advanced ability to explore the object. She demonstrates actions that are beyond his ability, and he seems to imitate her. It is as if she is thinking, "I know you cannot squeeze this toy now, but I will show you how to do it, so that you will begin to get the idea and so you'll know what to do when you're physically ready." Her behavior does not merely affirm the status quo but points the way to higher developmental levels. At the same time, her approach is facilitative rather than intrusive. She encourages him to engage with the toy in his own way and then tries to add to his experience.

We can see Rashid's mother's behavior in terms of both metaphors introduced at the beginning of this chapter. He is her young apprentice, and her actions provide scaffolding for his development. She provides him with experiences that promote his developing physical and cognitive skills, and at the same time she supports him physically and affectively as he exercises his abilities. Even at the age of 4 months the developing secure attachment with his mother encourages Rashid to engage his environment actively; already, their relationship is becoming a secure base from which to explore (Grossman et al., 1999).

AGE 6–12 MONTHS

During the second half of the first year, the infant advances rapidly in cognitive, motor, and social development. The baby's understanding of the world becomes more sophisticated, as she begins to understand cause and effect and intentionality, and realizes that other people have minds of their own. During this half-year the infant's interests all seem to intensify. She becomes more interested in exploring the world, more compelled to develop physical and cognitive skills, *and* more involved in her attachment relationships.

At about 6 months the infant's interests begin to shift away from an exclusive focus on interactions with attachment figures to an increasing interest in objects and the external environment generally. Stern sees this as evidence that the infant's confidence in the attachment is established and also hypothesizes that the infant is developing internal "schemas" or representations of the parents and the attachment relationships that allow him to "keep the parent in mind" even when he is not interacting with her (Stern, 1985). Parents describe their 6- to 7-month-old infants as more self-reliant. For example, when the baby wakes in the morning, he may not cry for the parent to come but instead will play—with objects in his crib or with his own voice—for up to half an hour before becoming fussy and alerting the parent to come. The baby at this age is not less interested in his relationships with parents. Rather, his interest in the external world, spurred by cognitive and motor development, becomes nearly as compelling as his involvement with caregivers. In spite of this increased capacity for autonomy and self-regulation, however, parents also describe the 7-month-old as intensely involved with them. Preferential attachment reaches its height between 7 and 9 months. This is demonstrated by the baby's pleasure in extended play with the parent, as well as by the emergence of stranger and separation anxiety.

The emphasis of the 6-month-old's play and social interactions also changes. In the first 5 or 6 months, interactive play in which infant and parent take turns is at the center of the infant–parent relationship. As the infant's interest in objects increases, the relationship gradually focuses more on "joint-attention activities" in which the parent and infant share experiences of objects or events. This particularly involves sharing affects and the parent's communicating an understanding of the baby's feelings. Strikingly, after 6 months, the infant becomes more of a leader in interactions with parents. Instead of primarily following the parent's lead, the baby initiates interactions more frequently. This behavior is intentional in the sense that the infant tries to elicit particular responses from parents. The infant's behavior is becoming goal-directed, reflecting cognitive advances in the understanding of cause and effect. For example, the baby who was a happy participant in peek-a-boo when the parent put a diaper over his face now begins the game by trying to pull the diaper over his face himself.

Physical Advances

One of the primary thrusts of infant development is toward increasingly full control of the body. As the infant's muscles strengthen and as she works to master control of bodily movements, she becomes more capable and independent. Infants take pleasure in mastery and are strongly motivated to establish control of their bodies. Physical abilities develop in a progression "from top to bottom." This progression follows the maturation of the central nervous system and muscular system. Between birth and 6 months, babies develop control of head and neck movements, then hand movements and hand–eye coordination, and then initial control of the upper body. By age 5 months, these accomplishments begin to interact to allow for more skillful motor functions. Any given motor skill, from reaching to walking, is really a complex of coordinated abilities (Thelen, 1995). Consider reaching for and grasping objects at 6 months. Control and balance of the upper body creates a stable base for arm and hand movements, while steadier head control and increasing hand–eye coordination allow for more accurate reaching and grasping. As a consequence of the coordination of all these accomplishments, the 5- to 6-month-old can usually grasp objects that are within his reach (Bertenthal & Von Hofsten, 1998). During the second 6 months of life, there are dramatic developments in physical abilities and control involving the trunk, arms, and legs, including sitting, postural control and balance, crawling, standing, cruising (walking while holding onto furniture), and walking.

These new abilities support the growth not only of new actions but also of new perspectives. Sitting is a good example. By about 8–9 months, the baby's back muscles are strong enough to allow him to sit erectly without support for long periods. From the erect sitting position, he can see more. He is higher and can turn his head and twist his trunk to see in all directions. His hands are free for use in grasping objects and bringing them close for examination. At 4 months, he could only sit supported and had more limited control of head and neck movements. He was far more passive and dependent, in the sense that what he looked at was determined by the position his caregiver had placed him in. Now he scans his environment following his own interests. His physical control affords him more autonomy in choosing what he will pay attention to. Similarly, by 8–9 months the infant's adeptness at crawling allows him to be more independent in realizing his wishes (Adolph, 1997).

Motor Skill Development and Infant Stress

Between 8 and 12 months infants practice motor skills with particular intensity. All of the skills they are working on add up to a big spurt in motor development. As in other periods of rapid development, infants typically experience emotional disequilibrium and anxiety, which shows up now as lower tolerance for frustration, poorer affect regulation, increased attachment behavior, difficulty in falling asleep, and waking in the middle of the night, apparently from frightening dreams. These reactions derive not only from the driven effort toward mastering physical skills but also because the new skills themselves create new experiences of anxiety (Campos, Kermoian, Witherington, & Chen, 1997). Mobility is not only exciting but causes uncertainty and fear when the infant finds she has crawled too far away from her parent, into an unfamiliar room, or to the bottom of a stairway. The infant who is practicing standing, cruising while holding onto furniture, and walking will often fall and will frequently be aware of the discrepancy between what she wants to do and her body's ability to do it. Gradually, the baby does master these skills and again becomes more confident and settled. Practice strengthens her muscles and leads to more and more frequent experiences of feeling proficient (Adolph, Vereijken, & Shrout, 2003). The acquisition of physical control in sitting, crawling, and walking gradually permits the infant to take those abilities for granted, freeing her to become more curious and interested in her environment. By 1 year of age the infant, while continuing to work on mastery of motor skills, is increasingly concentrating on cognitive explorations (Campos, Anderson, Barbu-Roth, Hubbard, Hertenstein, & Witherington, 2000).

Cognitive Advances

Memory

The development of memory and other cognitive functions follows the maturation of the brain. Experimental studies have shown surprising memory abilities in infants 2–6 months of age. By 3 months they can recognize stimuli they saw a few weeks before, if they are given a cue to jog their memory. For example, experimenters tied a ribbon between a 3-month-old baby's foot and a mobile above the crib. When the baby moves his foot, he sees that the mobile moves. Three weeks later, after the experimenter cues the baby by moving the mobile, the baby begins kicking his foot to make the mobile move, apparently remembering what he had learned previously (Rovee-Collier, Hartshorn, & DiRubbo, 1999).

Between 8 and 12 months, the infant's memory abilities show rapid development (Rovee-Collier & Hayne, 2000). An example that provides evidence for maturation of memory functions is "stranger anxiety," which shows up in infants across cultures at about 9 months. The infant begins to react with frightened expressions, withdrawal, or distress when an unfamiliar person comes near. Kagan (1984) explains stranger anxiety in terms of the infant's new ability to compare the face of the stranger with images of familiar faces he holds in his memory. This new ability to make comparisons based on memory leads to feelings of uncertainty when the infant does not recognize the stranger, and so the infant becomes anxious.

Similarly, the separation anxiety that also becomes prominent at 8–9 months can be seen as related to memory and anticipation. The baby is able to remember previous separations and recognizes the immediate signs that the parent is planning to leave. She also remembers feelings of distress associated with previous separations and anticipates feeling them again. As this awareness becomes clearer, reactions to separation intensify (Kagan, Kearsley, & Solano, 1978). Separation protests—crying, clinging to the parent, attempting to crawl after the parent—also represent a new level of coping behavior. The baby becomes aware of an impending loss of proximity to her parent and takes active steps to change the situation. While memory gives rise to separation distress, memory gradually helps the infant learn to regulate affects in response to separation. The baby learns that the parent who leaves also comes back. This remembered awareness makes brief separation understandable and bearable. The infant's distress lessens as reunion following separation becomes established in consciousness as a predictable experience.

Memory and Mental Representation

The infant's memory now includes generalized and specific images of objects and people. Infants under 7 months treat objects that disappear as "out of sight, out of mind." If an object is hidden from them, they will not look for it, even though they watched the parent hide it. At around 8 months, they will search for an object that is hidden (Rosser, 1994). For example, if a parent hides a toy under a diaper, the baby will pull the diaper off to find it. This ability is called *object permanence,* which means that the infant has a mental representation of the toy and can not only remember how it was hidden but also imagine where it is without being able to see it (Piaget, 1952b).

The infant also forms representations of caregivers, which is thought to lead to a concept of *person permanence.* This is a difficult concept to grasp because it seems so obvious that a person can recognize another person he or she is familiar with, even when that person's behavior and moods are somewhat different. However, this ability to internally represent another person develops gradually in infancy through repeated interactions with attachment figures. Internal representation involves being able to hold the person in mind when he or she is not present (Stern, 1995b; Bretherton & Munholland, 1999). It is not clear exactly when this ability develops. Stern (1983) argues that infants probably can evoke memories of the parent during the first 6 months. Nevertheless, separation anxiety at 8 months does suggest that infants have the ability to think about their parents when they are not there and to miss them. Stranger anxiety at about the same time suggests that infants have clear representations of their caregivers and other familiar people, and find it confusing and jarring when a person who does not match any of these representations comes close to them.

Awareness of Other Minds

A shift in cognitive awareness of others occurs near the end of the first year, which is consistent with the development of internal representations. Infants become aware that others have their own point of view and intentions. They also realize that "their subjective experiences, their attention, intentions and affective states can be shared with another" (Bretherton, 1987, p. 1079). This leads to a new perspective on the behavior of others. Infants observe the actions of their caregivers and begin to learn from them. New behaviors that illustrate this shift in awareness include the following.

Joint Attention. Older infants begin to look at a caregiver to see where she is looking and then look in that direction or at that object. If an infant follows the gaze of an adult and then cannot tell what is drawing her attention, he checks back with the adult, trying to discern what she is looking at. The infant "is now not only aware of an object but simultaneously aware of the mother's attention to the object" (Schore, 2001). The caregiver's awareness of the infant's growing capacity for joint attention encourages her to provide the infant with more chances to share experiences and to begin to communicate about them.

Social Referencing. The infant looks at a caregiver to see her attitude toward a new person or situation. By 1 year of age, when infants meet a new person or encounter a new event or object, they often look back at their parent for help in assessing the new situation. If the parent's affect is approving or positive, they will approach the new person or situation, but they will not approach if the parent registers concern or disapproval

(Thompson, 1998; Repacholi, 1998). The need for social referencing develops in connection with the infant's developmental progress. As the infant becomes more perceptive of reality, she feels uncertain more often and needs help in appraising new situations (Emde, 1992). For example, uncertainty increases when her developing motor skills put her in potential danger. A 10-month-old may crawl to the top of a flight of stairs, look down, and then look back at the parent for help in assessing the danger she senses. A look of alarm or a sharp "No!" from the parent will stop the baby from going down the stairs.

Social referencing has also been demonstrated experimentally. Researchers created an ambiguous situation that caused uncertainty in infants over 6 months of age. The infant was placed on a table that was extended by a piece of Plexiglas. The see-through extension created a "visual cliff" where the wooden part of the table no longer existed. The infant's mother was standing at the end of the Plexiglas extension, that is, on the other side of the "cliff." When infants approached the visual cliff, they looked at their mothers with uncertainty. If the mother registered fear, the infant would not cross the Plexiglas panel; if she expressed encouragement and smiled, he would crawl across the cliff (Sorce, Emde, Campos, & Klinnert, 1985).

Following (and Giving) Directions. At about 9–10 months infants begin to do simple things their parents ask them to do. Soon after this development, infants begin to consciously direct their caregivers to do things for them. This represents a new level of intentionality. At 6 months, for example, parents had to intuit their infant's wishes. During the second half of the first year the baby learns to intentionally signal a wish to the parent. For example, a 1-year-old can point to a toy, then look at her mother, signaling that she wants her mother to get it for her, or she can lift her arms toward her father while whining or vocalizing "uh-uh," which conveys the command "Pick me up."

Imitative Learning. Infants begin to watch their caregivers with the aim of understanding how they are doing something. They can be seen trying to do the same thing that the caregiver is doing with an object (Tomasello, 1995). Imitative behavior also provides evidence for improving memory. Piaget (1952b) coined the term "deferred imitation," which refers to imitation of something that happened in the recent past. This type of imitation, as opposed to immediate imitation, requires that the infant remember what she observed. In experimental conditions, infants as young as 6 months can imitate facial expressions they were exposed to 24 hours earlier (Rovee-Collier & Hayne, 2000). By 14 months, they demonstrate increasing power of memory by being able to imitate actions that occurred up to a week earlier (Meltzoff, 1988)

These cognitive developments reflect the infant's awareness that both the behavior of others and their own behavior have meaning. Over the next year, this awareness that others have a point of view leads to a direct awareness that they also have reactions to the child's behavior. A parent who says about a 6-month-old infant that, "He's crying because he's trying to upset me" is suggesting something that is developmentally impossible, because a 6-month-old is not yet aware the parent has a perspective. By contrast, one can observe a 2-year-old beginning to cry while obviously checking to see what impact his crying is having on an adult. But even by 1 year of age, the new awareness that others have a point of view that may be influenced creates a new understanding of communication and its utility. This realization increases his motivation to communicate and express himself in understandable ways. This sets the stage for language learning in the second year of life.

Language and Communication

When the infant speaks her first few words between 9 and 12 months, language development has clearly begun. However, a look back shows that the infant has been preparing to speak since birth. During the early weeks of life infants can discriminate between speech sounds as their parents talk to them. In the first few months the infant develops a repertoire of sounds—grunts, cries, and single syllable vocalizations. The infant vocalizes experimentally, repeating sounds in varying patterns, clearly listening to herself and enjoying the different sounds she makes. After age 6 months, brain maturation makes possible the more complex consonant–vowel combinations heard in babbling (Locke, 1993). The increase in vocal abilities has a self-reinforcing quality. Babies, like older people, enjoy hearing themselves "talk." Parents also respond to these language-like sounds by talking more and more to the infant. Thus, the ability to "speak" derived from maturation becomes reinforced by the parent's enthusiastic responses to babbling. In turn, the infant's babbling increasingly mimics the parents' speech sounds and patterns.

While early babbling cannot be considered language, it is a precursor of language, as demonstrated by the observation that between 6 and 10 months babbling focuses imitatively on the sounds used in the parents' native language (Cheour et al., 1998). Although all infants are capable of producing the range of sounds used in all human languages, by 10–12 months the baby has learned the favored sounds of his caregivers' language and less frequently uses sounds that are not included in that language. Through imitation and practice he has developed a map of the sound system of his parents' language, which provides a foundation for the emergence of spoken language in the second year (Kuhl, 1999). Parents often actively shape this process of sound learning by "translating" the baby's babbled sounds into the closest equivalent words (Locke, 1993). Playing with sounds also becomes integrated into interactions with caregivers. Vocal play is an important aspect of infant–parent interaction that develops between 4 and 6 months.

By 9 months, gestural forms of prelanguage communication also develop. Some examples include (1) the infant looks at something she wants—a toy or food—then looks at the parent for help in getting it; (2) to get help from an adult, the 9-month-old repeats "requests" by fussing and looking at the object, then back at the adult; and (3) the infant shows or hands objects to the adult (Bates, Camaioni, & Volterra, 1975). By 1 year of age, the infant communicates actively by pointing at objects.

By 10 months, the infant regularly imitates parents' gestures in ritualized games like patty-cake and by waving bye-bye. This ability to imitate behavior coincides with evidence that the baby is beginning to comprehend the parents' words. Shortly after this the baby shows the beginnings of true language when he says words intentionally. As has been true for previous development, the infant's relationship with parents provides the context for the development of communication based on *words*—sound combinations that mean the same thing to the speaker and listener. Through repeated labeling of objects and actions, caregivers teach the infant his first words. At this early stage, the infant can say only a few words, although experimental studies have shown that already the infant's receptive vocabulary exceeds his speaking vocabulary (Bloom, 1998). The parent and baby, through attachment behavior and social play, and with joint-attention activities as the infant matures, have been practicing communicative exchanges for many months. When the child's cognitive development reaches the point of comprehending and speaking words as intentional communication between 9 and 13 months, the continuing exchange between parent and infant becomes the scaffolding for actual language learning (Bloom, 1998).

A Developing Sense of Self

As the infant passes the age of 6 months, her increasing social competence and intentionality can be taken as signs that she is aware of her needs and how to express them. These qualities have been described as signs of the emergence of a subjective sense of self (Stern, 1985). During the first year, the sense of self derives particularly from the infant's feeling an increasing sense of control. In the early months of life, the caregiver provides the structure that helps the infant organize expectations. The caregiver provides "more" at the outset but gradually creates room for participation by the infant. The infant, in turn, gradually has more capacity for participation. If parents are sensitive to the infant's signals and initiatives in the early months, the infant begins to feel effective and in control, even though the parent is making this possible (Keller, Lohaus, Volker, Cappenberg, & Chasiotis, 1999).

> For example, a responsive mother watches her 4-month-old while feeding him and delivers the rice cereal each time he opens his mouth. At first, she feeds the baby rapidly because he shows that he is hungry by eagerly taking the food, swallowing it, and opening his mouth again. Over the course of the feeding, the parent slows the pace in response to the baby's signs of satiation. While the parent is orchestrating the feeding, the baby feels in charge because the parent is responding contingently. Over time this has an impact on his view of himself: "An infant whose mother's responsiveness helps him to achieve his ends develops confidence in his own ability to control what happens to him" (Bell & Ainsworth, 1972, p. 1188). By contrast, an infant whose parent pushes food at him too rapidly is likely to choke, spit up, or turn his head. Feeding becomes not just an unpleasant struggle but also an experience where the infant feels that he lacks influence to control what happens.

Self-Esteem and Self-Efficacy

Infancy researchers have been particularly interested in the emergence of the self and how the infant's view of self is shaped in interactions with caregivers. Two aspects of the sense of self have been particularly studied: self-esteem and self-efficacy. Self-esteem involves feeling good about oneself. Self-efficacy involves feeling effective and competent in one's actions and interactions. Many studies have found links between the quality of the infant's sense of self and the quality of attachment relationships. When parents are responsive and sensitive to the infant's behavioral cues and to her experiences of distress, the infant's self-esteem increases because the parent's responses are contingent and empathic. The infant feels valued and understood. When the infant experiences the parents' responsiveness as "evidence" that her efforts to communicate, share affects, gain attention, or express distress are effective, her sense of competence increases (Keller et al., 1999).

The infant's sense of self-efficacy is more likely to develop strongly "when a caregiver's behaviors are contingent upon the affective and behavioral cues coming from the infant, rather than geared to a schedule or to the caregiver's convenience" (Demos, 1986, p. 59). At the same time, as noted in Chapter 1, sensitive parents are not always optimally responsive, and therefore the infant at times has negative feelings because the parent is preoccupied, unresponsive, or simply misunderstands the infant's signals. These "mismatches" present the infant with chances to act to restore a positive or attuned interaction. The sense of competence is increased when the infant and parent are able to overcome these periods of dyssynchrony (Tronick & Gianino, 1986b). Researchers studying self-efficacy have found that it is self-reinforcing. The infant who has many experiences of success feels more and more effective (Harter, 1998).

Parental Support and the Infant's Experience of Mastery

The infant's experience of success depends a great deal on the quality of parental scaffolding. This issue has been illuminated by studies of "mastery motivation" of 6- to 12-month-old infants. The desire for mastery is an intrinsic motivation reflected in the infant's push to explore the environment, to solve problems, to learn, to exert control, to develop competence, and to succeed in developmental tasks (Harter, 1998). Mastery motivation is perhaps most obvious in the infant's persistent work on developing physical skills. Dramatic examples are the precrawling baby who exerts tremendous effort as she pulls herself across a room with her elbows or the 9-month-old repeatedly trying to pull herself to a standing position. However, older infants also show the same degree of interest and work just as hard to influence their parents to interact with them. They will smile, make noises, and touch or pull on the parent to get his or her attention.

Mastery motivation can increase or decrease depending on whether the infant feels successful in her efforts toward mastery. Parental support for the infant's efforts at mastery and competence allows her to feel more successful and contributes to self-esteem. Support includes not only hands-on help or structuring the infant's activities but also the parent's emotional encouragement and expression of pleasure when the baby succeeds at a task.

> A mother watches her precrawling 7½-month-old, Nisha, pulling herself with her elbows and pushing with her feet, intent on reaching a bright orange ball over 10 feet away. She becomes her baby's cheerleader, saying, "That's it, keep going, uh, it's hard, uh, but you're going to get there," with her voice expressing both encouragement and empathy for the struggle. When Nisha touches the ball, her mother says, "You did it! You went all that way and you got it!" Nisha laughs in triumph.

Such encouragement has effects on later attitudes and abilities: "Caregivers who are emotionally available and who promote . . . exploratory behaviors have infants who demonstrate greater task persistence, greater pleasure in goal-directed behavior, and greater subsequent social and cognitive competence" (Lyons-Ruth & Zeanah, 1993, p. 27). A consistent lack of support, as occurs in neglect, may result in feelings of incompetence, lowering the infant's self-esteem and perhaps over time creating an internal model of "learned helplessness," where the child believes that she cannot succeed by her own efforts (Aber & Allen, 1987). In social interactions, the infant whose behavior succeeds in eliciting a positive and sensitive response from the parent feels encouraged to continue the behavior. Such infants learn to expect to be successful in their actions. During the first year, interaction patterns, coping experiences, and resulting views of self are the building blocks of the child's working models of self and relationships.

APPENDIX 5.1. Summary of Infant Development, Birth–12 Months of Age

This chart on infant development follows a chronological sequence rather than developmental lines. Since development in infancy unfolds more rapidly than in later stages, this organization provides a clearer view of how an infant develops. Since there are individual differences in rate of development in children, I have indicated time ranges encompassing normal development.

Overall Tasks

- To develop attachments and dyadic strategies for maintaining them
- To gradually gain control over motor skills
- To develop a beginning ability to regulate arousal and affect

Neonatal Period: 0–4 Weeks

- Perceptual abilities are present at birth
- Orientation to sounds and sights within range of visual acuity (1 week+)
- Orientation to human face and voice (1 week+)
- Recognition of primary caregiver (1–4 weeks)
- State modulation begins: alternating states of alertness and habituation to stimuli (1–2 weeks)
- Discrimination between novel and familiar stimuli (2–3 weeks)
- Cross-modal perception and integration of senses (3 weeks)

Age 1–3 Months

- Developing capacity for self-regulation of body rhythms (with help of caregivers): regulation of sleep/wake and feeding/elimination cycles (1–2 months)
- Beginning capacity for regulation of arousal, including dyadic strategies and self-soothing (1–3 months+)

- Orientation to external world: using the senses to take in impressions of the environment (2 weeks–3 months+)
- Interactions with caregivers: beginnings of preferential attachments; focusing attention on caregivers for longer periods; social smiling; cooing (1–3 months)

Age 3–6 Months

- Development of attachment: consistent recognition of primary caregiver(s); clear preferences for interacting with them; responsiveness to parents' playful behavior; ability to use attachment relationship to regulate arousal and affect (3 months+)
- Play develops: within the attachment relationship (interactive play and baby games); exploratory play, utilizing the senses; both forms of play gradually become more elaborate and complex (3–4 months+)
- Memory develops, as indicated by the infant's preference for certain types of pleasurable interactions and play sequences (3 months+)
- Motor skills: gradual development of control over upper body functions, including head and neck control (3 months+), reaching for objects (4 months+), grasping objects (4–5 months+), eye–hand coordination 4–5 months+), coordinating hand movements by bringing the hands together (4–5 months+)

Age 6–12 Months

- Initiates play interactions, rather than depending on parent to initiate them; this is evidence for the beginnings of intentionality, goal-directed action, and awareness of cause and effect (6–7 months)
- Intensification of interest in relationships, own body, and the physical world (6 months+)
- Ability to "entertain" self for brief periods, due to interest in the physical world and own body (6 months+)
- Beginning ability for mental representation: the infant apparently can keep the image of the parent in mind for longer periods by remembering him or her (6–7 months+)
- Language and communication: vocalizing and babbling (4–6 months); gestural communication expressed via looking and pointing (8–9 months); understands first words (8–9 months); speaks first words (9–12 months)
- Persistent motivation to develop physical skills, especially locomotion, in a progression of creeping, crawling, cruising, and walking (7–14 months)
- Feelings of autonomy and pleasure based on the development of physical skills; also feelings of frustration and anxiety while the infant is working to master physical skills (6–12 months+)

- Memory: beginning awareness of connections between past and present, and predictability of repeated events, as indicated by reactions to separation from parents; awareness of differences between familiar and unfamiliar events and people, as indicated by stranger anxiety (8–10 months)
- Object permanence: looking for a hidden object shows the infant can keep an object she has seen in mind, even though it is no longer in sight (8–9 months)
- Beginning awareness of others' point of view: joint attention and social referencing (9–12 months+)
- Following simple directions: responding to parents' words and gestures (9–10 months)
- Imitative learning: watching caregivers to learn how to do things (9–12 months)
- Sense of self begins to develop, based on feelings of self-efficacy (a beginning sense of feeling control over action and communication with caregivers) and self-esteem, when the infant feels successful at accomplishing a goal. The development of a positive sense of self is strongly related to responsive caregiving (6–12 months+).

CHAPTER 6

Practice with Infants

Infant mental health is an approach that derives from the rich research knowledge on parent–infant interaction presented Chapters 1 and 5. Essentially, this research demonstrates that when parents are attuned to the infant's signals and feelings, encourage and take pleasure in communicating with the infant, and respond to the baby's needs in a timely way, the baby's development as an individual self and social person is supported and enhanced.

Infant mental health practice applies this perspective to situations where quality of interaction is compromised or at risk. Risk can emerge from a range of sources, including factors that compromise parenting ability, and infant factors, such as prematurity or developmental delays, which pose challenges for parents in learning to relate to their baby (Lyons-Ruth, Zeanah, & Benoit, 2003; Minde, 2000). In infant mental health practice both the parents and the baby are seen as clients. Intervention aims to promote strengths and resolve difficulties in their interaction, and to improve goodness of fit. Very commonly, infants and parents are seen in their homes. Home visiting allows the practitioner to see infant, parents, and interactions in their "natural" setting, where they are likely to be most comfortable and most open and real. The home visit also allows the parent to feel that the worker has seen things "as they really are" and in a broader context, compared with meetings in a clinic office (Seligman, 2000).

The baby is present when the parents meet with the infant mental health worker, and "baby watching"—the collaborative observation, wondering about, and interpretation of the baby's behavior—is a primary focus. The infant mental health worker invites the parents' questions about the baby's actions, and sometimes "speaks for the baby" in order to help the parents think about meanings and intentions in the infant's non-verbal behavior. The worker also puts the observations she and the parents make about the baby's behavior into a developmental context, which becomes the basis for forecasting future developmental steps (Weatherston, 2002). In cases where negative interactions have developed between parents and baby, the worker attempts to help the parents reflect on how their current stressors, the history of their relationship with the baby, their personal history, and their working models may contribute to the problem (Fraiberg, Adelson, & Shapiro, 1975; Lieberman & Zeanah, 1999). Through this focus on the baby and on the evolution of the interaction, the baby becomes comprehensible to the parents. Developing the capacity to understand the baby in turn supports the parents' sense of competence and enables solutions to the problems to be generated (Fraiberg, 1980). When the parent's conscious and unconscious views of the baby have been shaped by the parent's own difficult history of early relationships, treatment becomes more complex, linking the parent's past with her current caregiving (Lieberman, Silverman, & Pawl, 2000). Selma Fraiberg (1980) who, with her colleagues, founded infant–parent psychotherapy, states:

> In treatment, we examine with the parents the past and the present in order to free them of old "ghosts" who have invaded the nursery, and we must make meaningful links between past and present through interpretations that lead to insight. . . . We move back and forth, between past and present, parent and baby, but we always return to the baby. (p. 61)

ASSESSMENT ISSUES

The practitioner who works with infants and parents needs to be particularly attuned to the infant–parent relationship. Given the centrality of attachment as an influence on early development, the worker especially observes caregiving behavior, parent–infant interactions, the parent's statements about the infant and herself or himself as a parent, as well as taking a broader look at the quality of relationships and systems that surround the infant–parent relationship (Weatherston, 2002; Zeanah et al., 2000).

Infant mental health work frequently requires collaboration with a range of professionals. Especially when an infant is born with a combination of mental, sensory, or physical disabilities, practitioners from such disciplines as physical therapy, occupational therapy, communication therapy, vision services, early education, as well as mental health services, may be needed. In 1987, the U.S. Department of Education implemented the Individuals with Disabilities Education Act (IDEA). Part C of IDEA provides for comprehensive, multidisciplinary, and "family-centered" services for infants and toddlers with developmental delays, physical or mental disabilities, or at-risk conditions as defined by individual state programs (Gilkerson & Scott, 2000). In recent years, these multiple approaches to the child and family have increasingly been integrated into overall service planning, with the result that collaboration between practitioners with different perspectives has been increasing. Early intervention programs have increasingly embraced an infant mental health perspective by emphasizing the support of parent–infant relationships as the fundamental context for encouraging optimal development for young children with delays and disabilities (Hirshberg, 1998). Frequently mental health practitioners are called upon to provide assessment of infant–parent relationships and to collaborate (and effectively divide up) intervention on behalf of infants and toddlers. For example, an infant with regulatory and sensory-integration problems receives direct intervention from an occupational therapist, who also models techniques for his parents; his parents use sessions with an infant mental health specialist to reflect on their feelings about their child's difficulties; and the two professionals consult frequently with each other and with the parents to monitor the treatment (Ribaudo & Glovak, 2002). In cases like this, the practitioner needs to be sensitive to the expertise of other professionals and to the limits of her own perspective, yet maintain a focus on the relationship of the infant and parents.

When there are concerns about the infant's developmental status, a number of standardized assessment instruments can be utilized, such as the Bayley Scales of Infant Development–II, and the Mullen Scales of Early Learning (Bayley, 1993; Mullen, 1995). The Bayley is the most widely used standardized assessment. Although not predictive except in cases of serious developmental delays, the Bayley provides a useful snapshot of an infant's current strengths and weaknesses in the cognitive and motor areas, identifying areas that may require intervention (Gilliam & Mayes, 2000). Other assessment tools, such as the Infant–Toddler Developmental Assessment (IDA), the Ages and Stages Questionnaires (ASQ), and the Ages and Stages Questionnaires: Social Emotional (ASQ:SE) ask parents to report on their infant's development (Provence, Erickson, Vater, & Palmieri, 1995; Bricker, Squires, Mounts, Potter, Nickel, & Farrell, 1995; Squires, Bricker, Yockelson, Davis, & Kim, 2002). These tools help the clinician organize her view of the infant, and may identify, or at least raise questions about, whether the infant's development is on track. The IDA is a comprehensive assessment that synthesizes information about family, development, and health, through observation of the infant and detailed interviewing of parent, often by members of a multidisciplinary team (Erickson, 1996). The ASQ instruments were designed for parents to fill out independently, but they can be particularly useful when included as part of an interview. The parent's information about the baby can be reflected on by worker and parent and can become the starting point for collaborative work on behalf of the infant.

Specialized tests should never be the sole evaluation procedure. Testing, when indicated, should be part of a comprehensive evaluation that includes observation of the infant–parent relationship, since quality of attachment and the infant's social abilities are better predictors of developmental outcome than are specific aspects of infant development (Bernstein, Hans, & Percansky, 1991). Similarly, a questionnaire or checklist is not a substitute for careful observation. Observing in an open, curious manner, the clinician allows her knowledge base in infant development and her mental repertoire of "pictures" of infants she has seen previously to help her frame questions and ideas about the particular infant she is observing (Seligman, 2000; Fraiberg, 1980).

In all clinical work, but especially in work with infants, because it focuses on supporting and increasing the quality of relationships, the relationship the worker develops with the family during the assessment becomes the basis for effective treatment. It is helpful for the practitioner to state at the outset that she hopes to "form a team on behalf of the infant" (Seligman, 2000, p. 213). A statement like this affirms the parents' importance in the assessment of their baby, and emphasizes that they and the worker share common goals. Parents often begin an evaluation with worries that they will be judged and blamed for their baby's difficulties. A respectful, curious stance by the clinician, as well as explicit statements about collaboration, helps reduce parents' anxiety.

Seligman (2000) points out:

> Progress in clinical formulation and the evolving therapeutic relationship can be mutually reinforcing: To the extent that the parents feel that they have been collaborative partners in the assessment, they will be better able to embrace the treatment process. (p. 213)

The following case example of infant mental health practice illustrates the use of observation and relationship building in the assessment of transactional issues between an infant and her parents.

ASSESSMENT AND BRIEF INTERVENTION WITH AN INFANT AND HER FAMILY: A CASE EXAMPLE

The case of 1-year-old Julie and her parents illustrates an infant mental health assessment conducted by a social worker with training in this specialized area. My account focuses particularly on the transactional context of infant development, showing how an infant's early, probably normative difficulties in self-regulation stimulated a negative pattern of caregiving that compromised her attachments and threatened her affective and social development. The case also illustrates a brief intervention that was incorporated into an assessment. I will present the process of the assessment in detail so that the reader will be able to reflect on the material as it unfolds.

Referral

Julie Bryan's pediatrician referred her a few days after her first birthday. Almost since birth, Julie had cried for 6–12 hours every day. During her first year four different medical specialists had evaluated her, finding no physical causes for her crying. Julie's mother had twice rejected the pediatrician's suggestion for an infant mental health referral, but she accepted it this time because the baby's problems had not abated.

Initial Telephone Contact

Mrs. Bryan said immediately that Julie had been screaming many hours every day since she was 2 weeks old. The problem had waxed and waned but had recently worsened. Julie was very anxious with strangers and even avoided her father. Mrs. Bryan said: "I know they're supposed to be scared of strangers at this age, but this is just too much. Sometimes I have to be rough with her. I just put her in the crib and let her scream, because I can't take it anymore. How can I stop her from crying? She's got to shape up." She described times during the summer when she had put Julie in her crib and gone outside, to get away from her crying. I empathized with how hard it was to have a baby who cried constantly. I said that I had no immediate answer to stopping Julie's crying but hoped that a careful evaluation would provide some answers.

Mrs. Bryan's tone was anxious and exasperated. However, it was important to avoid answering her urgent questions with quick, formulaic answers based on general knowledge of infant development. By saying that I wanted to understand the problems thoroughly, I was conveying that I would think about Julie as an individual. This stance helps parents view the worker as someone who will try to provide thoughtful information about their baby. As it turned out, it was especially important that I did not try to answer Mrs. Bryan's pressing questions, because I learned later that she had already received many prescriptive but unsatisfactory answers from physicians, parenting books, and neighbors.

I asked if there had been any difficulties or medical complications with the pregnancy and birth. The pregnancy had been without problems and full-term. Julie had been a healthy child whose developmental milestones of the first year had emerged at normal times. For the first 2 weeks, Julie had been "a good baby." Then the screaming began. As I listened I wondered what had originally caused Julie's crying—perhaps an irritable temperament, perhaps early difficulties in self-regulation; but it seemed likely, given the duration of the problem, that the original difficulty had shaped parent–infant interactions in a way that perpetuated Julie's screaming. Mrs. Bryan noted, reflectively, that after the pediatrician had suggested counseling, when Julie was 8 months old, she had done a lot of reading about infants and that Julie had cried much less. I asked how she accounted for that change. She said, "I really don't know, but I must have done something. But then it started up again after about a month." This was a hopeful statement, suggesting that Mrs. Bryan could still imagine doing something to change the interaction.

I said that I could understand Julie best by seeing her in her home environment with her family and asked if there was a time when Mr. Bryan could be home. Mrs. Bryan was hesitant, saying that her husband worked every day from 7 to 7 but that he could get off if it was really necessary. I said I felt it *was* necessary because I wanted to get Mr. Bryan's views of the problem and to observe Julie as she related to all family members.

Commentary: Including the Father

Mrs. Bryan's uncertainty about her husband's participation and her comment about Julie's avoidance of her father raised questions about the degree of his involvement with her. In assessing children in two-parent families, it is critical to include both parents. Research on resilience consistently finds that family stability and mutual support between parents are protective factors for children's development. The father's emotional support of the mother influences the quality of caregiving she provides to the infant (Crockenberg, 1988). In families where traditional sex role divisions prevail (whether the mother works outside the home or not) and fathers are not highly involved in caregiving, the father's influence is indirect, through support for the mother. When fathers are highly involved caregivers, their influence is more direct, and infants establish strong preferential attachments and mutually regulating patterns of interaction and play with fathers (Grossman et al., 1999). Mrs. Bryan's hesitancy to involve her husband in the evaluation might have a number of different meanings. However, I would not be able to learn about his influence on his wife's caregiving or his relationship with Julie without seeing him directly. This point may seem obvious, but too often in practice fathers are excluded, at times by their own preference but also sometimes by their partners with the acquiescence of practitioners.

THE FIRST TWO HOME VISITS: LEARNING ABOUT THE FAMILY

Mr. and Mrs. Bryan voiced many complaints about Julie's constant crying. She would cry whenever Mrs. Bryan left the house, or even the room. Mr. Bryan said Julie avoided him, though he amended this to say that she had been more willing to play with him recently. I asked if there were times when Julie did not cry, and Mrs. Bryan said with exasperation, "Oh, yes, as long as I'm right there every minute, she doesn't have any trouble. She's stuck on me, and I can't seem to break her of it." She said that physicians and neighbors had told her to let Julie "cry it out" and eventually she'd "outgrow it." However, when she tried to follow that advice, Julie would cry in her crib for at least an hour, and Mrs. Bryan would feel a failure as a mother. Nevertheless, leaving Julie alone had been Mrs. Bryan's primary strategy ever since the crying began at age 2 weeks. I asked how she had explained the crying to herself. She responded, "Well, I just call it her getting mad at me for not being with her every minute." She said that her first child, Erica (now 3 years old), had been such an easy baby that she wasn't prepared for Julie. I said, "I don't know yet why Julie cries, but I do know from seeing babies with similar problems that letting them cry it out usually doesn't work." Mrs. Bryan said, "It relieves me to hear that."

Observations of Julie

Julie struck me as a pretty and appealing baby. She had brown curls around her ears and was still nearly bald on top. I could see her two new lower teeth but noted that her most frequent expression was more a strained grimace than a smile. When I said hello to her, she looked at me warily and curiously, but did not cry, as her mother had said she would. Later she approached me several times without anxiety. Julie was just beginning to walk and still felt more comfortable cruising along the furniture. She could climb up on the couch and get down on her own. She was adept at crawling. These observations told me that her motor skills were appropriate for age. Her language development appeared behind. At 1 year, one expects an infant to be babbling expressively using a wide range of sounds, using pointing and other gestures, and beginning to use a few real words. Julie's language was limited to grunting noises during this visit.

Three-year-old Erica was playing at her mother's feet. When Julie crawled near, Erica pushed her away, then crawled up onto her mother's lap. Julie pulled herself up next to her mother, who extended her arm. Julie wanted to climb onto her lap. Mrs. Bryan did not move to accommodate her, and Erica, in response to Julie's advance, molded herself closer to her mother's body. Julie tried to climb up, and Erica spread her body out to cover Mrs. Bryan's lap and thighs. Julie whined and grimaced and continued to stand as close to her mother as she could. Mrs. Bryan did not remark on the rivalry between the children. In observing this scene I remember thinking that there's not room for two babies in this family. It appeared that Erica was the favored child and Julie was the outsider. I also felt sad that Mr. Bryan did not offer to take Julie but left his wife to cope with two needy children. I asked Mrs. Bryan how it felt to have two young children wanting her attention at the same time. Mrs. Bryan laughed and said that Erica was pretty independent, so that it was not much of a problem. This led to a discussion by both parents of what an easy child Erica had been, how little rivalry Erica had shown, and how much more difficult Julie was. That response seemed incongruous with the scene I had just observed, and also felt defensive, in that a question about Mrs. Bryan's feelings was deflected into a positive description of Erica. The parents seemed to be saying that Erica is not needy or rivalrous—she is our good child. Neither of them remarked on Julie's whining bid for attention. This observed interaction raised questions about whether Mr. and Mrs. Bryan had been able to "make room" for Julie. However, since this was our first meeting and my question had brought a seemingly defensive response, I decided to continue to observe rather than ask more questions about this issue.

History Taking

I asked Mrs. Bryan how she had felt during the pregnancy. She sighed and said she was worn out and felt cooped up. Her husband was working long hours, and she was home alone with Erica. She said that she had not had a postpartum depression after Julie's birth. This led to a description by both parents of her depression after Erica's birth. Mr. Bryan said, "It lasted for about 8 months. She wouldn't talk to me about it. I thought we were going to get a divorce." Mrs. Bryan sounded wistful as she said the depression had been caused by having to give up her job: "After I had Erica, all of a sudden I didn't have anything to do, and I felt cooped up and lonely." By contrast, she had not been depressed after Julie's birth. She recalled feeling happy and energetic for the first few weeks, before Julie's crying bouts began. She described how she tried to stop Julie's crying by changing her environment, moving her from room to room in the house. She said, "She wouldn't have cried if I'd held her all the time, but I couldn't do that 24 hours a day. After a while, I had to get a little rough with her." This was the second time she had used this phrase, and I asked her to clarify. Again she said, "Just put her in the crib and leave her there. . . . You know, I've never cuddled her much. She hasn't been the kind of baby that you just want to come up and cuddle, and that may have had some effect."

A Demonstration of the Problem

As I was leaving, Mrs. Bryan said, "She's made a liar out of me. She hasn't screamed once since you've been here!" I said that sometimes a baby does not behave in her usual way when a new person is present. She said, "Maybe I can show you." She got up and left the room. Julie saw her mother leave and immediately crawled after her. As she passed her father's chair, he reached out to her, but she crawled past him and began to cry in a fearful tone. Mrs. Bryan reappeared smiling and said, "That's the scream." She picked Julie up and Julie stopped crying. Mrs. Bryan said, "If I hadn't come back, or if I'd put her in her crib, she'd really be screaming now."

Mrs. Bryan's Story

Mrs. Bryan asked to schedule the next home visit in the early afternoon because Julie's screaming was worst then. Mr. Bryan had said that he didn't need to be there because the problem was primarily between Julie and her mother. I agreed to meet at the earlier time but told them that Mr. Bryan's point of view and his relationship with Julie were important to understanding the problem and that I would want him to be included in future visits.

During the second home visit 2 weeks later, Julie did not cry at all. Mrs. Bryan commented that she was coping with separations more easily and was going to her father more often. Julie had also been waking up crying at night, but Mrs. Bryan said she just needed to pat her a few times and she would go back to sleep. This was a different image of Julie, as a more manageable child. It is not unusual for such progress to occur during an assessment. This is not a "miracle cure," but rather reflects that the parents, with the worker's support, are paying attention to the child's problems in a different way. A conscious focus on the problem often subtly changes the interactions that have grown up around the problem. For example, in response to a new development, Julie's crying in the middle of the night, Mrs. Bryan was comforting her immediately rather than leaving her to cry it out, and Julie was going back to sleep. Mrs. Bryan's reporting of progress in only the second interview also made me feel that she was investing in the assessment as a vehicle for change.

The family had been on a week's vacation, and Mrs. Bryan said that they all had enjoyed the time together. This break in the family's routine also contributed to Mrs. Bryan's more hopeful attitude. She said the children really liked it when her husband had time off. This led to a discussion of Mr. Bryan's work schedule. He was away from home for 12 hours each day, and his schedule required him to work for 21 days at a stretch, followed by 2-week periods when he had weekends off. She presented this information with clear ambivalence: her tone was matter-of-fact, but her facial expression was strained and unhappy. He had always worked this intense schedule, but before the children were born she had also worked long hours and had arranged her work schedule to match her husband's, so they had spent more time together. He had been present at Erica's birth, but a day later had gone into a 21-day work period. She came home from the hospital with her first baby and had received little help from her husband. They had no relatives in the area. I commented that it sounded difficult. She said, "There was nobody to help me out. I was depressed for about 6 months. It's a lot of work to take care of a baby." I agreed and said, "And even more work to take care of two." Mrs. Bryan felt she adapted to the new role of parent, especially as Erica got older and became more social and fun to play with. Erica had been an even-tempered infant who was happy going places outside the home. After Julie came home from the hospital, Mr. Bryan again had to work 3 weeks straight. Mrs. Bryan began to feel trapped again. Two children were not as portable as one. She had felt increasingly trapped after Julie's crying began. She also complained that Julie's crying had made it hard to feel comfortable about leaving her and hard to get babysitters, so that since Julie's birth she and her husband had rarely gone out and were spending even less time together.

As we talked, Erica and Julie played together near Mrs. Bryan. Julie climbed onto the couch next to me and pointed out the window. She babbled expressively. When I asked if she was showing me the pretty blue sky, she smiled broadly and babbled more. (This small incident points to the importance of making multiple observations of infants and young children. During the first home visit I had been concerned that Julie's language development was behind. However, her expressive babbling and pointing at the sky made me revise this first impression and see that her language ability was developing normally.) In response to Julie's insistent babbling, Erica called out to Julie and they played with their voices, one shouting and the other shouting in response. Mrs. Bryan asked Erica to play with some blocks, and the shouting stopped. Later the children frolicked on the floor, rolling on top on each other and laughing. But when Julie was on top momentarily, Erica became angry and began hitting her. Julie grimaced but did not cry. Mrs. Bryan allowed the hitting to continue for a long time—by my subjective response—before she asked Erica to stop.

At the end of this meeting, I made a few comments. First, I suggested that we focus on how difficult it was to feel trapped again after Julie's birth and on how Julie's problems had affected their marital relationship. I said that stress can circulate within a family—that the stress she felt over being trapped and less involved with her husband could have spilled over to Julie and made her more anxious. Mrs. Bryan was unsurprised by this interpretation and said, "You could be right." Second, I said that it would be important for Mr. Bryan to be involved in subsequent meetings, since the problem involved interactions in the family rather than just interactions between her and Julie. Mrs. Bryan was skeptical but looked pleased and relieved by this suggestion.

Impressions

Julie was developing adequately in the motor and cognitive areas, but her social development, as reflected in her ambivalent attachment, anxious demeanor, and intense reactions to separation, was compromised. Although separation anxiety is common between 8 and 12 months, Julie's seemed atypically intense and also part of a pattern of anxiety about her attachments that dated back to the early months of life. It was not clear what had caused Julie's crying originally. According to Brazelton (1992), between 3 and 12 weeks about 85% of infants go through a period of fussy crying at the end of the day. In the past, this fussing and irritability was called "colic" and was attributed to gastric distress. Although some babies do cry because of gastrointestinal pain, the irritable colicky crying of most young infants does not have obvious causes.

Brazelton (1992) recasts this phenomenon in developmental and maturational terms:

> Whenever a certain behavior is so predictable and widespread, we assume that it is adaptive and look for the purpose it serves. This fussing began to look like an organizing process. An immature nervous system can take in and utilize stimuli throughout the day, but there is always a little bit of overload. . . . Finally, it blows off steam in the form of an active, fussy period. After this is over, the nervous system can reorganize for another twenty-four hours. (p. 63)

Brazelton suggests that if parents can strike a balance between providing comfort and allowing the baby to cry for brief periods (5–10 minutes), babies will gradually become better organized and the fussy periods will become less frequent and disappear within a few months. Some infants with difficult temperament are more sensitive to internal and external stimuli and take longer to outgrow the fussy times. The more distress-prone an infant is, the more challenge she presents for parents. When parents repeatedly cannot soothe an irritable baby who cries excessively, or when they react negatively to her distress, insecure attachment patterns may develop (Rothbart & Bates, 1998). Recent research has found links between persistent crying and maternal depression and lack of positive responsiveness to the infant (Pauli-Pott, Becker, Mertesacker, & Beckmann, 2000).

Julie, however, did not seem to fit the profile of a child with a difficult temperament. At present she did not appear to be a globally hypersensitive infant. Her ability to accept the falls and bumps of learning to walk and to tolerate Erica's aggressive play without becoming seriously distressed suggested adequate internal affect regulation. Her one area of hypersensitivity focused on the presence or absence of her mother. Julie's crying for a long time had been a transactional response. When her mother left her alone, she would cry. Hearing her cry caused Mrs. Bryan to avoid her for longer periods, increasing Julie's anxiety and insecurity. It seemed that Mrs. Bryan did not want Julie to depend on her at a time when dependency is normal. Essentially, Julie "trained" her mother to avoid her, and Mrs. Bryan's avoidance had reinforced Julie's insecurity (van den Boom & Hoeksma, 1994). As this negative spiral persisted, Julie felt less and less secure in her family, and Mrs. Bryan became resentful and more distanced from her.

I wondered whether Mrs. Bryan had brought negative expectations to Julie's infancy based on her painful memories of her loneliness and depression during Erica's early months. Perhaps Julie's crying at 2 weeks had felt like a confirmation of those expectations. Had Mrs. Bryan felt helpless and defeated? It was clear that her early attempts to cope with Julie's crying minimized her own potential power to change things. Instead of offering more comforting, she hit on the idea of moving Julie from room to room, hoping that the change in environment would calm her. I wondered if Mrs. Bryan had been angry with Julie when she did not stop crying, and if her strategy of leaving Julie alone might represent an attempt to protect Julie from her anger and to defend against her own guilt about being angry. Her repeated statement "Sometimes I have to get a little rough with her" seemed to reflect her fear that she might hurt Julie and her guilt over hostile impulses toward her.

In these first two sessions I had observed and learned enough to hypothesize that Julie's crying represented a transactional issue that involved the whole family. I decided to focus this issue by exploring Mr. and Mrs. Bryan's memories and understandings about how the crying originated and what perpetuated it.

THE NEXT TWO HOME VISITS

I was pleased that Mr. Bryan was not only present but very active during the next two sessions. Mr. Bryan reported that Julie was coming to him more since they had been on vacation. I said that he had been able to spend more time with her then and perhaps that made it easier for her to come to him. He agreed. When Julie saw me she began babbling exuberantly as she had when she was looking out the window during the previous visit. I said, "I remember you showed me the sky last week. You're really trying to tell me something." Then I explained to Mr. Bryan how impressed I had been when Julie pointed at the blue sky and babbled so expressively, as if it was the most exciting thing she had ever seen. He said he too had noticed that she was babbling more and getting ready to talk. As we talked Julie came up to him, and he took her on his knee. He said, "See, she never used to do this." When I said that it must feel good, he agreed but emphasized that this was a recent development. I said, "It must have been frustrating to have a daughter who wouldn't come to you." Mr. Bryan did not respond, and Mrs. Bryan said ironically, "Oh, but she would come to me!"

As Julie bounced happily on her father's knee, I asked them to think back to when Julie's crying started. Mr. Bryan said, "I think she had a bad colic at the beginning." I said that a very fussy baby who cries a lot is really stressful for parents. I added that something had happened that kept Julie's crying going long after infants outgrow colic. Addressing both parents, I said, "I've wondered if a pattern started out of your responses to her early crying. She was not an easy baby and her crying really got to you, so much so that it was hard to be with her. I remember you told me you didn't know what to do and that you decided leaving her alone to cry it out would help. I wonder if her crying for long periods with no one to comfort her made her feel anxious and insecure. And then, after the colic was past, she would get anxious if she was away from you and begin to cry. I'm not blaming you for feeling like getting away from her when she cried, but when you weren't there I imagine she became more worried and cried more." Mr. Bryan was thoughtful about this idea and said, "I think that's possible." Mrs. Bryan also agreed but looked anxious. She said, "Maybe Julie wanted me all the time then, because that's the way she is now." She described her frustration when Julie's crying had persisted: "I'd thought, if I could just get through the first 6 months, when you've got to pay attention to the baby all the time, I'd have it made. But Julie's crying threw a monkey wrench into that plan." I empathized with how difficult that had been for her.

Instead of continuing this discussion, she shifted her focus to Julie, whom she had taken on her lap. For the first time I had seen, Mrs. Bryan began to play a game with her. Julie tossed her empty bottle onto the coffee table. Erica, sitting on Mr. Bryan's lap, laughed at Julie's performance. Mrs. Bryan retrieved the bottle and handed it to Julie, who tried to push it off the table repeatedly. Each time, Mrs. Bryan, prevented the bottle from falling. As the game proceeded, both children were laughing excitedly and both parents were enjoying the game. I enjoyed it too, because it showed the family's ability to have fun together. Although this was a typical "baby game," I was struck by the latent content of the scenario: Mrs. Bryan was actively preventing the bottle from disappearing from sight, much to Julie's pleasure.

At the end of this visit, I pointed out that Julie seemed to be doing better. She was allowing her father to hold and play with her, was becoming more expressive, and was tolerating separations better. I asked them to think about what they had done to make things go better. I asked them to pay attention to what they were doing and what Julie was doing when things were going well—that would help us figure out what would help during difficult times.

I felt encouraged after this session, particularly because Mr. and Mrs. Bryan had given thoughtful and undefensive responses to my formulation of Julie's crying, even though it must have been difficult to hear. I was also encouraged by Mrs. Bryan's acknowledgment that Julie's problems involved wanting her mother, by Mr. Bryan's deepening engagement in the assessment process, and by the family's shared pleasure during the game with the bottle. Seeing the strengths in these parents gave me confidence that they could do the painful work of looking at their early feelings about Julie.

In the next session, I asked Mr. and Mrs. Bryan to describe their feelings when Julie's problems first began. Mr. Bryan said he had tried to comfort her, but when she continued to cry, "I just gave up." I asked what he did after he gave up, and he described putting Julie in her crib and then going down to the basement so he wouldn't hear her cry. He said he tried not to worry about her, yet felt bad about giving up on her. I was impressed with his honesty. I commented, "It didn't sit well with you to give up. It must feel better now that Julie is improving and she's coming to you."

Mrs. Bryan answered the question with a story I had not heard before. She had decided not to nurse Julie, and Julie had thrown up her formula feedings while she was still in the hospital after birth. Mrs. Bryan said, "She threw up all over me. It was all over my hands. I wondered if she had an allergy, and I asked her doctor if it would have been better if I'd nursed her, but he said it wouldn't have made any difference." She described taking Julie to several specialists, and how each simply told her that she would grow out of her crying. She said, "We kept trying, but when she got to be 6 months old and was still crying, I stopped taking her to them and tried to figure things out myself. I kept telling myself, it's got to get better." I said, "You've been concerned parents and it's all the more frustrating that you tried so hard to solve the problem but weren't able to." After I said this, Mrs. Bryan took Julie on her lap and held her. (This response was encouraging. It is fairly common in infant work to see that when a parent feels understood and supported, she can turn to her infant.)

I also said that "It's got to get better" sounded like a hopeful feeling, but I wondered if she had other feelings that were more negative. Mrs. Bryan smiled anxiously and did not reply. I said, "I'm trying to put myself in your place and think how I might feel if I had a baby who cried all the time and I couldn't comfort her. I think I would get angry at a baby like that." Mrs. Bryan replied, "Oh, I've been angry with her a lot. Sometimes I just put her in her crib, because I was afraid I was going to hurt her." I said that her anger was understandable, but that it is very hard on a parent to feel angry at a little baby—it can make a parent feel terribly guilty. Mr. Bryan said that his feeling was not so much anger as giving up. He said, "If I can't solve a problem, I try to ignore it." I said that their feelings seemed justified, given how hard it was to comfort Julie, but that feeling either angry or resigned could complicate a parent's relationship with a baby. I suggested that each of them had reasons based on their own feelings for drawing back from Julie, and that even though Julie was improving, those feelings continued to influence how they saw her. I added that Julie had her own feelings as well, that she seemed mad at her mother and distant from her father. Mr. Bryan said, "Her cry does sound mad now." Mrs. Bryan had previously expressed frustration that Julie had demanded her attention when she was trying to write a letter earlier that day. I referred back to that and said, "It seems like you and Julie are mad at each other a lot because you can't seem to please each other. This is the feeling that's grown up between you, and it's kept going, even though her feeding problems and colic are long past." Mrs. Bryan agreed that she and Julie were mad at each other. She said, "I really wasn't attached to Julie, not for the first 6 months. I could have given her away at any time."

This was an important session. The assessment process was gradually creating a story that made sense of Julie's crying and their reactions to it. Both Mr. and Mrs. Bryan had described their negative feelings toward Julie, and we had begun to link their feelings to their behavior toward her. Julie's crying was being redefined from her own internal problem to a transactional issue with a long history in the interplay between her behavior, her parents' difficult feelings, and their defenses against negative feelings toward Julie, which had taken the form of trying to distance themselves from her. The formulation of Julie's problems had been a shared endeavor between the parents and myself. Although an experienced practitioner might be able to understand the dynamics of the problem and interpret them very quickly to the family, it is better to engage the parents in a shared process of discovery. Parents who have reflected on the evolution of a problem are more likely to accept the worker's formulation and intervention recommendations.

OFFICE SESSIONS: VIDEOTAPING AND INTERPRETIVE SESSIONS

The family came to our agency for a videotaped session. I had told Mr. and Mrs. Bryan that I wanted to make a videotape of Julie for use in consulting with colleagues. I also told them we could watch the tape together at our next meeting. Julie and Erica enjoyed the toys in the playroom while Mr. and Mrs. Bryan watched from the couch. Julie crawled rapidly, taking pleasure in moving around the room. She also took a number of steps without holding on. She and Erica played independently of their parents. Julie's affect was curious and good-natured. A critical incident occurred midway through the session. Julie climbed onto a child's chair and sat for a moment, proud of her accomplishment. However, as she started to get down, she lost her balance and fell off. She began to cry and crawled over to her mother. Mrs. Bryan visibly shrank back from her and then stood up and crossed the room to get Julie a bottle. Julie crawled after her, whining. Even though Julie accepted the bottle, she pulled up by holding onto her mother's pant leg and raised her arms to signal she wanted to be picked up. Mrs. Bryan stood there for a few moments, then put the bottle in Julie's mouth and returned to the couch. Julie sucked on the bottle for a minute, then resumed playing. Later she climbed up on the couch between her parents, and again Mrs. Bryan folded her arms and leaned away from Julie.

Mr. and Mrs. Bryan came without the children the following week, and we viewed the tape together. Videotape has been widely used in infant mental health practice (McDonough, 2000). Video is a non-threatening medium that offers concrete visual data that can become the basis for an individualized guidance process directly relevant to the parents' concerns and to the child's particular developmental stage. The practitioner can use the tapes to point out the infant's current tasks, celebrate recent accomplishments, and forecast upcoming steps in development. Viewing videotaped sessions allows parents to see strengths and vulnerabilities in their infant and in their parenting abilities that they might not otherwise see (Share et al., 1992).

Mr. and Mrs. Bryan were pleased with the image of Julie on the tape. They noted her interest in the new toys and her independence. Mr. Bryan said, "She looks like a normal 1-year-old." As we watched her work to get up on the chair, I commented on her persistence. When she sat on the chair, Mrs. Bryan said, "Yay, you did it!" When she fell off the chair, Mr. Bryan said, "Oh, now she's going to want some sympathy." As Mrs. Bryan saw herself shrink away from Julie on the tape, her expression became somber. When she watched Julie reaching to be picked up and herself standing above her unmoving, Mrs. Bryan spoke for Julie, saying, "Pick me up, you idiot!" Mrs. Bryan's reactions to observing her own behavior and her ability to speak for Julie were encouraging. She acknowledged the validity of Julie's request for comfort. She saw her own refusal to provide comfort clearly, without resorting to defensive distortions.

Afterward I suggested that the tape showed Julie's strengths and age-appropriate development, as well as the problem that had prompted them to request an assessment. I said that after meeting with the family several times I had seen a lot of progress in a short amount of time. Julie was crying less and was coping with separations better. She was becoming more playful and more involved with Mr. Bryan. I said I thought that

Julie's improvement was due to her becoming aware of their concern about her. Their concern and determination to help Julie had made the biggest difference so far. I was optimistic, I said, that their concern would allow them to change their ways of responding to Julie before her problems became worse. There was a problem—one we had just seen on the tape—that would require more work to resolve. I pointed out that neither of them had been able to comfort Julie when she fell, but said I was very impressed by Mrs. Bryan's ability to speak for Julie and say what she needed. In order to understand how the problem evolved, I said, it had been very helpful to learn the early history of Julie's crying. When Julie could not be comforted, they found that very hard to cope with and put distance between themselves and her by leaving her to cry it out. This made Julie anxious and fearful that they didn't care, which made her cling and cry all the more. A problem that began as colic became a problem in their relationship. On their side, because Julie was such a difficult baby, they felt she could never be satisfied and that she was making them feel like bad parents, which made it harder to reach out and comfort her. Mrs. Bryan looked sad and said, "I could disagree with you . . ., " then began to cry. She said, "It was so hard when she was little. I don't want it to be this way. I was always more attached to Erica than I was to Julie. But Julie's my girl too." I said, "That's right, and I know you want to get this worked out. I know what I've said was painful to hear. But I wanted to tell you as clearly as I could, because it's not too late to do something about it. I am worried that if you don't make some changes in your relationship with Julie now there will be problems later on. Already by age 1 it's become like a battle between you and Julie, and there's a danger that could get worse as she gets older and that you'll always be fighting with her. But it really doesn't need to be that way if we can get the problems worked out now."

Mr. Bryan said that he had been worried about how Erica would react to a new baby, and so he had concentrated on paying attention to her. He remembered that when Julie's crying started he had turned even more toward Erica when he was home. I said that both of them had helped Erica cope with the intrusion of a new baby, but I suspected that Erica had gotten a lot of love before Julie came along, and so she already had a secure place with them. Mrs. Bryan said, "And Julie just got rebuffed."

Mrs. Bryan opened the next session by saying, "After last time, I really wanted to disagree with you. But I thought about it a lot. I decided to watch myself when I was with Julie. I did catch myself getting mad at her when she was fussing and wanting to come to me. I caught myself sort of flinching away like I did on the tape. So I tried something different. I opened my arms, and Julie came and wriggled up against me and she was so happy." I told her she had been courageous to look at the problem in their relationship and that it was great to hear that welcoming Julie had made her so happy.

Mrs. Bryan's ability to observe herself and change her behavior was very encouraging. However, when a relationship problem has persisted for a long time, it is not sufficient to focus on behavioral change alone. Both Mr. and Mrs. Bryan had acknowledged during the assessment that their attitudes toward Julie had been shaped by their inability to console her. They had begun to examine their anger toward her and to reflect on the defensive strategies they had adopted. Just as Julie had begun to internalize a working model of her parents as inconsistently available and at times rejecting, her parents had built up images of her as a demanding, never-satisfied baby. The ongoing power of these images and defensive behaviors could potentially undermine the parents' sincere attempts to respond differently to Julie. Consequently, I suggested that our work focus in part on their memories of how they felt when Julie was inconsolable in early infancy. I said, "Though those times are behind you now, they still influence how both of you feel about Julie, especially when she's clingy or crying." Mrs. Bryan responded by saying that she remembered wanting to get away from Julie because she was afraid she would lose control and hurt her. Mr. Bryan said he was so frustrated and angry that he wanted to throw her against the wall. I said, "That helps me understand why both of you would walk away from her. Really, you didn't want to hurt her, but it was hard not to stay angry at her. I think it would help to remember and talk about how you felt, about your understandable anger and how it has influenced your relationship with Julie." I believed that their attitudes toward Julie would change if they could reflect on their "unacceptable" anger and how it caused them to distance themselves from Julie. Exploration and validation of their anger could be a pathway to diminishing their defenses against getting close to her, which in turn could lead to a more consistent responsiveness to Julie.

DISCUSSION

The assessment of Julie and her family was informed by a knowledge of infant development in its transactional context. Julie's difficulties probably started in the young infant's typical fussiness at the end of the day. However, her parents were not able to tolerate her crying and responded in ways that decreased rather than increased her ability to regulate arousal. When an infant has to wait too long for relief of distress repeatedly, she begins to feel fearful and anxious in the face of mild distress, which increases the distress. It was likely that for Julie as a young infant the experience of anxiety was constantly reinforced by her parents' solution of letting her "cry it out." Her anxiety and disregulation, expressed in frequent bouts of crying, alienated her parents from her, so that the mutual regulation of arousal so helpful to young infants was not available to her. This affected her confidence in her attachments and probably kept her focused on keeping her mother close. However, this preoccupation with her mother's proximity, combined with both parents' tendency to avoid her when she was crying, prevented the full development of the pleasurable activities that emerge in a secure attachment between 3 and 6 months. Julie and her parents did not learn to play together or to find mutual pleasure in interaction that is characteristic of this age. (It was encouraging that both parents were beginning to play with her more at age 1.) Although she could play independently and showed normal interest in the world when her mother was present, these capacities seemed to disappear when her mother was not present.

"Goodness of fit" was poor between Julie and her parents in the first month of life. This set the stage for difficulties in Julie's ability to cope with stress. From the parents' side, there were several factors influencing their difficulties in helping Julie regulate arousal. Mrs. Bryan was under stress from having become a parent for the second time. In a parent who is already stressed, having another child is a risk factor for further stress. Mrs. Bryan's loneliness and depression during her first child's infancy promoted negative expectations of how she would feel during Julie's infancy. She felt unsupported by her husband, who also felt alienated from Julie. They were unable, until the period of the assessment, to come together to support each other. Prior to that Mr. Bryan had resigned himself to Julie's problems and had implicitly withdrawn support for his wife's attempts to cope with those problems.

Julie had come to be seen by her parents as a demanding, impossible-to-please baby. Their view of her, colored by their anger and anxiety, made it difficult to see what was normal about her. For example, they could not see her stranger anxiety, separation anxiety, and increased fussiness in response to working to master motor skills, all characteristic of 9- to 12-month-old infants, as aspects of normal development. Rather, they could only see these responses as continuing evidence of her earlier problems. Fortunately, over the course of the assessment, they began to see Julie's behavior in more normative terms. Throughout the assessment I supported this changing view by pointing out Julie's normal behavior and underscoring their descriptions of how Julie was improving.

The assessment prepared the family for more extensive work, yet it was an intervention in its own right. The assessment served to do the following:

- Define the original problem of crying in developmental terms
- Frame Julie's difficulties in a transactional context
- Focus the parents' memories and observations of their current feel-

ings and behavior on *interactions* rather than on Julie as an individual

- Help the parents distinguish between their images of Julie and her current actual behavior
- Lead the parents, through a gradually deepening examination of their behaviors, feelings and defenses in relation to Julie's problems, to a more empathic understanding of themselves and Julie
- Bring Mr. Bryan into a more supportive role and a fuller partnership with Mrs. Bryan on behalf of their children

The assessment also constituted a prognostically hopeful beginning, in that the Bryans showed determination to cope with Julie's difficulties, were responsive to initial interpretations (as shown by observation of Julie and their behavior between sessions), and demonstrated a capacity to work on understanding themselves in relation to their infant. Their ability to form a positive alliance with me was another positive sign. During the course of this assessment and beginning intervention, the relationship between myself and Mr. and Mrs. Bryan showed increasing depth and trust, as indicated by their willingness to share painful memories of their early relationship with Julie with me. Their courage in telling me about their fantasies of hurting Julie (which are perhaps the most painful and "blameworthy" thoughts a parent can have) signaled that they were increasingly willing to enter a real and collaborative relationship with me on Julie's behalf.

Observation Exercises

1. Spend 20 minutes observing a 5- to 6-month-old infant with one of his primary caregivers—either mother or father. Focus your observation on the following issues:

   a. Affective tone of parent and infant.
   b. Parent's physical handling of the infant.
   c. How well does she or he know the baby?
   d. Attunement and responsiveness to each other: eye contact, smiling, sharing perceptions, and attention.
   e. Parent's responsiveness to the baby: ability to see baby's needs, read his signals and cues, take his perspective, see him "as he is."
   f. Dyadic regulation: if mismatches or distress occur (e.g., the infant becomes fussy, or the infant reacts to the parent's attention shifting away from him), how do they restore a sense of synchrony?
   g. Play: If the observation includes play between the parent and infant, what is the content and process of the play? What do they do together, and how do they keep the play going?

2. Spend 20 minutes observing a 10- to 13-month-old infant who is on the verge of being able to walk, preferably in her home. Focus your observation on the following issues:

   a. Interaction—What is the balance of independent and attachment behavior? What does the infant do to gain the parent's attention? Does she use babbling, gestures, smiles or glances? Does she approach the parent? Does she share experience/objects with the parent by showing and pointing? How does the parent respond?

   b. Motivation—How intently does the infant practice physical skills such as crawling, pulling up, and cruising by holding on to furniture?

   c. Affective style/temperament—What affects and attitudes does the baby show as she practices physical skills? Descriptive terms might include exuberant, pleased with herself, determined, excited, reckless, self-contained, calm, irritable, easily frustrated, and the like.

   d. Dyadic and self-regulation—Observe how the infant responds to frustration. For example, how does she react when she falls repeatedly? Does she become affectively disorganized? Does she remain task-focused? Does she turn to a caregiver for emotional support?

   e. Reflect back to your observation of a 5- to 6-month-old. What differences do you see between that baby and the 10- to 13-month-old?

CHAPTER 7

Toddler Development

As the infant enters the second year of life, she becomes a toddler. The name of this developmental period, which covers 12–36 months of age, comes from the verb "toddle," to walk with short and wobbly steps. The image of the transition into toddlerhood is an infant pulling herself up, standing, looking around expectantly, taking several steps, falling down, and then repeating the process over and over, with gradually less wobbling and uncertainty. Toddlerhood is marked by the child's increasing ability to do things on her own and with gradually improving skill. The upright posture presents her with a new and wider view of the world. Walking permits her to move more easily and to cover greater distances. The toddler's increasingly effective motor skills make possible all sorts of new actions. Cognitive advances, combined with curiosity and will, intensify her desire to experience and understand everything she sees. Before she can use words to ask about the world, she uses actions to explore her environment and to raise questions about what she is experiencing. The new theme of the toddler is exploration.

The toddler moves into the world, but she is not ready to move out of the attachment system that has provided security during infancy. The need for secure attachment is carried along and transformed as the infant evolves into a toddler. *Toddlers have a dual orientation: toward maintaining attachment and toward exploring the world and the self* (Bowlby, 1969). The direction of toddler development, however, is toward individuation, toward a sense of the self as capable of autonomous thought and action. There is a corresponding shift in the toddler's motivation and goals. During the first year, the infant generally wants to interact with her parent. During the second year, the toddler increasingly wants to realize her own inner goals (Sander, 1975). By about age 2½, the toddler has begun to be self-aware, as indicated by correct use of the pronoun "I," to think of herself as able to take action and to evaluate how well she has done something. The toddler's growing self-awareness and knowledge is paralleled by growing awareness of how the world—her family, immediate environment, and, implicitly, her culture—is organized. The toddler period marks the child's gradual internalization of parental standards and expectations, as well as the construction of internal understandings of how the world works. The 2-year-old works very hard to make sense of her experience. Increasingly, she thinks her own thoughts and expresses her own ideas, using her developing capacity for representation, through play and language.

PHYSICAL DEVELOPMENT

Toddlers continue to grow at a rapid rate, though not nearly as fast as during the first year. Between ages 1 and 3, American toddlers, on average, increase in height from 29 to 38 inches and in weight from 20 to 33 pounds (Cole & Cole, 1989). Motor abilities, most dramatically symbolized by walking, increase considerably. Control of hands and hand–eye coordination improve so that, for example, a 2-year-old can stack three blocks and use a spoon, fork, and cup efficiently (Bayley, 1993). Between 2 and 3 the toddler develops sufficient control of bladder and bowel muscles to be toilet-trained.

Even though toddlers are gaining motor skills rapidly, they often must concentrate intently to maintain control of their bodies, especially between 1 and 2 years of age. The gap between what a toddler wants to do and what he *can* do physically is a frequent source of frustration. However, by age 3 the toddler walks with ease, runs, climbs stairs, and can peddle a tricycle.

Brain development continues rapidly up to age 2, then slows, since by that time length and branching of neuronal circuits has nearly reached adult levels (Nelson, 2000b). The theme of brain development during the toddler period is integration of functions. As myelination insulates the circuitry linking the brain stem, cerebral cortex (and different parts of the cerebral cortex), and frontal lobes, integration of perceptual and cognitive functions increases, processing speed in thinking improves, and self-awareness begins to develop (Nelson, 2000b).

ATTACHMENT AND SECURE BASE BEHAVIOR

During the second and third years, the toddler's ability to regulate affect and behavior and to organize experience continues to depend to a large degree on parental responsiveness and mutual regulation. A secure attachment during the first year predicts the child's continuing ability to use the parent's help to regulate affect and behavior in the face of frustration or stress (Vondra, Shaw, Swearingen, Cohen, & Owens, 2001). This capacity to utilize the attachment relationship on a continuing basis promotes mastery, social competence, and the development of autonomy (Sroufe, 1989). Working models of attachment develop. Although the toddler continues to depend on the actual relationship with the parent, she is also constructing representations of the caregiving relationship that allow her to gain comfort by thinking about the parent or by symbolizing the attachment through play (Bretherton & Munholland, 1999). For example, as pretend play develops midway throughout the second year, its themes often involve caregiving.

> When her mother was away for part of the day, an 18-month-old girl, playing with a little baby doll, kissed the doll, gave it a drink, put it in an infant seat that had previously been her own, and put a blanket over it. This child's play demonstrated an organized schema of good caregiving; at the same time her caregiving play probably helped her cope with a separation from her mother.

When the parent has been consistent in helping the child feel secure, helping the child cope with situations that arouse anxiety, and helping the child appraise situations that may be dangerous, the child internalizes these capacities as part of her working models: "Reliable protection by the mother allows the child to become self-protective" (Lieberman & Pawl, 1990, p. 379). Toddlers who have secure attachments with both parents show more positive affects, better frustration tolerance, and better problem-solving abilities than do insecurely attached toddlers (Kochanska, 2001).

Transitional Objects

Transitional objects (or comfort objects) exemplify the toddler's ability to symbolize the attachment relationship (Winnicott, 1958). Toddlers use transitional objects such as blankets, teddy bears or other stuffed animals, or dolls to help them cope with separations from parents and other potentially stressful situations, and with their growing sense of separateness. A transitional object is a single preferred object that the toddler takes to bed. After the parent leaves, the child may suck on it, snuggle with it, or talk to it. A toddler often takes his comfort object when he is going away from home or is going to be separated from his parents. The transitional object symbolizes the relationship with the mother, but also the toddler imbues it "with magical powers to soothe, protect, and empower the toddler to continue to explore the world" (Gemelli, 1996, p. 238). The transitional object is under the child's control, and he can use it to play out comforting aspects of the attachment when the parent is absent. The use of transitional objects is more common in Western cultures where infants and toddlers sleep alone. Parents encourage transitional objects and children value them because they help with the tension involved in an actual nightly separation. In cultures where young children sleep with their parents and breastfeed longer than is typical in the United States, comfort objects are much less prevalent (Steir & Lehman, 2000).

Secure Base and Exploration

The attachment relationship forms a context for the exploratory behavior that is so characteristic of the toddler period. A secure attachment creates a secure base from which to explore (Bowlby, 1969). Toddlers with secure attachment may spend relatively long periods playing by themselves without demonstrating any attachment behavior. Young toddlers are so interested in learning about the world, exploring the properties and functions of objects and toys, and experimenting with and practicing physical skills that they often appear surprisingly independent and self-absorbed.

> A 14-month-old examined all the toys in a play room while interacting very little with his mother. Yet, when the box with a crank on the side that he was turning exploded a doll into his face (a jack-in-the-box), he looked shocked and ran to his mother. She cuddled him for no more than a few seconds. They looked at the jack-in-the-box together, and she demonstrated how it worked while he watched. Then, although he was still wary of the jack-in-the-box, he went back to playing, with little interaction with his mother.

This brief example illustrates the interaction between the attachment and exploratory systems in the early toddler period. If the toddler is feeling comfortable and secure, his interest in exploring his immediate world dominates. However, if he becomes distressed, this activates the attachment system, and he "returns to base" and receives comfort or explanation from his parent until his sense of security is restored (Bowlby, 1973).

The secure base phenomenon so prominent in the behavior of toddlers as they move away to explore and then return to the caregiver is actually established in the attachment period during the first year. Infants play with objects or with their own bodies and look around curiously, studying their immediate world. In this sense they are already exploring "away" from their caregivers. In the first year, they have also learned how to return to base, or more precisely have learned how to bring the base back to themselves. They have practiced disengaging and re-engaging. If infants and parents have been able to work out effective ways of restoring attachment security after the infant has been focused on other things or after a separation or period of distress, the infant develops a sense of having a secure base, which will be put to use more obviously when she is a toddler. Attachment security translates into a sense of personal security and self-confidence in exploration (Grossman et al., 1999).

Additional Functions of Attachment during the Toddler Period

In addition to providing a secure base, the attachment relationship takes on some other new functions in supporting the child's development during the second and third years, including the following:

• *Providing modeling for behavior.* Toddlers watch their parents carefully and imitate their behavior, mannerisms, and words. When a toddler's relationship with a parent is secure and positive, she *wants* to do what the parent does. Toddlers imitate their parents in many ways, including wanting to join in household tasks:

> Two-year-old twins watched their father mopping the kitchen floor. They asked to help. Lacking toddler-sized mops, their dad gave them sponges and poured small puddles of water on the floor. These children spent the next 10 minutes wiping the floor, encouraged by their father.

• *Social referencing.* As toddlers encounter new situations, objects, and people, they turn to the parent for help in evaluation. If a stranger kneels down to talk to the toddler, he is likely to reach for his parent's hand and catch her eye in order to learn whether this is a safe person. The toddler relies on the parent to mediate between himself and new experiences and people.

• *Helping the toddler construct an understanding of the world.* The parent increasingly is an explainer and clarifier for the child—putting things into words in order to help the toddler understand her experience and feelings (Fivush, 1998). Parental explanations often include preparing the child in advance for unfamiliar or stressful experiences, describing in words what is going to happen. Everyone, including toddlers, appreciates advance preparation. But toddlers in particular benefit, because they encounter so many things that seem new and confusing. Providing information and clarification can be seen as a cognitive and affective dimension of providing a secure base. This function of attachment has implications for the treatment of toddlers (and older children) who have had stressful or traumatic experiences. Parents can help the child master a difficult experience by putting it into words, locating it in the past, and providing reassurance (Bennett & Davies, 1981).

• *Encouraging and scaffolding the toddler's language and communication skills.* The parent helps the toddler learn language and construct images of the world by "filling in" connections, asking questions, and adding elements to help the child create narratives. Dialogues between parents and toddlers have similar formal qualities to infant–parent play at 4–6 months in that the parent tends to take the lead and structure the language situation so that the child can participate. When toddlers begin to speak, parents talk to them using simplified grammar, frequent repetition, and a slow pace in the service of making language accessible to the toddler. Recordings of ordinary conversation between toddlers and parents reveal that they are "co-constructing" accounts of recent events (Engel, 1995). Conversations between toddlers and parents help toddlers create narratives of their experience, essentially helping the toddler organize and remember what he has seen and done and strengthening his sense of self as the central actor in his experience (Fivush, 1998; Harter, 1998).

• *Providing encouragement for progressive development.* Parents play a powerful role in supporting the toddler's practicing of developmental tasks by offering praise, asking questions that require the toddler to think about his experience, and pointing out when a toddler has succeeded at a new thing. The parent's encouragement and positive affect convey to the toddler that he is not only valued but also on the right track.

> The mother of an 18-month-old girl watched her push a 4-wheeled plastic "shopping cart" down the sidewalk and took pleasure in her accomplishments by saying, "You go! You're so fast." Her daughter smiled, then with a look of concentration began pushing faster. Then she stopped and lifted the cart completely off the ground, and her mother said with a mixture of pride and surprise, "Hello, girlfriend! Look at what you are doing!"

• *Continuing dyadic regulation of affect and impulse.* The parent, through comforting, setting limits, and putting things into words, helps the child learn to regulate feelings, especially helping him cope with powerful feelings, such as anger in tantrums, or frustration over not being able to accomplish a task. The attachment relationship "expands" to contain a wider range of affects, including negative feelings that arise in conflicts between the parent and toddler. The toddler's need to assert himself and to be in control poses a challenge for the parent, who may find herself struggling with her own anger as she tries to help the toddler cope with his strong feelings. However, toddlers particularly need limits and support from parents in regulating affects because their internal controls are not well developed: "The internalization of rules and prohibitions actually *empowers* toddlers, allowing them to regulate their own behavior and to resist temptation in situations where the caregiver is not present" (Harter, 1998, p. 563).

Relationships and Social Development

Both within the family and in interactions outside the family such as in day care, the toddler begins to learn about social tasks and expectations as they are defined by his culture. Mastering skill and understanding in the following tasks will continue to dominate social development throughout childhood

- Sharing and reciprocity
- Controlling impulses for social reasons
- Status, roles (including gender roles) and social rituals

Increasingly, learning how to be a social person will be negotiated in interaction with peers, not just parents. By age 2, toddlers have begun to engage in social play with peers, especially if they are in day care. Toddlers alternate between solitary play, parallel play (playing side by side, without direct interaction), and social play. Early social play lacks the imaginative role taking of 4-year-olds. It revolves around imitation of each other's behavior, shared interest in toys, and simple games like chasing each other. Older toddlers show the beginnings of cooperative pretend play by taking on different roles, for example, with one child playing the parent and pretending to feed another child. Through these interactions toddlers begin to learn social skills of engaging another person, coordinating actions with another child's, and sharing feelings. These beginning social skills reflect the 2-year-old's dawning awareness that others have their own ideas. This awareness allows the toddler to choose to coordinate her play with another child's (Brownell & Carringer, 1990).

Although toddlers' play with peers and sharing behavior display a motivation to be social, this motivation competes with the toddler's wish to be autonomous and in control. Spontaneous sharing of toys or food is very common between ages 1 and 2. At this age sharing is a sign of early sociability, and young toddlers enjoy it while showing little of the possessiveness that develops after age 2 (Hay, Castle, Davies, Demetriou, & Stimson, 1999).

A 15-month-old eating grapes alternated between popping one into her mouth and offering the next to her grandmother, for the pleasure in sharing and without any evident awareness that the grapes would be gone sooner.

Between 2 and 3 years of age, however, sharing declines somewhat in response to the toddler's awareness of being an autonomous self. This development is signaled in language by the emerging use of "I," "me," "my," and "mine" and in behavior by increasing insistence on having things his way. These normal developmental steps mean that 2-year-olds have much less ability than do older children in subordinating their own wishes in order to share or to maintain reciprocity and harmony in play. Consequently, their play together is often not sustained and is conflictual, as when two toddlers shift from sharing a toy to competing for it. Toddlers often become possessive of toys. They apply the word "mine" to whatever toy they happen to have. To a toddler "mine" means "I have it" or "I want it." They regard objects they possess as extensions of themselves (Elkind, 1994), regardless of who the actual "owner" is. Parents and caregivers sometimes fail to understand the importance of the toddler's developing an autonomous sense of self during the third year, as manifested in possessive behavior, and scold or punish toddlers for "not sharing." However, children of parents and caregivers who model sharing, empathize with their two-year-old's possessive actions while still encouraging sharing, and refrain from punitive discipline are likely to internalize the value of sharing over the long term (Hay, 1994).

COGNITIVE DEVELOPMENT

Toddlers' rapid cognitive development is interwoven with other areas, such as development of language and the sense of self. Details about cognitive advances will be highlighted in the context of other areas of development throughout this chapter. The following brief discussion presents some major themes of cognitive development.

Toddlers show an intense interest in learning to understand their own bodies, the physical world, and the social world. They seem to notice everything. By age 18 months they want to know how things work and how to use objects, such as a comb or washcloth, "correctly." They have begun to internalize the standards of their parents. They have learned to notice if a toy is broken and have constructed an internal map of their home environment, so that they notice and may even become distressed if something is dirty, missing, or out of place. They become aware of gender differences and around the age of 2 for the first time identify themselves as female or male.

As toddlers become capable of observing patterns and regularities in their lives, they develop conscious cognitive expectations. For example, a toddler who has regularly been comforted when she has been hurt is likely to come to her caregiver and ask her to kiss the hurt to make it well. The toddler develops a sense of sequence and rudimentary ideas of cause and effect. She becomes capable of thinking ahead, wondering about what will happen in the near future, and imagining possible outcomes. This cognitive advance allows the toddler to predict and anticipate what is going to happen, but it can also be a source of uncertainty and anxiety when a toddler correctly understands that *something* is going to happen but does not know what. For these reasons, toddlers sometimes show fear in novel situations and distress over transitions from one activity to another.

The toddler's improving cognitive abilities are demonstrated by his capacity for observation and imitation. Toddlers watch their parents and others carefully and are capable of imitating sequences of behavior. When a parent is cooking, they enjoy stirring with a spoon in an empty pot. If a toddler sees his parents dancing, he will try to dance like them. Most parents have occasional disconcerting experiences when their toddler imitates them too well. A toddler riding in a grocery cart said "Shit!" when his father made a loud noise by dropping a can into the cart. This little boy was not trying to embarrass his father but rather was saying what his father had said earlier that morning when he dropped and broke a cup.

The toddler's persistence and determination, which can be very frustrating for parents, is also a sign of cognitive development. Specifically, by about age 20 months, toddlers persist at activities, whether playing with a toy or repeatedly climbing up to forbidden places, because they can now formulate a conscious goal *and* keep the goal in mind (Kagan, 1981). Consequently, they are no longer as distractible as they were earlier. A 1-year-old can be deflected from pushing the buttons on the TV set if a parent shows him an interesting toy. He evidently stops thinking about the TV buttons. But a 2-year-old keeps the TV buttons in mind and keeps pushing them until *he* is satisfied or until a parent stops him.

LANGUAGE AND COMMUNICATION

From the first birthday to 18 months, the toddler's language acquisition proceeds gradually. Then, at about 18 months, the child's wish to communicate in language takes on new urgency. Language development seems to be driven by an inherent "urge to convey" one's thoughts (Locke, 1993), as well as by the toddler's awareness of the uses of language, as a social tool, a means of expressing her intentions, and a way of conveying her interpretations of reality (Bloom, 1998). Adults create the interactional context for the toddler's motivation to communicate. When parents encourage toddlers to express themselves, respond to what they say, and carry on "conversations" with them, the child is more likely to meet language milestones somewhat earlier and to show superior skill in using language expressively and pragmatically (Tamis-LeMonda, Bornstein, & Baumwell, 2001).

Neurobiological studies suggest that the burst of language learning between 16 and 24 months is made possible by a surge of growth in the cortical areas of the brain related to language. The rapidly increasing density of synapses in these areas, particularly in the left temporal lobe, increases the memory capacity and information processing ability that is necessary for learning large numbers of words and linguistic structures (Johnson, 1998).

For younger toddlers gestural communication and the first use of words are often combined. A 1-year-old enjoyed turning on light switches—when the light went on, he would point at it and say " 'ight! 'ight!" Understanding of words precedes the ability to speak them, and therefore receptive vocabulary accumulates ahead of speaking vocabulary. Toddlers can understand about 50 words between 13 and 15 months, but they are not able to speak 50 words until 18–22 months (Locke, 1993). During this period, toddlers often become skillful at using symbolic gestures that, like words, have a similar or the same meaning each time they are used.

> At 16 months a little boy regularly used a gesture (learned from his parents) to communicate perplexity or that something was missing. If he was asked, "Where did Daddy go?" or "What happened to your shoes?" he would raise both hands, palms upward, and open his eyes wide, with a serious look on his face. Within 2 months, he was accompanying this gesture with the words it signified, "Dunno."

At about 18 months, there is a burst of language learning marked by the toddler's wanting to know the names for everything. By 20 months, toddlers are beginning to combine two words, using verbs and adjectives in addition to nouns ("play ball," "dirty bugs"), and to string contextually related words together ("roll ... mah bush"—"my push," meaning I want to push the stroller) in rudimentary sentences. Evidence for the role of brain development in preparing a child to learn language comes from studies of deaf children. A deaf child who is being taught to use sign language shows a surge of vocabulary at the same time as children who can hear and speak (Lillo-Martin, 1996).

Toddlers are particularly drawn to learn words that are relevant and functional in their immediate experience, such as the names of objects in the environment, common events and actions, and words that have been emphasized by their caregivers. Relevance also influences which words children remember as well as the tendency to assimilate new words that are contextually related to the words a child already uses (Ninio, 1995).

> A somewhat precocious 17-month-old could say at least the following 60 words: "Mama," "Daddy," "Papa," "nursey" (to nurse), "Nana," "more," "water," "car," "hat," "truck," "bus," "shoe," "La-La" (a Teletubbie character), "ball," "yes," "no," "bye-bye," "hi," "dog," "bird," "baby," "poopy," "snotty," "that," "up," "down," "bubbles," "eat," "cheese," "cracker," "diaper," "nose," "eye," "walk," "shut," "rama" (for grandma), "kitty," "whee!," "light," "duck," "socks," "bottle," "book,"

"cup," "opitul" (for hospital), "back" (as in coming back), "star," "flower," "butter," "vroom-vroom" (for car). She was beginning to combine these words, and said a three-word sentence: "Daddy vroom-vroom opitul." Of course, she understood many more words than this and demonstrated a rudimentary understanding of English sentence structure, as indicated by her responsiveness to the questions and statements of her parents.

Although the vocabulary of toddler increases faster when their parents talk directly to them, they also pay great attention to what others say and learn many new words by hearing adults use them in the context of word meanings and situations they already understand (Akhtar, Jipson, & Callanan, 2001).

During the third year of life, vocabulary continues to develop rapidly, as do grammar, syntax, intonations, and pronunciation accents that are particular to the parents' culture. The transition from single words to two- and three-word sentences occurs normatively at around age 2. The child's use of verbs increases at this point, and toddlers use them to express actions they want to do: "running outside," or "read book." More complex sentence structures, involving subject, verb, and predicate, some connecting words such as "and," and, often, correct use of verb tenses, emerge between ages 2½ and 3 (Bloom, 1991).

After a 2½-year-old overheard his grandparents worrying about an old and sick cat they could not find in the house, he said, "I don't know where that cat went. Maybe she's hiding down in the basement."

By age 3, the child has a large vocabulary and command of present, past, and future tenses, enabling her to follow conversations and understand narratives. She has come to rely on words—as opposed to gestures and actions—as her main way of communicating.

Language as Organizer of Experience

This increasingly complex use of language is paralleled by other developments, including the emergence of symbolic play, improving memory, improving cognitive organization, and verbally mediated thinking—thinking in words. Language acquisition should be seen not simply in terms of increases in the number of words or complexity of grammatical structure but rather as a fundamental shift in the child's ability to process and organize experience. Language allows the child to construct representations of his experience and to locate them in a narrative or time sequence (Thompson, 1998).

Language, combined with a beginning understanding of how narratives are organized, provides the child with a way of sharing her inner life in an active way. Older toddlers begin to tell stories about their everyday life. Storytelling, symbolic play, and combinations of the two become a way of organizing experience through the use of narrative. The stories of 2- and 3-year-olds begin to show the quality of all narratives, in that they have characters (often the child herself), a beginning, a sequence of happenings, and an ending, as well as some element of tension, excitement, or humor (Engel, 1996). When older toddlers tell stories about their experience and receive interested responses from adults, their sense of power increases. Rather than having to depend on parents to intuit what has happened to them, they can now convey directly what happened and how they felt about it. Engel (1996) points out that "children tell stories as a way of solving emotional, cognitive and social puzzles and to sort out problems and concerns" (p. 8).

Language also becomes a tool for understanding emotions. By age 18–24 months toddlers begin to use words that name feeling states, such as "happy," "sad," "good," "hungry," "angry," "tired," and "sleepy" (Saarni, Mumme, & Campos, 1998). Language about emotions gives the young child a new and clearer way of understanding subjective states—her own and others'. Toddlers acquire words describing emotional states more readily when parents talk openly about feelings. For example, a parent says, "You were sad just now when I got mad when you put your car in the toilet." In this statement, the parent names feelings, helps the child make sense of what he is feeling, clarifies the parent's reaction for the child, and models the use of emotional language as a means of understanding conflict and distress (Dunn, Brown, & Beardsall, 1991).

Language and the Construction of Meaning

Toddlers also begin to think in words and to use thinking as means of constructing a view of the self and the world. Studies of narratives told by very young children demonstrate that they are often trying to "talk through" something they do not understand or find troubling. The stories of 2-year-olds go beyond merely trying to objectively describe the world in language; rather, they use narrative language to bring a personal sense of order and understanding to their experience. It is useful to think of toddlers' brief narratives as often reflecting questions about experience (Engel, 1995). What is the ocean? Is it dangerous? Why did Mommy yell when I went near the edge of the dock? Was I bad? For the toddler, there is a great deal to understand.

Many toddlers (though not all) demonstrate thinking in words by talking to themselves when they are alone, especially at naptime or bedtime. This is an extension of vocal play of infants when they are in their cribs. Crib talk gives the toddler practice with words and linguistic structures, just as vocal play represents the infant's practice with sounds. But toddlers' monologues before they go to sleep demonstrate a new dimension: they are thinking about and processing the events of the day. Katherine Nelson and her colleagues have analyzed the crib speech between the ages of 21 and 36 months of Emily, a child whose parents audiotaped what she said after they had tucked her in and left the room. Emily's monologues were often organized around questions of memory and anticipation: What happened? What is going to happen? The content frequently focused on variations in routine and novel situations—in other words, on events that Emily was trying to understand and put in perspective. The raw transcripts of Emily's monologues provide a fascinating window on a young child's attempts to make sense of the world. Here is an example from age 28 months. As he was tucking her in, Emily's father told her about a trip to the beach they would be taking the next day. Emily later talked to herself about the trip, clearly trying to anticipate what it would be like:

"We are gonna at the ocean. Ocean is a little far away . . . I think it's a couple blocks away. Maybe it's . . . down downtown and across the ocean and down the river . . . The hot dogs will be in a fridge. And the fridge would be in the water over by a shore. And then we could go in and get a hot dog and bring it out to the river, and then the sharks go in the river and bite me, in the ocean. And ocean be over by . . . I think a couple blocks away . . . we could find any hot dogs, um the hot dogs gonna be for the beach. Then the bridge is gonna, we'll have to go in the green car, 'cause that's where the car seats are." (in Nelson, 1989, pp. 66–67)

The parents' notes indicate that Emily had never seen the ocean, nor had she ever eaten a hot dog. Not surprisingly, she keeps going back to these two elements of her father's description trying to make sense of them. In her statements about the ocean and hot dogs, many questions are implied: Where is the ocean? Is it far away? Is it like a river? Will we drive across a bridge? Where will the hot dogs be? Since hot dogs are food, will they be in a refrigerator? Will the fridge be in the water? (Perhaps this reflects a previous experience with a cooler submerged in water.) Will sharks be in the water? Emily is trying to prepare herself for a new experience by constructing some pictures of it in advance. She combines her father's statements with her general knowledge, attempting to assimilate unknowns into what she already knows. For example, it is plausible to think there will be a fridge at the beach because that is where food is kept at home.

Emily's out-loud monologues demonstrate several functions: practicing language skills, recounting memories, anticipating experiences, processing emotionally difficult events, solving problems and questions, and reflecting on interactions between herself and others (Nelson, 1989). The young child's nighttime monologues have the same function Jean Piaget

(1951) ascribes to symbolic play: to sort out and contain experiences that have been stressful or hard to understand. Emily's overriding aim, according to Nelson (1989), is to construct "an understandable world within which she can begin to take her place . . . [and that is] a coherent representation of her experience" (pp. 27, 34). Crib talk tends to disappear around age 3. The child continues to think in words, but speaking out loud is replaced by inner speech, or silent thinking in words (Bruner & Lucariello, 1989).

Language and Self-Regulation

Toddlerhood marks the beginning of the child's ability to substitute words for action. Language allows the 2-year-old to say what she wants instead of merely acting. To understand this development, contrast a 14- to 18-month-old with a 2- to 3-year-old. The 14-month-old is attracted by a doll another toddler is playing with and simply grabs it. In response, the other child bites the first child. In this exchange neither child announces her intentions in words. Each one acts immediately following an impulse. An older toddler, however, may say, "I want the doll." She not only communicates a wish, but she also uses words to delay action on her impulse. Containing an impulse in language, "I want that," inserts a thought between impulse and action that may allow the child to think about the consequences of the action. Representing thoughts and feelings in language has a "cooling function." That is, putting an idea or feeling into words, whether out loud or in thought, "helps to 'cool' or reduce some of the uncertainty and emotionality in the child's world just by its displaced mode of representing that world in memory and thought" (Bruner & Lucariello, 1989, p. 76).

Even though this ability is developing, toddlers do not use it consistently. They still want to fulfill their wishes and express their emotions immediately, and frequently they act on impulse. It is important to recall that, although a 2-year-old can understand a great deal of what is said to him and may be speaking in sentences, representation in language is *only beginning* to help him delay impulses. Toddlers with intrinsic or environmentally based language delays often show problems in self-regulation, specifically because they are unable to use language to contain impulses, and tend to express themselves behaviorally, often through aggression that is at least in part based on frustration over not being able to communicate (Dionne, Tremblay, Boivin, Laplante, & Perusse, 2003).

Language as Communication

Toddlers are excited about their new ability to communicate about experience in words. The child begins to discover that language is a much more precise and predictable means of communication than gesture or action. Language allows children and parents to share awareness on a new level, because they are communicating through words that mean approximately the same thing to each of them. The parent's verbal confirmation of the toddler's perceptions and feelings validates them and contributes to the development of a sense of self. To express her thoughts in words and then have them confirmed in words gives the child the feeling that her ideas are real and valuable. This awareness provides the toddler with a powerful motivation for learning language.

Limits of Toddlers' Language Abilities

In spite of toddlers' dramatic progress in language development, they have important limitations in their language and cognitive abilities. Because the wish to communicate is very strong, toddlers can become very frustrated when they cannot express themselves clearly. This can occur because they are unable to pronounce the words clearly or because they do not yet know the words. The frustration is also a product of growing self-awareness. The toddler is more frustrated because he *knows* that others are not understanding him. Frustration over not being able to communicate is a common source of angry or aggressive behavior in normal toddlers. Even when a toddler has a good command of words, limitations in cognitive and affective development often cause the words to mean different things to the toddler and the parent. For example, an older toddler may use words that denote complex ideas and relationships, such as "truth," "share," and "promise," yet not fully understand their meanings (Leach, 1978).

Toddlers' use of language, especially when they are under stress, is often less a vehicle for describing "objective" reality than a way to convey thoughts influenced by wishes and magical thinking. If a toddler is accused of doing something wrong, she is likely to "lie." These lies by adult standards are, from the toddler's point of view, attempts at self-protection. The toddler who expediently says "I telling the truth!" may not be and further does not understand the meaning of "truth." She is not yet motivated by an internalized belief in the importance of truth telling. Rather, she shapes what she says to try to gain the parents' approval and avoid their disapproval. Wishes easily overcome logic and "truth" in the thinking of toddlers.

SYMBOLIC COMMUNICATION AND PLAY

During the early part of the toddler period, the child's play with objects is consistent with play in infancy. The younger toddler is interested in the properties and functions of objects. He plays with toys by learning what they feel like, what noises they make, how they look, what they can do.

Piaget (1951) labeled such use of toys and objects *sensorimotor play*. Play in the kitchen—banging pots and pans, fitting them together, or pouring water between them—is typical sensorimotor play for a toddler.

Between 1 and 2 years of age, sensorimotor play is increasingly associated with figuring out how things work and learning about cause and effect. Toddlers watch parents to see the correct way to use objects and try to imitate them. They learn through observation and then experimentation that knobs and buttons turn on the TV set or radio. Similarly, they act out the rituals of caregiving—patting, hugging, combing hair, feeding. Sometime between 12 and 18 months, toddlers' imitations of caregiving or eating behavior take on a pretend quality. For example, a 16-month-old takes an empty cup, looks at her father to signal he should pay attention, lifts the cup and "drinks" from it, says "ummm," and then laughs. In this sequence, the child has carried out an ordinary behavior, drinking, but since she has done it knowing there is nothing in the cup, she has transformed the behavior into play. Imitation has evolved into pretend play.

Midway through the second year *imaginative or pretend play* begins to alternate with sensorimotor play. The toddler begins to use toys symbolically and to integrate them into play scenarios. One of the earliest types of symbolic play occurs when the toddler substitutes one object for another. For example, as a 16-month-old boy was playing with pots and pans, he stepped into two pots and said "shoes." Then he tried to shuffle across the kitchen and laughed. Toddlers even at this age *know* they are pretending. Increasingly, if they are sharing a pretend scenario with an adult, they show their pleasure in pretend by smiles, laughs, and knowing looks that convey "we are pretending together" (Walker-Andrews & Kahana-Kalman, 1999).

Between ages 2 and 2½, toddlers make a more dramatic substitution by pretending they are someone else. Toddlers enjoy pretending to be animals. Piaget (1951) described his 26-month-old daughter's pleasure in walking on all fours and saying "Meow." Pretend play in normal toddlers often imitates adult behavior, with the toddler in the adult's role. A 2-year-old may pretend to feed his teddy bear, brush its teeth, and put it to bed, a sequence that demonstrates an organized view of his caretaker's behavior.

A 20-month-old boy watched his grandmother making tea. She noticed him watching and handed him a tea bag. A few minutes later they were in another room, and he was taking apart some wooden Russian nesting dolls. He took the cup-shaped base of one of the dolls and put his tea bag in it, then pretended to drink. Then he pointed to a wooden duck on a shelf and said "duck." His grandmother got it down for him, and he dipped the duck's beak into the cup to give it some tea.

Gradually toddlers' play becomes more complex and comes to represent the child's commentary on her experience. Play takes on a psychological function for the 2-year-old by giving her the freedom to explore experience through pretend. Piaget and Inhelder (1969) describe the new function play fulfills. The toddler is

> obliged to adapt himself constantly to a social world of elders whose interests and rules remain external to him, and to a physical world which he understands only slightly. . . . It is indispensable to his affective and intellectual equilibrium . . . that he have available to him an area of activity whose motivation is not adaptation to reality but, on the contrary, assimilation of reality to the self, without coercions or sanctions. Such an area is play, which transforms reality by assimilation to the needs of the self. (pp. 57–58)

Play becomes a vehicle for expressing strong feelings, a way of raising and answering questions about stressful and confusing aspects of reality, a mode of solving problems through "trial action," and even, within limits, a space where normal social rules do not apply. One of the developmental tasks of the toddler is to establish a compromise between his own wishes and the rules and expectations of his parents. The need to shape one's behavior to meet social demands is not easy for toddlers, who, as part of establishing a sense of self, want to follow their own desires. Toddler negativism and willfulness reflect this conflict. Symbolic play provides the toddler with relief from the demands of reality.

Play as Coping Strategy

Play provides the toddler with a nonverbal means of coping with confusion or stress. Older toddlers in child care, for example, regularly play out caretaking scenes, with themselves in adult roles, as a means of coping with the stress of separation from parents. Piaget (1951) noted that symbolic play offers the young child a vehicle for reliving and assimilating the stressful aspects of reality, at a distance, through fantasy that is under the child's control. Piaget underscored this aspect of play when he said that a young child's doll play in the evening would reflect all the child's pleasurable and difficult experiences of the day.

It is noteworthy that pretend play emerges at the same time as language, suggesting that a more general representational ability underlies both (Thompson, 1998). However, Bowlby (1980) noted that "because a child's use of language lags far behind his nonverbal modes of representation, there is a persistent tendency for adults to underestimate a young child's cognitive capacities" (p. 429). It is important for practitioners to realize that the play and behavior of very young children is a representation of cognitive and affective processes and that observation of such play provides us with a window on experiences and feelings that the toddler cannot yet represent in language.

Play as Representation of Experience

Symbolic play is referential: it refers back to the child's experience. It has a narrative quality and a point of view that conveys the child's perspective on her experience. This type of play begins at about age 2 and continues to develop into the complex, rich, and sometimes fantastic imaginative play of the preschool child. The symbolic play of toddlers often appears as fragments of narrative elements strung together. As in the crib narratives of Emily, the elements that are emphasized often represent aspects of the child's experience that have been perplexing or stressful. The following example illustrates the analysis of symbolic play in a toddler who was showing symptoms reactive to witnessing domestic violence.

JARED: A BRIEF CASE EXAMPLE

Jared, age 2½, had been referred because of aggressive behavior at his family day care home. He hit and bit other children and often hurt himself intentionally, running his head into the wall and then laughing. For a 6-month period, when Jared was between 10 and 16 months old, he had witnessed many episodes of his father's aggression toward his mother. The parents separated when he was 16 months old, but he witnessed more such episodes until the father moved out of state when he was 20 months old.

I wanted to assess possible links between family violence and Jared's symptoms. As the first interview began, I told Jared that my job was to help boys with their worries and explained to Mrs. Taylor that by observing Jared's play together we could learn what worried him. Then we could begin to respond in a reassuring way to his concerns. Jared repetitively pushed a car fast until it crashed and each time said, "It's broken." I asked Mrs. Taylor about this play, and she immediately associated to his father's pleasure in driving fast. Then she told a story of how the father, while hitting her in the car, accidentally hit Jared. She said he was only 5 months old then, so she doubted he would remember it.

As she told this story, Jared had found a small baby doll and put it in a little crib. I asked Mrs. Taylor if there were experiences he might remember. She described an incident after the separation, when Jared was 18 months old. She had closed the door in her husband's face. He kicked out the glass in the door, and it sprayed over Mrs. Taylor and Jared, whom she was holding. Jared screamed and began hitting her. As Mrs. Taylor described this event, Jared lowered a roaring plastic dinosaur into the baby's crib, saying, "Monster bite baby." I called her attention to this play as Jared continued to repeat it, noting that the monster appeared while she was telling the frightening story about the father's violence. In the second session Jared elaborated the symptomatic play, this time having the dinosaur repeatedly break down a Lego door and bite the baby inside. Mrs. Taylor said, "This is obviously about the night Al broke the door." I commented that Jared was showing us that he experienced his father as a frightening monster, and suggested that we were learning very specifically what Jared worried about—that something like that incident could happen again and he could be terrified and hurt. Mrs. Taylor said, "Every night he goes to the front and back doors to make sure they're locked." She had not previously connected this ritual with the door-breaking incident.

Jared's symptomatic play conveyed his anxiety that the violence he had seen might occur again. When the issue of his father's violence was raised in his presence, he quickly moved from diffuse crashing play to a stark and exquisite representation of his frightening experience when his father broke the door and he and his mother were showered with glass. From this clearer vantage point afforded by observation of Jared's play, it was possible to read his presenting symptoms of aggressiveness, fearlessness, reversal of affect, and self-hurting behavior as attempts to cope with tremendous anxiety about being hurt. He was hyperalert to danger and, like so many young children who have witnessed violence, was quick to attack in order to ward off imagined aggression. Play became a vehicle for expressing concerns Jared could not yet express in words. The observation of his play clarified for his mother and the therapist that he was preoccupied with fears of repetition of violence, and enabled them to collaborate on a treatment plan that would directly address his fears and traumatic memories (Davies, 1991).

REGULATION OF AFFECT AND BEHAVIOR

The toddler gradually develops capacities for self-regulation. During infancy, regulation of arousal was a dyadic process. Although we can see many elements of self-regulation in infancy and many examples of the toddler's need for the parent's help in regulating arousal and behavior, in toddlerhood there is a gradual shift toward more autonomous self-regulation that is part of the toddler's overall movement toward an autonomous self. It is typical for a toddler to try first to cope with a challenge by using her internal resources. If the toddler feels successful in this, her ability to recover from upset or stress increases. When internal coping devices do not work, the toddler quickly turns to external supports, particularly her attachment relationships with caregivers.

The toddler's cognitive characteristics present challenges to effective self-regulation. Her egocentric perspective prevents her from viewing reality objectively. Her difficulty in understanding the causes of events may lead her to confuse cause and effect. The urgency of her wishes and affects may lead her to believe that feelings and thoughts can cause things to happen. So the toddler, because of normative limitations in the level of cognitive development, is prone to interpret experience in concrete, egocentric, and magical ways that confuse cause and effect and fail to distinguish between thought and action (Piaget, 1952a). These cognitive limitations, as well as immature mechanisms for dealing with stress, leave the toddler vulnerable to stressful experiences. Parents play a critical role in supporting toddlers' capacity for affect regulation by explaining and clarifying their experiences, particularly those that are stressful for the child (Bennett & Davies, 1981).

Sources of Anxiety for Toddlers

Although the toddler wants very much to be in control of his own affects and impulses, the reality is that his capacity for self-regulation is not well established. Consequently, toddlers need parental limits and support for help in controlling impulses and allaying anxiety. Table 7.1 presents typical sources of distress and anxiety for toddlers.

TABLE 7.1. Sources of Anxiety for Toddlers

- *Difficulty in understanding what is happening,* based on lack of knowledge and unclear ideas of cause and effect. Egocentrism and magical thinking can cause misconceptions that create anxiety.
- *Difficulty in communicating.* Toddlers can think better than they can speak. There are questions they want to ask and statements they want to make, but their language has not developed to the point that they can find the words. Lieberman (1993) points to the frustration this engenders: "Often what passes for negativism is really the toddler's desperate effort to make herself understood" (p. 38).
- *Frustration over not being able to do what they can imagine.* For example, a 2-year-old boy watched his 5-year-old sister put on her jeans and then tried to imitate her. He tried to lift one leg up as his sister had done and lost his balance and fell down. He tried a few more times and became angry, kicked at his pants, and then went whining to his father for help.
- *Conflicts between wanting to be on their own versus wanting parent's help.*
- *Separation or threat of separation from caregivers.* This is connected with a more fundamental source of anxiety—"that the parent will not be reliably available at times of need" (Lieberman, 1992, p. 563).
- *Fears of losing the parent's approval and of being unloved, rejected, or abandoned.* This is particularly common during the toddler period because the child's wishes and behavior frequently clash with the parent's expectations. "Toddlers' anxiety over losing the parent's love is fueled by their experience that they no longer love the parent when they are angry at her. Because of their cognitive limitations, young children find it difficult to understand that others may feel differently than they do in a given situation" (Lieberman, 1993, pp. 130–131).
- *Reactions to losing self-control.* Although toddlers often appear to lose control of their impulses, they do not like to. It feels frightening to dissolve into a temper tantrum, or to hit or bite a peer and see the distress of the other child.
- *Body anxieties.* Examples include fear of body damage, anxiety about parental demands for toilet training, and concern about observations of differences in the genitals of boys and girls.

The "Terrible 2's" from a Developmental Perspective

The toddler's many sources of potential distress, difficulties in autonomous regulation, and determination in asserting herself often lead to behavior that appears willful and negative, as implied in the phrase "the terrible 2's." Toddler behavior is sometimes distressing to parents and other adults because it appears irrational and out of control, both affectively and behaviorally. A 21-month-old boy, Patrick, demonstrates behaviors that may occur during this phase:

> Patrick, age 21 months, had an active and intense temperament. He loved movement and activity. He expressed his feelings intensely and at this age was having frequent tantrums, especially when he was frustrated or told "No." He was quick to anger and would sometimes hit his parents if they prevented him from doing what he wanted to do. He was speaking very little, which made him rely on action to express himself. Patrick was sitting in a high chair at a restaurant, with his extended family, who were on vacation together. He was eating while adults around him talked. When he finished eating, he picked up a fork and threw it the length of the table. It bounced once and landed on his grandmother's plate. His parents were shocked and scolded him. Perhaps Patrick had felt excluded from the adult conversation. Perhaps this active child felt confined in the high chair, and throwing the fork was a signal of his displeasure. Acts like this are often intentional, not merely impulsive, and may represent the toddler's assertion of will, dissatisfaction, anger, or his sense of being affectively out of contact.
>
> After lunch, at the beach, Patrick splashed in the waves with his uncle. He was delighted. Later, when his uncle was dozing on the sand, Patrick threw a handful of sand in his face. Perhaps Patrick felt ignored and became angry, as had apparently happened at the restaurant. Perhaps his misguided aggression was an attempt to get his uncle to play with him again, a request he could not yet make in words. Such behavior angers adults and may provoke punitive behavior. Patrick's uncle did speak angrily, saying, "I don't like it when you throw sand in my face!"
>
> Such intentional aggressive acts perturb the equilibrium of the toddler–caregiver relationship. The adult's challenge is to reach out to the child and promote or acknowledge the toddler's attempts to restore the equilibrium following aggressive behavior (Sander, 1975). Patrick's uncle pointed to a pail and shovel and suggested they dig a hole and fill the pail. Patrick picked up the pail. His uncle said, "Let's go over there, away from the people, so we don't throw sand on them." Sander suggests that restoring the positive relationship after it has been violated by the toddler's destructive actions helps restore the toddler's inner equilibrium. By contrast, "should the caretaker ... fail to aid in restoring the facilitating self as the toddler had previously experienced it, the toddler's own familiar 'good self' as a constant frame of reference would be impaired" (Sander, 1975, p. 199).

Sources of Aggression in Toddlers

A more sympathetic view of toddler negativism, implied by Sander's analysis as well as Patrick's uncle's behavior, recognizes that toddlers face difficult developmental challenges that lead to frequent frustration, internal conflict, and conflicts with their parents. One of the possible responses to these conflicts is aggression. Lieberman (1993) lists three factors that may lead to aggression in the toddler or to expressions of anger, frustration, and anxiety that parents may perceive as aggression: (1) disagreements about what is safe; (2) the toddler's desire to have it all; and (3) opposition and negativism that go with wanting to have things their way. When a toddler's will is thwarted, he may become quickly frustrated and may have a temper tantrum, hit, or throw things.

Toddlers may also react strongly when parents or other caregivers expect them to function above their developmental level. For example, children can be ready for toilet training from age 15 months to 3 years. They signal their readiness by letting their parent know when they are urinating or defecating. Toddlers whose parents begin toilet training too early are often more angry and aggressive because they face the frustrating situation of the parent's exerting control over an internal bodily function. When toddlers are pushed to do something they are not yet ready or able to do, such as using the toilet, or picking up their toys, or happily sharing their toys with other children, they react with refusal, protest, and tantrums.

Strategies for Self-Regulation and Coping

Although the toddler faces a wider range of normal stressors than an infant, her range of strategies for coping with stress and self-regulation is also increasing. These include the following:

Mutual Regulation

Mutual regulation between parent and child continues, but in a new form, with the parent explaining and clarifying the toddler's fears of unknown or stressful events, setting limits that help the child contain her impulses, and remaining a secure base, available to comfort the child. The toddler can more easily elicit a parent's support by going to the parent and, during the third year, telling the parent what is wrong (Kopp, 1982).

Self-Stimulation as an Outlet for Tension

Toddlers may suck their thumbs, masturbate, or rub themselves and cuddle with transitional objects during times of fatigue or distress. These behaviors are normal responses to internal or external stress and occur particularly at the end of the day. They should not be seen as problematic unless they occur constantly. Caregivers should examine the child's life for sources of stress if self-stimulation is constant (Brazelton, 1992).

Play

Play—both interactive and with toys—becomes available during the toddler period as a vehicle for mastering stress and anxiety. For example, a 2-year-old who has a secure attachment can master separation distress by playing out a caretaking role with a doll.

Language

Language becomes available as a means of organizing experiences and feelings. The older toddler's capacity for thinking and expressing himself in words helps him delay actions. Between the ages of 2 and 3, the toddler begins to learn the names of feelings, including "negative" emotions such as anger, fear, and sadness, which allows him to convey feeling states more precisely (Ridgeway, Waters, & Kuezaj, 1985). The toddler who can say "I am mad" is likely to get a more empathic and focused response from a caregiver than one who expresses anger through aggression or a temper tantrum.

Internalized Standards of Behavior

Internalized standards of behavior develop in response to parental demands and modeling. Across the toddler period, parents gradually raise their expectations of the child's behavior and ability to maintain self-control. As the child accommodates to these increasing expectations, she internalizes ideas about behavior that is acceptable and not acceptable, and begins to regulate those behaviors, at least when a parent is present. She also learns the value placed on different emotions by her culture, and learns to inhibit "inappropriate" affects and emphasize "appropriate" ones (Saarni, 1999). By the third year, the child begins to use these internal standards to self-monitor affects, impulses, and behavior. When the older toddler can prevent herself from acting on the impulse to do something that is prohibited, her anxiety diminishes and self-esteem increases (Kagan, 1981).

"Effortful Control"

Effortful control refers to conscious attempts by the child to control expression of feelings, or alternatively to persist with an action in the face of interference or frustration (Kochanska, Murray, & Harlan, 2000). The older toddler begins to focus his attention "on purpose." Examples of effortful control, which can be cued from within the child or by someone else, include:

A toddler's parent says to a 2-year-old who is enjoying banging on the bottom of a pot, "Stop banging, I need to make a phone call," and the child stops.

A 2½-year old is working to pull a pair of shorts up on a doll. The shorts get stuck at the doll's knees, and the child continues to pull on them with an expression that blends frustration and concentration. She keeps working at it until she succeeds. She has been able to control her frustration in order to finish her task.

A 3-year-old who has been socialized to inhibit crying bumps his head on a closet door. His face crinkles, but then smoothes out, and he sits down in the closet for several seconds, breathing heavily, until he has gained control of his feelings.

Familiarity

Familiarity decreases stress. As previously unknown events, such as going to a child care center, are repeated, the child's anxiety diminishes simply because he knows what to expect. The child's ability to respond more neutrally to familiar situations is in turn based on memory development in the toddler period. By the end of the second year, memory has improved sufficiently to capture and hold "event representations" and scripts of actions that are repeated. The awareness of repeated sequences allows the child to predict what is likely to happen and also to begin to generalize about what to expect in different sequences of events that have similar elements. For example, a 2½-year-old in child care is told that his group is going on a field trip. Even though he has not been to the particular destination of this outing, the words "field trip" cue him to predict major elements of what will happen. Familiarity with the "script" helps contain anxiety about the uncertain aspects of the trip (Hudson, 1993; Thompson, 1998).

Sources of Difficulties with Self-Regulation in Toddlers

Anxiety is signaled by physiological arousal. Variations in young children's arousability can be due to temperamental factors, intrinsic regulatory disorders, sensory integration disorders, or previous anxiety-producing experiences (Posner & Rothbart, 2000). Toddlers who are more vulnerable to frustration, hyperarousal, or negative affects may have difficulty developing strategies of self-regulation. For example, a child with sensory processing difficulties may quickly feel overstimulated in a noisy, crowded situation and react by tantruming or becoming aggressive. He will need adult help to decrease arousal (DeGangi, 2000). A less reactive child in the same situation may not become aroused to the point of becoming distressed. Children who have not been helped to regulate arousal by parents during infancy may also become highly reactive because they quickly feel helpless and anxious in response to stressors. In Chapter 6, I noted that Julie did not seem to be a globally hyperreactive infant; however, out of repeated experiences of overarousal because she was left to cry, she became highly reactive in situations when her mother left her. Toddlers with histories of insecure attachment demonstrate problems in self-regulation by showing more anger and physical aggression; at the same time, because the attachment relationship has not adequately helped them regulate arousal as infants, they tend not to rely on the parent for mutual regulation (Vaughn & Bost, 1999). By contrast, toddlers with histories of secure attachment show more positive affects and more internal ability to cope with stress (Kochanska, 2001).

Similarly, toddlers who have had repeated stressful or traumatic experiences, such as witnessing domestic violence, are often highly anxious and reactive in situations (e.g., competition for toys) that contain mild elements of threat. Such toddlers often have difficulty regulating arousal and anxiety in new, ambiguous, or mildly stressful situations, because the experience of arousal itself has become associated with the previous trauma. Toddlers exposed to harsh and coercive discipline, maltreatment, or parental fighting also show more difficulties with self-regulation and aggression than do other toddlers (Thomas & Guskin, 2001).

MORAL DEVELOPMENT

During the second year, as the toddler becomes more mobile, he begins to have conflicts with his parents. His climbing onto the kitchen counter, for example, brings a quick and possibly sharp rebuke from his parent. At this point the conflict is external, between the child's wishes and the parent's prohibitions. However, through experiences of parental disapproval and approval, and through a new cognitive awareness that others have expectations and standards, the child's moral development begins.

As the second year proceeds, toddlers gradually internalize ideas of standards and deviations from expected norms, based on what they have learned from their caretakers. For example, a 1-year-old boy notices a tear hole in his T-shirt, considers it interesting, and sticks his finger through it. The same child at age 18–24 months, on discovering a hole, looks worried and says "Oh, oh," points out the hole to his parent, and may even ask to change the shirt. The infant notices the hole as a discrepancy, whereas the toddler sees it as problematic or incorrect (Kagan, 1981).

A 19-month-old was enjoying watching her father and uncle shoot baskets. But when her uncle threw up a big yellow ball and it stayed on top of the rim because it was too large to fit through, she scowled and said "No." Her uncle knocked it down and threw it up again, and she became more distressed when it got stuck again. Her father said, "That ball doesn't go there, does it, Anna? It's too big." Several hours later, she pointed out an upstairs window at the hoop on the garage and said, "No, no!"

This toddler's reaction reflects important shifts in cognitive development. Toddlers are working very hard to "construct," or make sense of the world. They are generalizing from one experience to another, looking for common elements. They are beginning to perceive and expect regularities in their experience, and these perceptions lead to schemas of what "should" happen.

Toddlers have also begun to internalize parental standards. Consequently, by about 18 months they become more acute in noticing deviations from what is expected, particularly when the norm violated is associated with their parent's disapproval. The toddler's concern with deviation and damage is reflected by common words in his vocabulary— "dirty," "messy," "missing," "yucky," "boo-boo," "broken." Kagan (1981) attributes this concern to the toddler's new awareness of cause and effect: "When the child sees a crack in a toy, he infers that the crack was caused by someone's action. Because that class of actions is associated with adult disapproval, he responds affectively" (p. 124). The toddler's worry may also be linked to his egocentric view that if he sees the broken toy he is somehow involved in its breaking.

Development of Evaluative Abilities and Standards

By 18 months and with increasing frequency up to about age 26 months, toddlers focus intently on evaluating their environment. Evaluative words such as "good," "bad," "hard," "easy," "nice," and "mean," reflecting standards of behavior and performance learned from adults, appear in their speech. By age 20–24 months, toddlers begin to evaluate their own behavior, as indicated by their pleasure in mastery and by their frustration when they cannot accomplish a task. A toddler who has worked to stack five or six blocks smiles broadly, looks to her parent for approval and recognition, and says, "I did it!" This toddler has developed the ability to make judgments about her behavior and to feel pride when she succeeds. The toddler is particularly likely to feel pride and self-approval when a parent notices her success. The same toddler may cry in frustration when she is unable to put on her socks. In both cases she has an internal representation of a goal and of the behavior required to realize it, a model of "correctness" or "success."

Two-year-olds *know* when they have done something well; they also know when their actions have not been successful. In a series of experimental, observational, and cross-cultural studies, Kagan (1981) and his colleagues demonstrated that toddlers become distressed when they are confronted with a task they believe they cannot do. If an adult modeled a series of actions with a toy that the toddler could not understand or that seemed too hard, the toddler was likely to become upset. At 14 months, younger toddlers did not become distressed when a "difficult" action was modeled. But by 23 months a significant majority became upset. Kagan (1981) interpreted the toddlers' distress as reflecting a self-evaluative awareness of their level of competence, as if the 23-month-old was thinking, "I feel I should do what this grown-up is showing me, but I know I can't, and it is upsetting to realize that I am confronted with a standard that I can't meet."

The Parents' Point of View and Internalization

Added to these cognitive elements, toddlers are learning from their parents concepts of correct and incorrect, proper and improper, permitted and prohibited (Kagan, 1984). The older toddler reflects this development when he looks up at the kitchen counter and says "No! No!" This may not be enough to stop him from climbing up again, but it shows that he has begun to incorporate the parent's point of view. He is experiencing a conflict between his wish to climb up and his wish to please his parent. Another indication that the toddler remembers his parent's prohibition is that he looks to his parent and checks her reaction when he has the impulse to do something forbidden (Lieberman, 1993). The toddler's developing capacity for representational thought means he can now recall and think about what kinds of behavior the parent approves or disapproves (Kochanska, Casey, & Fukumoto, 1995).

The development of a clearer understanding that others have intentions also supports early rule learning. For example, the toddler who has learned from the parent's strong reaction that she is not to allow the bathroom sink to overflow inhibits that particular action in the future. In inhibiting a forbidden action, the toddler implicitly acknowledges her parent's point of view, as if she is thinking "I want to do this, but my father does not want me to." Internalization supports moral development especially through the child's imitation of parental behavior. Through observing parents' behavior, including how a parent copes with stress, sets limits on her, and acts consistently or inconsistently, the toddler learns, imitates, and begins to internalize the "rules" of acceptable and unacceptable behavior. By age 2, this process is also supported by the toddler's understanding of language. Her understanding of words and tones that set limits—"No," "I don't want you to do that," or "Get down right now!"—helps make internalization possible. Her understanding of language also enables parents to increasingly set the limits through words alone. When the child is motivated to please her parent, verbal limit setting becomes increasingly successful.

The crib monologues of Emily provide some wonderful examples of a toddler in the process of internalizing parental rules and prohibitions. At 29 months, on a day when she and a friend were scolded for waking up her baby brother, Stephen, Emily produced the following monologue:

> "And we don't do it that much. But sometimes you go rinky-dinky all over the house. And do *that*. And go running away. And Stephen says I don't like *it*. Why do you do *that*, says Pooh-Bear. And my mom says you look like a . . . Why why why why. Why did you do *that*? [repeated five times]. Why did you go flying about getting out of bed. Why do you do *that*? I think maybe you wanna do that. But you can't. Over and over you can't . . . Why were you running around in Stephen's room and the other room and another room. Children, what are you doing? Why did you two do that? You can't do *that*. You can't. . . . " (in Nelson, 1989, pp. 164–165)

Emily's intense tone conveys distress over being scolded. She is replaying a stressful experience in words as a means of coping with it (Posner & Rothbart, 2000). However, this remarkable monologue clearly demonstrates how a child works to take in parental injunctions. The form Emily imposes on her experience reflects her mother's affects and point of view. It sounds as if she is repeating exactly what her mother said. Implicitly, she is identifying with her mother's prohibitions and attempting to internalize them. It is noteworthy that her mother's affects—apparently exasperation and anger—made a powerful impression on Emily. In the learning of rules and prohibitions, strong parental affects—anger, disgust, irritation, shock—play an important role in signaling to the toddler what is important (Dunn, 1987). Emily does not like her mother's disapproval, and it appears that she is working extra hard to take in the content of the rule "Don't make noise and wake Stephen up" in order to avoid disapproval in the future. Such experiences are the building blocks of later conscience development. Phrases like "You can't" and "Why did you do that?" become enshrined in "inner speech" as prohibitions that older children (as well as adults) use to criticize themselves when they have violated their internalized expectations and rules.

Although Emily's dramatic reaction illustrates how parental scolding contributes to conscience development, it is a mistake to assume that emotionally charged disciplinary situations are the only (or best) way for toddlers to learn parental expectations and values. Children with secure attachments are more likely to comply with parents' expectations: "Conscience emerges not only from . . . parental discipline but also from the incentives provided by a harmonious, mutually-cooperative parent–child relationship" (Thompson, 1998, p. 81). From the foundation of a secure relationship, the toddler is oriented toward gaining her parents' acceptance. She learns moral values by imitating parents' behavior, and takes in "moral lessons" by talking with parents about daily experience, creating "shared understandings of behavioral standards, moral values, and compliance" (Thompson, 1998, p. 82).

Recent research on moral development emphasizes the importance of nondisciplinary information, as when parents help the child anticipate what will happen in a new situation and convey their expectations for a child's behavior. A parent who talks with a toddler when he has calmed down after misbehaving may have more impact in conveying moral expectations (Thompson, 1998).

A young mother who had yelled at her 2-year-old son when he had opened the refrigerator for the fifth time, after she had told him not to several times, later said to him, "Remember when I got mad when you opened the fridge? I don't want you to do that. If you want something from the fridge you can tell me. But when Mom tells you not to do something, I want you to listen. That way I won't have to get mad and you won't have to get upset." The little boy listened with wide eyes. Then his mother hugged him.

This toddler is more likely to take in his mother's prohibition because (1) the child is not in a state of distressed arousal and therefore is more able to think about the content of the parent's statement; (2) the parent states her "lesson" calmly and rationally; and (3) the context of the lesson is reassuring—the child is aware that the parent loves and values him in spite of his misbehavior. A child whose parent treats him with respect and empathy is more likely to internalize the parent's values. By contrast, a toddler disciplined in a punitive and derogatory manner has more difficulty accepting parental standards (even though he may outwardly comply) because he associates them with fear, negative arousal, and the parent's unjust use of power (Kochanska & Murray, 2000).

Prosocial Behavior

Although this account so far has emphasized toddlers' internalization of standards and prohibitions, another critical aspect of morality that begins to emerge during this period is "prosocial behavior," defined as "acts that include provision of comfort or sympathy, helping, sharing, cooperation, rescue, protection and defense" (Zahn-Waxler & Smith, 1992, p. 229). Underlying these behaviors are prosocial thoughts and feelings, including "empathy or emotional incorporation of the other's emotional experience . . . [as well as] moral reasoning and cognitive comprehension of the others' internal states and needs" (Zahn-Waxler & Smith, 1992, p. 229). Parents influence the development of prosocial behavior by modeling prosocial acts, praising the toddler's positive behavior, modeling positive regard for others by being warm and supportive of the toddler, and directly stating their expectations of prosocial values and actions (Eisenberg & Fabes, 1998).

As toddlers develop the cognitive ability to comprehend others' perspectives, they also become capable of empathizing with the feelings of others. Many observational studies have demonstrated prosocial behavior in 2-year-olds (Zahn-Waxler & Smith, 1992). For example, a toddler in a child care setting sees another child fall off a slide and begin to cry, and goes over and pats or hugs her. This toddler empathizes with the other child's distress and, drawing on memories of being comforted himself, offers concern and comfort. Empathy is an essential element of later moral development. The toddler who responds to the distress or pain of another child is not acting in response to rules or prohibitions but rather to feelings of identification with the other child. The capacity to empathize with what it feels like to be hurt begins to play a role in the older toddler or preschooler's ability to inhibit aggression (Kagan, 1984). Through empathy and imaginative role taking, an older toddler can sometimes control aggressive behavior, as if he is saying to himself, "I would not like to be hit or kicked, and so I will stop myself from kicking this kid." Toddlers who demonstrate good capacities for empathy and prosocial behavior generally have histories of secure attachment with parents who have modeled empathic perspective taking (Kochanska & Murray, 2000). Overall, the young child's internalization of morality is founded on a history of the child's secure relationship with the parent. Young children are motivated to comply with parents' wishes and to make them part of an internal value system because "they are confident that the behavior expected by [the parent] is in their own self interest" (Grusec, Goodnow, & Kuczysnski, 2000, p. 207).

Limits of Toddlers' Moral Development

The toddler period marks only the beginning of moral development. Consequently, the toddler's internalization of rules, self-control, and capacity for empathy are subject to frequent breakdown. It remains hard for a toddler to inhibit a strong wish or impulse. Although internalization is proceeding, toddlers are not yet able to consistently comply with parents' expectations simply because it is the "right thing to do." Egocentrism and self-preoccupation impose limits on the toddlers' ability to empathize with another's point of view. In Kohlberg's (1984) formulation of moral development, the toddler's motivation for doing the right thing derives from wishes to gain approval and to avoid punishment, rather than from well-established internalized values or a sense of self as a good person.

For these reasons, contemporary books on parenting caution against having overexpectations about the toddler's moral abilities and self-control, suggesting that parents avoid control battles as well as coercion by structuring the child's choices and combining firm limits with diversions and alternatives. They suggest that parents be ready to move in and pick the child up when she does not respond to verbal limits (Sears & Sears, 1995).

The discussion thus far describes the first steps in the internalization of a positive morality. However, early socialization may also teach "immoral" values or create moral confusion. If parents fail to set limits on toddlers' aggression or rule breaking, give direct or implicit approval for impulsiveness, permit intense competition and aggression between siblings, model negative behavior, or present contradictions between their own behavior and moral injunctions, the toddler is likely to internalize those values and is unlikely to develop strong capacities for empathy and prosocial behavior. The development of self-control will also be attenuated (Dunn, 1987).

THE DEVELOPING SELF

The concepts "sense of self" and "development of the self" are abstractions. Whereas language or motor development can be tracked definitively, the evolution of the self is not so easily observable. However, several milestones in the second half of the second year convince us that the toddler is developing a sense of self and beginning to differentiate that self from other selves. Between 18 and 24 months, toddlers begin to recognize themselves in a mirror. Prior to this, they may show interest in the reflected image but not be aware it is their own image (Lewis & Brooks-Gunn, 1979). *Self-recognition* is one of several indicators of the child's developing sense of self at this age. By age 2, toddlers have begun to take in a view of self, or *self-representation*, that is strongly based on attachment experiences and the views of them that their caregivers have communicated to them: "Children perceive themselves through the lens of others' regard" (Thompson, 1998). Another clear sign of a developing self is *self-assertion*. Between 14 and 20 months, the toddler's behavior is increasingly directed by her own wishes and goals. She is clearly thinking more about what *she* wants to do and somewhat less about coordinating her behavior with her parent's (Sander, 1975).

A 19-month-old girl at a Chinese restaurant with her family finished eating and fussed about being in the high chair, saying, "Down!" Her mother tried to placate her by offering her broccoli, which she liked. This child, who was quite precocious in language, said angrily, "No! I no want it!" Yet, as soon as her grandfather took her out of the chair and walked outside with her, she began talking happily about cars and trucks going by on the busy street. This little girl was aware of how she felt and what she wanted, and asserted her wishes.

A child who disagrees with her parent implicitly asserts, "I have a self, with my own desires." The 2-year-old's awareness that other people have intentions, an awareness that probably arises out of experiences of conflict between his own intentions and his parents' wishes, contributes to the child's understanding that he has a self distinct from other selves. Awareness of self and awareness of other selves develop in tandem.

Mahler's Separation–Individuation Theory

Margaret Mahler studied the development of the sense of self in the context of the attachment relationship through longitudinal observations of infants and toddlers with their mothers. Mahler theorized that, up to about 16–18 months, the infant does not seem to have a full awareness that she and her mother are separate beings. Parental responsiveness has protected the child from having to rely on herself too much, and this has allowed her to experience herself as part of an adaptive unit, "my mother and me." Mahler argued that prior to 16–18 months the child's internal images or representations of the parents and the self are not yet separate and distinct (see Mahler, Pine, & Bergman, 1975). More recent researchers have criticized this formulation, since there are many indicators that infants can distinguish themselves from parents during the first year (Stern, 1985; Emde, Biringen, Clyman, & Oppenheim, 1991). Nevertheless, Mahler's descriptions of the toddler's "separation–individuation" process provide understanding of how the sense of self develops.

Mahler and colleagues observed that, beginning at about 16–18 months, toddlers regularly became more anxious about their attachment with the mother. They were more easily distressed, more reactive to brief separations from the parent, more clingy and controlling, and showed more negative affects such as depression or angry outbursts toward the mother. Mahler et al. (1975) explained these reactions as related to advances in the child's cognitive development that enable the toddler to understand reality ever more clearly. This includes being able to differentiate the intentions and feelings of others from one's own. Essentially, the toddler becomes aware that "My parent and I do not think the same thoughts, or always want the same things." When the toddler, intent on asserting his will or pursuing his own goals, runs into opposition from his parents, his awareness of psychological separation further intensifies. The toddler increasingly realizes that the parent has separate intentions and that he cannot control the parent.

Mahler theorized that this perturbed period, which she called the "rapprochement crisis," represented a struggle for the toddler overcoming to terms with his actual and psychological autonomy from his mother. She argued that the feeling of being separate and individuated was exhilarating, because of the increase in autonomy and power, but also frightening because of separation anxiety. Eighteen-month-olds seem to alternate between acting powerful and invulnerable and feeling very vulnerable and unsure of themselves. Consequently, the rapprochement crisis is characterized by ambivalence, "By the rapidly alternating desire to push mother away and to cling to her" (Mahler et al., 1975, p. 95). Parents of toddlers observe rapprochement as conflicting behavior. The toddler at one moment refuses help with something she is not yet capable of doing, such as buckling a seat belt, insisting "Me do it!" But when they arrive at a place the child has never been before, she refuses to walk on her own and whines, "Carry me." From the perspective of attachment theory, the toddler seems to be asking "How can I be an autonomous individual and maintain the attachment?" These conflicting feelings are expressed behaviorally through shadowing the parent everywhere, ignoring the parent, darting away (often with the hope that the parent will chase), being demanding toward the parent, and becoming more vulnerable to frustration and temper tantrums. This is the period when parents exclaim "I can't even go to the bathroom without him following me. If I lock the door, he sits against it and whines until I come out!" Yet, at many other times the toddler's loving feelings shine through without ambivalence, and he is responsive and interested in sharing feelings with his parents.

Steps in Mastering Separation Fears

What allows the young child to gradually master the frightening aspects of autonomy? First, when the parent remains a secure base, tolerates yet also sets limits on the toddler's demanding behavior, and welcomes his need for closeness, the child gradually understands that it is possible to be autonomous *and* connected. As in earlier periods of perturbation, the child is protected from negative psychological effects by the security and dyadic regulation of the attachment relationship (Sroufe, 1989). A second answer is found in the process of internalization. Mahler and others have pointed out that what allows the young child to tolerate the anxiety that comes with the awareness of being separate is the development of *object constancy*. This term refers to the internalization of a positive representation of the parent that is ultimately felt to be part of the self. The idea is that the child gradually takes into the self the caregiving and protective functions of the parents as well as aspects of the parents' ego functions, including the parents' defense mechanisms. Through this internalization the child gradually becomes able to use her own inner psychological resources to "take care of herself" and to become capable of regulating her anxiety without immediately needing to turn to the parent. This psychodynamic explanation has much in common with John Bowlby's (1973) description of working models of attachment.

Of course, if a parent responds negatively to the toddler's ambivalent behavior, there is risk that the "2's" really will be terrible. When parents react punitively or reject the toddler for being assertive, willful, and demanding, the toddler may feel disconnected and angry. Her separation anxiety may become more intense because of the parent's rejection. Consequently, her attempts to control the parent may also intensify, but with an angrier tone that in turn angers the parent. This spiral of negative interactions may lead to an attachment relationship characterized by mutual coercion and to the toddler's internalization of a negative self-representation.

Self-Awareness and Awareness of Other Minds

The shift to cognitive self-awareness around 18 months is paralleled by increasing awareness of the subjective states of others.

The toddler is beginning to feel differentiated from others and simultaneously becoming more aware of the possibilities of sharing mental experiences with others (Harter, 1998). The toddler begins to develop a "theory of mind," the awareness that others have *their own thoughts and intentions*, which may be similar to or different from one's own. After age 1, several new behaviors imply the beginnings of a theory of mind. The child increasingly notices and is curious about what others are paying attention to (joint attention). She notices and reacts to the emotions of others when they differ from hers. She reads adults' cues and uses them as guides to her own responses (social referencing). Her imitative behavior suggests curiosity about the behavior of others (Charman, Baron-Cohen, Swettenham, Baird, Cox, & Drew, 2001). The 18-month-old's ability to understand the intentions of others, even when those intentions are not expressed in words, has been demonstrated in experimental studies. For example, as the child watches, an adult tries and *fails* to carry out a simple action, such as pushing a button with a stick. The stick comes close to the button but does not touch it. When the stick is handed to the child, she touches the button with it, demonstrating that she has understood what the adult apparently intended to do (Meltzoff, 1995).

The development of a theory of mind makes possible new perceptions of relationships, new ways of appraising the feelings of others, and new ways of communicating that take into account the awareness that the other person's perspective differs from one's own. Theory of mind underlies the development of empathy and prosocial behavior. However, it also makes it possible for the child to get what she wants more easily (Jenkins & Astington, 2000).

> Chanitra, a young 3-year-old in a preschool, approached a child who was playing with toy pots and pans by herself, and said, "Can I play?" When the other child said, "No," Chanitra got some plastic carrots off the shelf and handed them to her, saying "We can cook these." The other child was pleased, and they began cooking together. Chanitra intuitively realized the other child's perspective was "I want to keep the toys for myself." This understanding allowed Chanitra to devise a strategy to induce the other child to share the toys, thus allowing her to realize her original goal.

However, the development of theory of mind also allows young children to apprehend another's child's threatening or negative behavior more clearly. Displays of anger, pushing, and hitting that occur when 2-year-olds play together often derive from one child's correct intuition that another child intends to take his toy. And most 2- and 3-year-olds are not yet as skillful as Chanitra at turning their understanding of another's intentions into a positive interaction (Hay, Castle, & Davies, 2000).

Like so many aspects of normal development, the concept of an emerging theory of mind seems unsurprising until the normal 2- to 3-year-old is compared with a child who is developing atypically. An autistic child shows a relative absence of the signs of a theory of mind (Baron-Cohen, 2001). Autistic children tend not to pick up on adults' affective cues and facial expressions. They seem unaware of the feelings of others, do not initiate or sustain joint attention, do not attempt to discern the intentions of others, and often have little interest in social imitation (Klinger, Dawson, & Renner, 2003).

> Luke, a 4-year-old autistic boy I evaluated with his parents present, showed no clear indications that he was able to mentally represent or intuit the perspectives of others. He played in an isolative and self-stimulating way, repeatedly pacing back and forth holding several playing cards in his hand. When his father demonstrated drawing on a paper with a marker, Luke did not imitate him. He did not respond to his dad's positive, mildly excited voice tone. His father worked hard to engage him in joint-attention activities. He rolled a toy car across the floor and motioned for Luke to roll it back. Luke glanced at the car, then turned away and continued pacing. His father commented, "It seems like he doesn't get it that I *want* to play with him."

The emergence of theory of mind in toddlers forms the basis for later advances in social and moral development. An older toddler can empathize with another child's emotional distress as well as feel guilt if he has hurt another child. In spite of these early capacities for role taking and empathy, it should be emphasized that the toddler is egocentric and preoccupied with self. He thinks about himself more than about others and tends to assume his point of view is shared by others. Studies of the verbal discourse of 2-year-olds show that they refer to themselves not only much more often but in more complex and varied ways than they refer to others (Budwig & Wiley, 1995). The capacity to see the world from another's point of view does not emerge fully until school age.

Self-Consciousness

Near age 2, the toddler is also developing self-consciousness, that is, becoming able to imagine how another person sees him.

A 2-year-old boy was brushing his teeth while looking in the mirror. He was enjoying watching himself doing what he had seen his parents do. His father was standing behind him, and several times he looked at his father. Each time when his father smiled and encouraged him, he looked very pleased and brushed more. It appeared that he was feeling, "I am doing what big people do, and my father sees that I'm doing it. He's proud of me, and that makes me feel proud of myself."

It is out of such experiences of seeing oneself from another's point of view that the toddler begins to feel the human emotions associated with self-consciousness—pride in success, pleasure in receiving praise, but also embarrassment at failing and shame over being scolded. Self-consciousness allows the toddler to evaluate his performance through another's eyes. This opens the way to internalization of parental standards and expectations (Kochanska, Aksan, & Koenig, 1995). Gradually, older toddlers begin to show the capacity to monitor their own actions, which suggests that they are taking an outside perspective on themselves. For example, 2-year-olds are self-aware enough to monitor their speech, as demonstrated when they spontaneously correct themselves after mispronouncing a word (Kagan, 1981).

The Intentional Self

The toddler's emerging sense of her self as an autonomous person is demonstrated by her urge to do things herself. She wants to feed herself, comb her own hair, and dress herself. The fact that she cannot do these things competently does not diminish her urge to assert control over her own activities and her own body. The toddler's behavior expresses the assertion "Do it myself!" even before she is able to say these words. By age 2, toddlers show considerable independence and persistence as they try to do things. They are more determined to do it their way and are not as easily deflected or distracted as they were at age 1. The toddler's insistence on doing things her way has been described as willfulness, oppositionalism, and a sign of "the terrible 2's." However, the toddler's having "a mind of her own" is a positive sign of cognitive development, indicating that she is now able to keep goals in mind, persist in pursuing them, and resist being deflected from them.

TODDLER PERSISTENCE: A BRIEF CASE EXAMPLE

An example of the toddler's persistence in pursuing her own goals appears in this vignette from a developmental testing. Tiffany was 2-year-old referred for testing because child care providers worried about developmental delays, particularly in the area of language. The Stanford–Binet testing was conducted in the playroom at a child guidance clinic. Tiffany sat at the table and did the first three or four items of the testing with ease. It is possible to see on the videotape, however, that her eyes kept darting to the corner of the playroom where the toy stove and cooking utensils were. After the fourth test item, she got up and went to play at the stove. The tester, who was knowledgeable about toddlers, waited while she played for a minute, then coaxed her back to the table. Tiffany came back as he presented an item that tested memory. He showed her a toy kitty, which she briefly looked at with interest. Then she got up and went back to the stove. He coaxed her back again and put the kitty under one of three small boxes. Then he put a sheet of paper in front of the three boxes and started counting to 10. The idea is to see if the child can remember where the kitty is after 10 seconds. However, by the count of 2, Tiffany was back at the stove. Her mother commented wryly, "She likes those toys better than yours." The tester asked her to come back, and she did, but brought a plate, knife, and fork, and pretended to eat, seemingly ignoring the three boxes. The tester repeated the sequence while her mother sat beside her to keep her from leaving the table. Finally, almost as an afterthought, she correctly found the kitty under one of the boxes.

In watching this sequence, it is a matter of one's perspective in judging whether Tiffany is a willful and oppositional child or a child who has a clear idea of her own interests and goals—which happen not to coincide with the tester's objectives.

The Self at Age 3

By the end of the toddler period the child's sense of self as an individual seems clearly established. The older toddler uses the pronoun "I" regularly. She describes her own actions—"I eating now"—and gives herself credit when she succeeds—"I did it!" She is capable of describing internal psychological states: "I am angry." She also uses the pronouns "you," "she," "he," and "we" appropriately, which indicates her ability to differentiate others from herself. She has learned her gender identity, can readily distinguish girls from boys, and has begun to internalize culturally based values and behaviors regarding gender (O'Brien, 1992). Her experiences in the attachment relationship, assuming they have been consistent, have promoted a sense of internal continuity, the sense of being the same person over time. Alongside the working model of attachment, a working model of the self has developed. The content of the toddler's sense of self depends a great deal on the patterns of regulation of affect and behavior that have been internalized from the attachment relationship (Sroufe, 1989).

APPENDIX 7.1. Summary of Toddler Development, 1–3 Years of Age

Information in parentheses shows when developmental features unfold and tasks become salient. Since there are individual differences in rate of development in children, I have indicated time ranges encompassing normal development. When a process is a salient part of development during the whole period, I have indicated this by including the whole period (1–3 years) in parentheses.

Overall Tasks

- Balancing attachment and exploration, with increasing movement toward autonomy and individuation
- Internalization of parental values and standards
- Developing the ability to symbolize, through mental representation, play and communication

Attachment

- Continuing transactional patterns of regulation of arousal and affect (1–3 years)
- Working models of attachment develop, allowing the toddler to develop some autonomous self-protective and self-soothing behaviors, especially between 24 and 36 months
- Use of transitional (comfort) objects for self-soothing and to cope with separation (16–36 months)
- Attachment relationship supports progressive development, including pro-

viding modeling for behavior, social referencing, helping the toddler understand the world, encouraging language and communication, and support for autonomous behavior (1–3 years)

Social Development

- Toddlers' egocentric view of the world, combined with their need to feel autonomous and in control, limits their ability to share or acknowledge others' different intentions (16 months to 3 years)
- Beginning understanding of reciprocity develops through play with peers (2–3 years)
- Imitation of parental behavior implicitly incorporates a beginning understanding of social expectations (2–3 years)

Cognitive Development

- Intense interest in understanding and learning about the world (1–3 years)
- Development of conscious expectations, based on memory of prior experiences; awareness of violations of expectations (18 months to 3 years)
- Ability to observe and imitate others facilitates learning (1–3 years)
- Conscious goals and plans: toddlers can formulate plans, consciously remember them, and persist in trying to realize them (18 months+)

Language and Communication

- Language learning: after gradual growth in vocabulary from 12 to 18 months, there is a burst of language development; this burst is motivated by the toddler's growing wish to communicate her experience (1–3 years)
- Two- and three-word sentences are used (18–24 months)
- Rapid development of vocabulary, syntax, grammatical structures, as well as idiomatic usage and pronunciation patterns used by parents (2–3 years)
- Beginnings of mental representation using words, narrative, and verbally mediated thinking (18 months to 3 years)
- Use of language to understand and "construct" the world: asking questions, telling about experiences, talking to oneself, crib talk (2–3 years)
- Social uses of language develop: using language to share experiences, putting wishes into words, and a beginning ability to slow down impulses by verbalizing them (18 months to 3 years)
- Limitations in language ability are a common source of frustration (and angry behavior) over not being able to communicate (18 months to 3 years)

Symbolic Communication and Play

- Sensorimotor play: exploration of properties and functions of objects (1–2 years+)
- Pretend play: imitation of ordinary activities (pretending to eat) or caregiving behavior (1 year to 18 months+)
- Symbolic play: substituting one object for another, sequences of actions in pretend (16 months+)
- Play becomes used as the child's symbolic commentary on his experience, as well as a means to represent and emotionally discharge reactions to stressful situations (18 months to 3 years+)
- Play of toddlers often provides a more complex representation of experience than they are able to express in words (18 months to 3 years+)

Self-Regulation

- Beginnings of autonomous self-regulation emerge; however, toddlers' internal means of coping with stress are limited and consequently they continue to rely on dyadic strategies of coping, based on the attachment relationship (1–3 years)
- Toddlers are subject to many sources of uncertainty and anxiety, and have difficulty exerting autonomous control over impulses; impulse control slowly improves during the toddler period (1–3 years)
- Coping mechanisms of toddlers include the following: dyadic regulation through attachment relationships; self-stimulation as an outlet for tension; play as a vehicle for mastering stress; language as a means for communicating distress; imitating and internalizing parents' ways of regulating anxiety (1–3 years)

Moral Development

- Young toddlers' mobility and strong motivation to explore inevitably causes parents to limit their behavior, often to protect them from danger; the toddler begins to experience a discrepancy between his wishes and his parents' limits (1–2 years)
- Parents' direct approval and disapproval, especially when accompanied by strong affects, supports internalization of parents' rules; at this point, the toddler tries to control his behavior in order to gain the parents' approval and avoid punishment (1–3 years)
- Internalization of standards: toddlers notice deviations from expected norms and become concerned if their expectations are violated; they evaluate their own performance, feeling good if they have done well and bad if they have not; they have learned their parents' expectations for behavior—

all these factors support the development of self-control (18 months to 3 years)

- Beginnings of prosocial behavior: beginning capacity for empathy may cause toddlers to comfort distressed peers and may help older toddlers inhibit aggressive impulses (18 months to 3 years)

Sense of Self

- Self-assertion: insistence on having things their own way and pursuing their own goals imply toddlers' increasing sense of self-importance (14–20 months)
- Self-recognition: midway through the second year, toddlers can recognize themselves in a mirror, confirming a new sense of consciousness of themselves (18 months to 2 years)
- Egocentrism dominates toddlers' view of self and others; they tend to emphasize their own needs and point of view over those of others (1–3 years)
- Separation–individuation: awareness of psychological differences and autonomy from parents; toddlers are more vulnerable to separation anxiety and more likely to activate attachment behavior during the most stressful period of separation–individuation, occurring at about 18–20 months (16 months to 3 years)
- Theory of mind: awareness that others have thoughts, feelings, intentions that may differ from one's own (16-18 months+)
- Beginnings of an autonomous sense of self, symbolized by independent behavior and in language by the emerging use of the words "I," "me," "my," and "mine" (2–3 years)
- Gender identity: sense of self includes awareness of gender identity (2–3 years)

CHAPTER 8

Practice with Toddlers

ASSESSMENT

As with infants, assessment of toddlers frequently combines observational with structured approaches. The toddler's capacity for symbolic expression through behavior, play, and—increasingly—words permits the clinician to observe how the toddler represents her experience. Observation of toddlers' representational play often becomes the vehicle for clarifying possible meanings of their behavioral symptoms. In the assessment of Jared (Chapter 7), for example, his repeated playing out of the incident when his father smashed the glass door demonstrated his ongoing fears and helped recast his "aggressive" behavior as symptomatic of anxiety about being attacked and hurt. Practitioners can also learn about the more immediate precipitants of toddlers' symptoms through naturalistic or structured observations at home or in child care settings.

Developmental testing of toddlers may be more difficult than at other stages of development because toddlers frequently do not cooperate with an agenda that differs from their own. The toddler's desire to assert herself and to explore on her own terms sometimes conflicts with the demands of structured testing. These are not insurmountable obstacles, however. Clinicians who test toddlers usually become skilled at adapting the pace and order of test items to achieve a compromise with the toddler. They learn to engage parents to help the toddler stay on task. While testing is useful, especially when the presenting problems include possible developmental delays, observation and interaction with the toddler often provide the most telling information about psychological, interactional, and developmental issues; see Table 8.1 (Meisels, 1996).

Assessing Secure Base Behavior

Although assessment must consider the full range of developmental tasks and accomplishments of toddlers, Lieberman and Pawl (1990, 1993)

TABLE 8.1. Summary of Assessment Issues for Toddlers

- A balanced assessment aims to identify optimal levels of functioning and areas of strength and potential, as well as areas of deficit.
- Observation, rather than testing, is often the most useful approach to the assessment of many toddlers, including those with developmental delays. As with infants, observation of the toddler in multiple settings—home, child care center, and office—provides a full picture of the child's range of functioning.
- Emerging representational abilities in the toddler permit the clinician to learn directly how she has constructed and given meaning to experiences, particularly stressful or traumatic ones.
- Since the attachment relationship remains essential to the child's capacity for adaptive coping, toddlers should be observed with their primary caregivers. These observations should focus on the quality of attachment, the balance of exploratory and secure base behavior, and the caregivers' attitudes toward the toddler.

argue that secure base behavior and the balance of attachment and exploration are especially sensitive indicators of the toddler's functioning. Since these issues can only be assessed in the context of the toddler's primary relationships, *toddlers must be seen with their parents.* The function of attachment is to provide the child with a sense of protection and security. A lack of responsiveness or inappropriate responses by parents can interfere with the toddler's ability to internalize adaptive ways of managing fear and anxiety. When the toddler does not feel secure, because of a history of unreliable protection in the attachment and the resulting failure of internalization of self-protectiveness, "the child's ability to engage in a confident exploration of the environment is disrupted, and alterations in the balance between exploration and attachment behaviors (secure-base behavior) are observed" (Lieberman & Pawl, 1990, p. 379). Lieberman and Pawl identify three patterns of distortion of secure-base behavior: (1) counterphobic recklessness and accident proneness, (2) inhibition of exploration, and (3) precocious competence.

Counterphobic Recklessness and Accident Proneness

The attachment history of toddlers who put themselves in dangerous situations involves a failure of protection. Parents have exposed the child to danger or have discounted, minimized, or ignored the child's distress. Frequently, the attachment figure has been subjected to domestic abuse and has implicitly shown the child that she cannot protect herself. This leads the child to rely less on the attachment relationship for a sense of protection. When such infants become toddlers and the urge to explore becomes paramount, they seems to court danger, "as if trying to discover how much risk they have to endure before the mother intervenes"

(Lieberman & Pawl, 1990, p. 382). These reckless toddlers have high levels of anxiety and reactivity to stress.

JARED: A BRIEF CASE EXAMPLE

Jared's presenting symptoms and the dynamics of his relationship with his mother illustrate the counterphobic reckless style. He was referred after a day care program threatened to expel him because of his wild, uncontrollable, and aggressive behavior. He often hurt himself and would reverse his affect, laughing instead of crying or registering pain. He climbed high on the jungle gym and jumped off. He ran into the street during a field trip. His provider said, "I try to restrain him, but there is no way to discipline him unless you are right there to keep him quiet." Jared's experience throughout his first 18 months included frequent exposure to his father's violence toward his mother. His mother reinforced his reckless, aggressive behavior by failing to set limits on it, simultaneously conveying to him through her lack of firmness that she could not protect him or help him control his anxiety-based impulses.

Inhibition of Exploration

These children, in a manner surprising for toddlers, avoid exploring the environment and instead appear as passive, vigilant, or unemotional watchers. They cling to the parent and are very distressed by separation. Two types of distorted parenting were identified to explain the behavior of these inhibited toddlers: parents who "needed" their infants and discouraged or punished autonomous exploration, and parents who were unpredictable and abusive, which seemed to encourage their toddlers to withdraw and to be cautious about making a move.

Precocious Competence

The toddler reverses roles with her caregiver, as shown in vigilance of the parent's moods and caretaking of the parent. The toddler gains a sense of security by staying close to and attending to the parent's needs, but at the cost of autonomous exploration. This pattern is associated with parents who are self-absorbed because of depression or other conflicts that make them emotionally unavailable. These toddlers perceive an emotional fragility in their parent that leads them to become precociously self-reliant because the parent cannot be depended upon. They direct their energies toward taking care of the parent and may become "compulsive caregivers" (Bowlby, 1980).

Observing Behavior in Context: Functional Assessment

The approach of functional assessment of behavior is commonly used in schools and can be used in child care settings and also be adapted for use by parents (O'Neill, Homer, Albin, Storey, & Sprague, 1996). Functional assessment of behavior is a simple but useful observational approach to understanding the behavior problems of toddlers and preschoolers. It is particularly relevant for toddlers because it relies on careful observation of behavior, as opposed to what the young child says.

Functional assessment starts with the assumption that behavior problems of young children are not random but rather have functions and meanings. From this perspective, difficult behavior represents a solution to a problem or need, may be an implicit communication, and is likely to represent a "chapter" in a longer and more complicated story. Understanding the function of behavior requires an "A–B–C analysis," A meaning antecedents, B meaning behavior, and C meaning consequences. This approach asks us to contextualize a child's challenging behavior so we can understand how it functions for a child (Arndorfer & Miltenberger, 1993).

When a behavior, such as hitting or emotional outbursts, is identified as a regular problem, the observer looks for antecedents—what is happening *just before* the behavior occurs. For an anxious young child at a child care center, the antecedent may be a transition from one activity to another; for a toddler with sensory processing problems who is easily overstimulated, the antecedent may be the increased intensity of play and hubbub that begins when a teacher announces that it is time to clean up (Fisher, Murray, & Bundy, 1991). It is also necessary to consider more remote antecedents, referred to as "setting events" or circumstances. Perhaps a child is more volatile on those days when his parent must go to work early, and he's dropped off at a family day care home at 7 A.M., and he knows the separation from his parent will be longer than usual. In some cases, a setting event may be extreme stressors such as witnessing domestic violence, a parental separation, or other events that disrupt the child's sense of continuity or traumatize him.

When we look at consequences, we ask, what happens after the challenging behavior? What reactions do caregivers and other children have? By looking at these reactions we can begin to understand what is reinforcing the behavior. For example, if one child pushes another child and takes her toy, and a caregiver ignores what happened, the first child may be reinforced in her use of aggression as a means of getting what she wants. For other children, especially those with ambivalent attachments to parents, a punishing, upset, or concerned response by the caregiver may be reinforcing because the child has learned that it is better to get negative attention than no attention at all. While the responses of others often make a child feel like her negative behavior has paid off, it is also important to go beyond learning theory and to consider that sometimes aggressive behavior persists because the child is angry, frustrated, anxious, or traumatized, not primarily because it is reinforced. In those cases it will be necessary to focus on understanding the immediate antecedents and setting events that contribute to the child's ongoing anger.

Note that this simple approach to assessment is helpful because of its power to *reframe* the understanding of behavior and to direct attention to the *meanings* of the behavior instead of to the behavior in isolation. Functional assessment calls attention to *A* and *C*, the two aspects of a three-part sequence that are more under adults' control than the behavior itself. By modifying the antecedents and consequences, we may be able to change the behavior (Kaiser & Rasminsky, 1999).

Functional assessment requires observation, preferably systematic observation across several days at regular intervals or particularly at times when a child is likely to be disruptive. Careful observation gives us a chance to develop hypotheses about the function of the behavior *before* we intervene. From these hypotheses, practitioners and caregivers can collaborate on interventions informed by a contextual understanding of young children's behavior. In the case described in the following section, I will illustrate the use of functional assessment in a clinical evaluation.

ASSESSMENT OF TODDLER DEVELOPMENT: A CASE EXAMPLE

The evaluation presented here illustrates issues of toddler development when a child is not functioning at the expected developmental level. Marcel, age 2 years, 8 months, presented with intrinsic developmental difficulties. Marcel's difficulties in navigating the developmental tasks of the toddler were primarily caused by his deficits in language and affect regulation, though the parent–child transactions that had been shaped by his mother's responses to those deficits also played a role in Marcel's presentation.

In assessing children with atypical or delayed development, it is crucial to examine the child's optimal level of functioning and areas of developmental adequacy, as well as areas of delay (Greenspan & Meisels, 1996). It is essential to identify areas where the child's functioning is age-appropriate or has the potential to become age-appropriate, because these areas of relative strength can become the basis of an intervention plan to address the areas of delay. This case example illustrates the uses of a careful developmental assessment. It also demonstrates how intertwined the toddler's developmental tasks are and how difficulties in one area can interfere with the accomplishment of tasks in another area. Marcel's development was very uneven, with age-appropriate functioning in some domains and severely delayed functioning in language and regulation of affect and behavior. These delays led to severe symptoms that overshadowed Marcel's areas of adequate functioning. Because of the severe language delays, it was difficult to assess his overall cognitive abilities. Between the ages of 2 and 3 years, cognitive progress proceeds in tandem with advances in verbal abilities. Marcel was moving ahead in

the development of awareness of self and others
wanted to communicate and was aware of the p
cation. However, he was tremendously frustrate
use words to communicate, and thus experien
between his cognitive abilities and desire for intera
and his ability to communicate what he was th
Finally, the case illustrates how consultation after e
important intervention on behalf of a child. Followi
was able to frame Marcel's difficulties and strengths i   .ay that helped
a school-based early intervention program plan services for him and his
mother.

Referral: A Toddler Out of Control

Marcel was the only child of his 24-year-old single mother. His father
rarely visited and was not involved in his life. Ms. Montgomery was supported by AFDC (Aid to Families with Dependent Children) and was not
working outside the home. The family was African American. Marcel and
his mother lived alone, but extended family members lived in their neighborhood. A school early-intervention program referred Marcel for evaluation at age 2 years, 8 months.

Presenting problems included severe language delays, short attention span, "hyperactive" behavior, and frequent severe tantrums. The
school district had attempted to evaluate him using standardized tests,
but he refused to cooperate with the examiners. His refusals were characterized as "lack of motivation." Estimates of his abilities were based on
observation and suggested delays in several areas. Language was estimated at 15 months, a very significant delay since it represented less than
half his chronological age. A normal hearing test had previously ruled
out hearing loss as a cause of his language delays. Cognitive abilities
were estimated at 20 months, while self-help skills were at the 24-month
level. His fine-motor coordination was seen as significantly delayed, at
about the 2-year level, while his gross motor abilities were judged to be
age-appropriate. His social abilities were seen as at the 10-month level.
This extremely low estimate was based on his "antisocial" behavior,
which the school program's report described in detail. Marcel ran around
the classroom, threw toys, opened desk drawers and threw the contents
about, pushed books and personal items off the teacher's desk, and tore
pictures off the wall. When the teachers tried to restrain him, he hit and
kicked them. He was, according to the report, "completely out of control." Apparently in desperation, a teacher put him on top of a tall file
cabinet, which stopped his behavior briefly. The school intervention program referred him for a pediatric neurology examination in order to discover whether neurological dysfunction explained his extreme behavior
and with the hope that medication could be prescribed.

physical examination showed no clear signs of neurological dysfunction. The medical report contained imagery and a tone similar to those in the school report. During the examination, Marcel ran against the door, hurtled around the room, and fell on the floor, constantly screaming and crying. He refused to cooperate with the examination and was "completely impossible to control." The pediatric staff could not capture his attention, and the resident evaluator commented, "Not much interests him." Marcel did not comply with his mother's demands, but it was noted that she was very patient with and invested in him. The report ended with the awed and decidedly nonclinical impression that neither the resident evaluator nor his medical supervisor had "ever seen anything like Marcel." A psychiatric evaluation was recommended.

Impressions of Referral Reports

These reports made clear that Marcel showed difficulties in several areas of development. It appeared that he had few adaptive strategies for coping with stress. I wondered if he might be unusually sensitive to novel situations. The previous evaluators were perplexed and awed by his intense, disturbed behavior. Their descriptions conveyed that he was incomprehensible and very difficult to empathize with. Both reports described him as lacking in motivation. This is a very unusual comment about a toddler, since so much of a toddler's behavior reflects the strong motivation to master his environment. The school report referred to his "destructive and dangerous acting-out behavior." Such language is commonly used to describe delinquent adolescents. It seemed extreme as a description of a 2-year-old. Because Marcel was African American, I was concerned about this characterization, since it might later contribute to stigmatization based on racist stereotypes of African American males (Canino & Spurlock, 2000).

The image of Marcel that emerged was a child who was incomprehensible, out of control, and dangerous. A child like Marcel understandably evokes in adults strong reactions that cause them to want to restrain and control him. The parent of a young child with serious behavioral problems often feels helpless and alarmed by the intensity of the child's behavior. However, a focus on the surface of behavior may prevent parents and others from understanding its potential meanings and may lead to controlling and punitive responses. But efforts at restraint, which ignore the sources of the child's distress, often elicit an escalation of the behavior. Marcel's behavior was so extreme that even seasoned evaluators were emphasizing the need to control him rather than formulating an understanding of his behavior.

Since Marcel seemed incomprehensible and possibly unreachable, the school had not been able to develop an intervention plan. Their request to our program was for intervention recommendations and medication. In my experience it is unusual for a request for medication to figure so prominently in a referral of a child so young. When such a request comes in, it is usually because the child's behavior is not only extreme but also unexplained. When extreme behavior in a toddler does not yield to a biological, developmental, or psychosocial explanation, parents and professionals, in desperation, may hope that a medication can be prescribed that will at least moderate his behavior.

Assessment Plan

I decided to spend my limited evaluation time observing Marcel in free play and interaction with his mother. This approach was consistent with current thinking on the developmental assessment of young children: "The cornerstone of assessment should be the observation of the child in interaction with trusted caregivers and the appreciation of the child's core functional capacities" (Greenspan & Meisels, 1996, pp. 25–26). The interview was videotaped so that I could carefully review Marcel's developmental abilities later.

Marcel's "deficits" had already been described in the two previous evaluations that attempted to impose structure on his behavior. Formal evaluation had not succeeded and had yielded only estimates of his developmental levels. There are a number of limitations in the use of structured testing for toddlers, not least of which is the toddler's frequent refusal to cooperate. Furthermore, formal tests, which have been standardized on samples of normal children, may not "bring out the unique abilities and potential of children with atypical or challenging developmental patterns" (Greenspan & Meisels, 1996, pp. 24–25). Since most test instruments designed to assess development after age 2 rely heavily on *verbal* directions and therefore on the child's ability to understand language, Marcel's language delays put him at a great disadvantage. I speculated that language-based tests—even assuming that Marcel would cooperate with them—would reveal his already known language deficits but perhaps obscure his capacities in other domains. I wanted to see what he was like in a more relaxed situation, without the pressure of formal testing. I wanted to see if his behavior told a story that made sense and to learn if he demonstrated areas of strength upon which an intervention plan could be built.

Parent–Toddler Interview and Observation

For the first 20 minutes of the 90-minute interview, Marcel did not fit the image of the previous evaluations. While I spoke to his mother and the school social worker who had driven them to my office, Marcel played with toys on the floor. He sustained his play and only approached his mother a few times to show her a toy. His preference for exploratory play was typical for a toddler. I did not observe any evidence of distress or attachment-seeking behavior. He seemed to regard his mother as a secure base and to feel comfortable exploring a new environment in her presence. However, other observations immediately raised questions of developmental delays.

- Marcel played exclusively at the sensorimotor level, looking at the toys, seeing what noises he could make with them. He moved from toy to toy in a restless way. I did not see any clear examples of symbolic play or imitation of adult behavior that would be typical for an older toddler.
- He said nothing. Toddlers often accompany their play with noises or verbal commentary, but Marcel was strikingly silent for nearly 20 minutes.
- He did not show evidence of understanding what we were saying. An older toddler with normal language development often responds to adult conversation about himself, especially when a parent expresses anxiety, concern, or negative feelings about him. His play may become more agitated, or he may become distressed and approach his parent. When Ms. Montgomery gave a concerned description of his frequent extreme tantrums, Marcel continued to play by himself. I suspected that his lack of reactiveness meant that he could not understand his mother's words.
- During his solitary play, his affect was serious and subdued. Playing did not evoke a range of affects. His affect did not change when he was spoken to. He seemed alone and out of contact with us.

History Taking

While I observed Marcel, I asked Ms. Montgomery about his development. I learned that pregnancy and delivery were normal, and, except for colic during the early months, she did not recall any problems during the first year. Motor milestones were on target. She said that her sister had thought that Marcel was not a very responsive infant. However, she had not been concerned during the first year because she usually knew what Marcel wanted and he seemed to enjoy being held and cuddled. During the second year, the capacity for imitation was present, but language and symbolic play did not develop. By 18 months, Ms. Montgomery had become concerned about Marcel's lack of social responsiveness and his lack of language. He was increasingly oppositional and began to have tantrums that she could not help modulate. Ms. Montgomery seemed highly invested in Marcel but perplexed and dismayed by his behavior.

Family history was positive for speech delays and severe stuttering by Ms. Montgomery during early childhood. Her younger brother was diagnosed with hyperactivity and learning disability in middle childhood. Ms.

Montgomery was poor but received emotional support from her mother and sister who lived nearby. However, she said that recently her mother had been pressuring her to spank Marcel when he had a tantrum. She said she was reluctant to do so because "I know there's something more wrong than just being contrary." Marcel's mother was a gentle woman who was trying very hard to understand him. She was a good informant about his development, which suggested she had come to know him well by being engaged with him over time. As she reported the developmental history, there were no holes in the information, as occurs when a parent has been neglectful, depressed, or abusing drugs or alcohol. Her descriptions of his development also seemed consistent with Marcel's current presentation, which suggested that her perceptions of him had been free of distortion. Her account was factual and free of attributions that connoted negative working models or unrealistic expectations of him.

Risk factors, including poverty and single parenthood, were present, but Ms. Montgomery had apparently been able to mediate the impact of these stressors up to this point. There was no evidence of risk factors such as parental psychopathology or substance abuse, which are particularly damaging to early development. Nor were there clear signs of physical or sexual abuse. These findings pointed away from a primarily psychosocial explanation for Marcel's difficulties and in the direction of intrinsic developmental problems.

Observation of Normal Behavior: Social Referencing

I noticed that as Ms. Montgomery began to feel increasingly comfortable with me during the first 10 minutes of the interview, Marcel's use of the play space changed. At the beginning of the interview, he played near his mother, a few feet from her chair. Gradually he moved away from her, while staying on her side of the room and at a distance from me. When his mother began to relate to me in a more warm and relaxed manner, Marcel moved to the center of the room and a few minutes later picked up a Fisher–Price house and put it on the table between us. He was relaxed and curious as I showed him how the house opened up and pointed to the small figures and furniture inside. Marcel's willingness to move closer to me as his mother became comfortable with me was another encouraging sign of a "normal" behavior, a clear demonstration of social referencing. Toddlers assess the safety of a new situation or person by paying attention to their parent's affective cues. If the parent expresses coolness or wariness, the toddler tends to avoid closeness or contact with the stranger. If the parent's affect is warm and relaxed, the toddler gets the message that the stranger is a safe person (Thompson, 1998). Social referencing has been studied in young toddlers who still understand very little language. The toddler's acceptance of the stranger depends not on language but on the affective tone the parent conveys to the new person (Emde, 1992). Marcel used his mother's responses to guide his own behavior, suggesting he saw her as a reliable beacon and secure base. Since such trust of the parent is based on a positive attachment, this was an encouraging observation.

A Critical Incident

As Marcel played with the house, he suddenly became upset. He screamed and banged his fist against the house. His mother thought he'd had trouble fitting a car into the garage and pointed to the garage opening, saying, "That car goes right there." Marcel looked at the house and screeched again. He tried to push the house off the table, then began to jump up and down. He jumped so hard he fell down. He began to cry loudly. He slammed the car against the house. Then he approached his mother crying very loudly and signaling gesturally that he wanted to be picked up. She picked him up, and for a few seconds he seemed to feel comforted. Then he arched away from his mother, crying harder and kicking. Ms. Montgomery held him for several seconds, trying to restrain him from bucking, then became frustrated and put him down. He lay on the floor, crying and kicking at the legs of her chair. She became angry and told him to stop it. He stopped kicking and began moving around the room in a "hyperactive" way, still crying. While this tantrum was going on, his mother confirmed that they occurred often, and she frequently did not know what caused these catastrophic reactions.

Marcel's tantrum was stunning in its intensity and duration. At first he had tried to use his attachment relationship to modulate his apparent frustration with the house. When that failed he was unable to regulate his own affects and became disorganized, collapsing into helpless, rageful jumping and screaming. He had almost no capacity to control the escalation of a negative feeling once it had started. His mother looked perplexed by his intense behavior and also demoralized because she did not know how to help him modulate it. I could identify with her sense of helplessness and with the reactions of professionals who had previously evaluated him. This was the behavior that had been seen as "completely out of control," dangerous, and inexplicable.

However, I had paid careful attention to the sequence of Marcel's behavior and formed a hypothesis about the causes of his extended tantrum. My position differed from that of an evaluator who assesses a child by trying to get him to do a structured task. I was free of the pressure— and frustration—an evaluator can feel when a child refuses to perform. It looked like Marcel's tantrum had been precipitated by his inability to do something with the garage door of the house. I wanted to assess whether he could regulate affect and behavior if he was helped to refocus on the point where things began to go wrong. I encouraged him to come back to the house, pointed to the garage, and said, "Let's figure this out. Did something go wrong with the house?" In response, he banged the car against the house and tried to push it into the garage. His angry response seemed a way of saying "Yes!" Already this was encouraging because his anger focused on a problem instead of being expressed in diffuse and aggressive discharge. When I helped him put the car in the garage, Marcel's affect changed dramatically. He calmed down and became interested in play again. For a minute we played together at the sensorimotor level, moving the car in and out of the garage. When he started another tantrum because he could not get the garage door closed, I helped him by showing him the small handle, and he quickly calmed again. Marcel could remain calm and focused if I physically demonstrated solutions to what had frustrated him and put into words what was happening. After the frustration was mastered, he was able to follow my suggestions about where to put people and furniture in the house. He also imitated me when I showed him how to ring the doorbell. As Marcel continued to play with the house, he said "Dee, dee, dee" in an excited and pleased tone and then said two words, "uh car, uh truck." Afterward, Marcel played independently with the house and other toys for about 15 minutes without the need for outside support.

Making Sense of Marcel

A different view of Marcel emerged from this interaction. His behavior was no longer incomprehensible. When I responded to him in terms of the actual source of his frustration (the car that wouldn't fit, the garage door he couldn't close) and helped him master a previously difficult task, his affect modulated and his behavior became much more organized. I immediately pointed out to his mother that his extreme behavior was a response to frustration with the house and that she had been correct in seeing that. His response to my help with the garage door made clear that he was not an "unreachable" child. On the contrary, he was very responsive to my support and suggestions. This suggested he could be open to instruction based on a reciprocal relationship. When I framed his tantrum as caused by a frustration with the house, he responded positively. This response suggested that it would be fruitful to think of his problems as based on a primary deficit in communication that had secondary effects on his relationships and his ability to regulate arousal and affects.

Functional Assessment of Marcel's Behavior

My observations of Marcel's behavior served as a spontaneous example of functional assessment. As I watched Marcel prior to his tantrum, it appeared that he was enjoying playing with the house. The antecedent event which seemed to set his tantrum in motion was his difficulty fitting the car into the garage. The "story" here seemed to be "I can't get the car in the garage, and it's so frustrating." Since Marcel had a severe language delay, a second, related, antecedent was that he did not have the verbal ability to communicate what was distressing him. The more remote antecedent, or setting circumstance, was a long history of difficulty in communication between Marcel and his mother. Consequently, he could not anticipate that his mother could help him regulate his intense arousal. The consequences of the tantrum were frustration and demoralization on the part of his mother because she could not understand what he was trying to communicate. This was followed by Marcel's frustration that his mother was unable to help him with the problem with the house and with his feelings. Frustration over the house escalated into frustration over not being understood. The consequence was that Marcel's tantrum intensified. With a theory about the cause, or antecedent, of Marcel's tantrum, I was able to test out an intervention on the spot.

Formulation

Marcel's behavior told a story that led to a clinical hypothesis that encompassed his intrinsic developmental problems and the transactional difficulties they created. Marcel was hyperreactive and easily distressed. He was motivated to communicate his distress. His approaches to his mother indicated that he saw her as a resource for dyadic regulation of affect. But his deficits in communication made this nearly impossible. His mother, who was strongly invested in him, frequently could not understand him. This made Marcel feel out of touch with her, which had a disorganizing effect on him and led to or at least intensified his tantrums. Unlike an autistic child, Marcel was clearly motivated to communicate and be understood by others, but he was unable to convey his internal states in understandable ways. He had so few words that he could not use language to help his mother and others understand his needs.

Interactive coping depends on the ability of the toddler to signal and engage a caregiver, who can then take steps to help the child cope with a stressor (Williamson, 1996). Marcel and his mother had not been able to evolve the more complex communication system one expects to see between toddlers and parents. As a result, their ability to use their attachment to help Marcel deal with distress was seriously compromised. The lack of dyadic regulation strategies led to many interchanges that were frustrating on both sides. For his mother and other adults, it was distressing to try to understand and fail; for Marcel, it was affectively disorganizing to try to communicate and fail. By the time of the evaluation at age 2 years, 8 months, this communication failure had a long history, resulting in negative expectations for both Marcel and Ms. Montgomery, not only about their ability to communicate but increasingly about the viability of their relationship.

The interactional sequence following Marcel's difficulty with the house was not only frustrating for Marcel and his mother but led to an escalation of mismatched responses and ultimately to demoralization in Ms. Montgomery and what appeared to be a profound sense of abandonment in Marcel. When Marcel first became distressed, he demonstrated secure-base behavior by turning to his mother for help. This was an appropriate use of their attachment relationship and was typical for a toddler who becomes anxious or encounters difficulty during exploratory play. However, Marcel was unable to communicate the particular meaning of his distress, which might be stated as "I can't get this car in the garage, and I'm feeling angry and helpless. I need help both with the car and to get control of my feelings." Lacking the linguistic means to convey this, he simply approached his mother for comforting. His mother then *thought* he wanted to be cuddled and picked him up. Marcel immediately became angry, feeling his mother had failed to understand him. His mother also began to feel helpless and responded by trying to control the symptomatic behavior by restraining him. Then she gave up and pushed him away. The desire of both to communicate was thwarted by Marcel's diffuse signals and by his mother's inability to decipher what they meant. The interaction became aversive for both, and the original tension, instead of being resolved, increased and was transformed into an interactional tension. In this type of interaction, there is no closure, and Marcel had to fall back on his own capacity for regulation of affect, which, when he was under stress, was limited to diffuse or aggressive motoric activity that others tended to view as "out-of-control" and incomprehensible behavior.

Assessing Areas of Developmental Adequacy or Potential

My observations confirmed the developmental deficits or delays found in the previous evaluations. Marcel showed serious delays in receptive and expressive language, which were likely related to deficits in auditory processing. He was hyperreactive to external stressors and internal frustration. His capacity for self-regulation even under mild stress was poor. Because of his difficulty in communicating in ways his mother could understand, mutual regulation of affect was also compromised. However, assessment must also define areas of developmental strength or potential. Identifying areas of normal development not only provides the parent with a sense of hope about her child but also helps the practitioner frame a treatment plan that uses the child's areas of strength to approach the areas of deficit.

A crucial aspect of my assessment of Marcel was seeing that he was capable of joint attention. In fact he was highly motivated to share my focus on the house. He could not express this interest in words, but he demonstrated it by looking where I looked and imitating my behavior.

Joint attentional behavior has been identified as an important condition for language learning (Baldwin, 1995). Typically, when parents look at an object or an event with a child, they talk about what they are seeing, implicitly teaching the child the names of objects and actions and gradually helping the child think about what she is seeing in words (Huttenlocher, 1999). This process had probably been derailed for Ms. Montgomery and Marcel because his language deficits prevented him from taking up the child's role in the process, which is to imitate the parent's utterances. Ms. Montgomery acknowledged that her behavior had been shaped by Marcel's lack of response. She had decided that he was "not ready to talk yet, or maybe he didn't like talking," and had talked to him less and less. I had engaged him as one might engage a very young toddler. Instead of relying primarily on words, I pointed out parts of the house and physically demonstrated how to do things that had previously frustrated him. I accompanied my actions with words but did not expect Marcel to grasp what I said. It was helpful to think of him as being like a toddler early in the second year, who is beginning to learn language but who needs concrete demonstrations as a bridge to language learning.

The assessment of Marcel's motivation was another crucial issue. It was very important to notice that, although he constantly struggled with feelings of failure and incompetence, he was still trying hard to communicate and master his environment (Eccles, Wigfield, & Schiefele, 1998). Marcel was not an unmotivated or apathetic child; rather, he appeared to have strong wishes to express himself and be understood. From this perspective it was possible to think about the intensity of his tantrums as a measure of his frustration about not being able to communicate. Further, seeing Marcel as motivated to make sense of the world and to communicate his feelings and ideas made him seem much more like a normal toddler rather than a child whose behavior was beyond comprehension. Marcel certainly was not "normal," because of his severely delayed language development and auditory processing skills as well as poor regulatory capacities; yet, his motivations were typical for a toddler. The observational assessment of Marcel illuminated several areas of developmental adequacy or potential. These included the following:

- Strong motivation to communicate and to master his environment
- Positive (though not always functional) attachment with his mother
- Interest in exploratory behavior
- Capacity for autonomous affect regulation when not under stress
- Capacity to use interactive coping to deal with distress
- Capacity for joint attention

These observations confirmed that Marcel's overall developmental maturation had been proceeding, even though one area, language and symbolic communication, was seriously impaired. Brazelton (1990) notes that "the force of the central nervous system as it develops is relentless" (p. 1664). Even in an infant or young child with deficits, the maturational thrust "tries to force around that defect, to push beyond what's holding the infant back" (Brazelton, 1990, pp. 1664–1655). Marcel's strong desire to communicate, marked by the intensity of his anger, frustration, and behavioral disorganization, could be seen as the force of development as it tried to overcome a defect. Brazelton (1990) also notes: "This is a critical force for recovery from a defect in an impaired infant, if it can be harnessed properly" (p. 1665).

An Intervention Plan Based on Developmental Understanding

This observational assessment, combined with the findings of the previous evaluations, suggested an approach to intervention that addressed Marcel's deficits by making use of his existing developmental strengths and potentials as well as the strengths in the parent–toddler relationship. To be effective, the intervention would need to address transactional issues between Marcel and his mother as well as Marcel's language and communication deficits. The following recommendations were offered to the early intervention program.

Toddler–Parent Developmental Guidance with a Specialist Trained in Infant Mental Health

This part of the intervention would attempt to build upon Ms. Montgomery's investment in Marcel and the adaptive aspects of their attachment relationship. Goals would include the following: helping Ms. Montgomery learn to observe and understand Marcel's behavior as reflecting attempts to communicate; helping her develop more empathic communication with him as she came to understand him better; and helping the two of them move toward an increasingly shared affective experience and "vocabulary" of gestures and words. The communication difficulties between Marcel and his mother had caused a relative failure in the functioning of the secure base. Marcel wanted to use his mother as a secure base when distressed, but since he could not communicate the content of his distress, he experienced his mother's caregiving as frequently off the mark and unreliable. On her side, Ms. Montgomery was baffled by Marcel's intense distress and consequently did not know how to help him regulate arousal. Although it is likely that Marcel had an intrinsic regulatory disorder (Zero to Three, 1994; Barton & Robins, 2000), it was clear that his mother was relatively unable to help him regulate intense affects. An additional goal, therefore, was to increase Ms. Montgomery's skill in dyadic regulation, both as an end in itself and as a bridge to self-regulation (DeGangi, 2000). The essential aim of the parent–child work would be to help Ms. Montgomery read Marcel's behavior accurately so that her responses would be more appropriate to needs implied by his nonverbal behavior. If Marcel could feel that his mother understood him more often, his ability to use her as a secure base would be strengthened (Lieberman & Zeanah, 1999).

Speech Therapy in the Context of an Intensive Early Intervention Program

Because of Marcel's severe language deficits and possible deficits in auditory processing, he needed speech therapy carried out at a basic language-learning level. I suggested in my report that "those who work with him will need to start where he is developmentally, responding to him much as one would to a young toddler. This will involve putting everything he does into words, providing a kind of running commentary, and being ready to provide concrete hands-on help if he becomes frustrated." I also suggested that if his progress in spoken language was slow, it would be useful to teach him some basic hand signing in order to give him some means of communication. This would lay the groundwork for verbal communication as his language skills developed.

Continuing Periodic Assessment

I suggested that I evaluate Marcel periodically to assess the effects of interventions and to provide consultation to the practitioners working with him and his mother. I hoped that periodic assessments—approximately every 6 months—would help Ms. Montgomery see Marcel's progress. During the first 3 years of life, development is rapid and responses to intervention are often more obvious than at later stages of development. Periodic assessments can provide a sense of progress and hope to the parent, since the evaluator can often point out real signs of developmental advances (Parker & Zuckerman, 1990).

No Medication

The request for medication to control Marcel's extreme behavior had figured prominently in the referral. This was a delicate issue, since the referring professionals hoped that medication would be recommended. In recent years there has been an increasing trend toward medicating very young children, especially those presenting with serious behavior problems. Recent research reviews have questioned the wisdom of this growing practice, because there have been very few studies of the safety and efficacy of psychotrophic medications for children under 4 (Zito, Safer, dos Reis, Gardner, Boles, & Lynch, 2000). Rather than simply focusing on symptoms, my report carefully detailed the dynamics of Marcel's extreme behavior. My intention was to provide a framework for understanding his tantrums and aggressive behavior in terms of developmental delays and interactional problems. I hoped that if Marcel's behavior could be seen as making sense and if the parent–toddler and speech therapy interventions began to show results, there would be less pressure to medicate him. In my report I indicated that I had consulted with our psychiatric staff and noted that we were unwilling to recommend medication for a child as young as Marcel unless other types of intervention were unsuccessful.

Follow-Up

Marcel entered a preprimary early-intervention program. He established a good relationship with his primary teacher and made steady progress in language development, with slower improvement in reactivity and affect regulation. His mother had attended school with him frequently and was borrowing some of the teacher's approaches to playing with him and setting limits. At the time of the follow-up assessment, 6 months after the first, Marcel's play was more organized and accompanied by more verbalization. He did not have any tantrums during the session. Ms. Montgomery played with him in a more sustained way, yet she said that she still often felt at a loss to understand his behavior. Significantly, the infant mental health referral had only just been made and Ms. Montgomery had not yet begun to receive the same level of intervention and support that Marcel was receiving at school.

INTERVENTION: PARENT–CHILD THERAPY

Intervention with toddlers involves an extension of the principles of infant–parent psychotherapy. Developmental attachment theory provides a rationale for seeing the parents and child together rather than either the toddler or parent alone (Lieberman & Zeanah, 1999). Even though the toddler is becoming an autonomous self, he still requires the support of the attachment relationship as it expands to include helping him understand the world. In joint therapy the therapist and parent can observe the toddler's play and behavior in order to learn about the sources of his distress or difficulties in the child–parent relationship. An important contrast with infant work, however, is that toddlers, because of their more advanced development, become more active participants in the therapy (Bennett & Davies, 1981; Lieberman, 1992).

Even though the toddler can't express complicated thoughts and feelings in words yet, he can increasingly represent his experiences through symbolic play. Toddlers' play often provides a more complex representation of their experience than they are able to express in words. Beginning between 18 months and 2 years, symbolic play and behavioral reenactments allow parents and therapists to learn about the child's perspective. Often the play of very young children is transparent, because it is less influenced by defensive processes than is the play of older children.

The toddler's growing facility with language also becomes available for therapeutic uses. After the burst of language learning beginning at age 18 months, words become increasingly available to the young child as ways of understanding and constructing images of the world. By age 2½ most children are well on the way to thinking in words rather than in imagery, and many older toddlers are becoming adept at expressing thoughts and feelings verbally rather than behaviorally. An awareness of the toddler's burgeoning receptive language skills is especially important in conceptualizing treatment of toddlers. The toddler's growing ability to understand the explanations of adults can be used to further the goals of treatment. Language offers new ways of organizing experience, and in traumatized young children holds the potential for reorganizing the experience of trauma. With words a toddler can begin to create narratives and learn about cause and effect. Therapist and parents can name the toddler's feelings and describe stressful experiences in simple terms so that the toddler is helped to make sense of them.

"Dialogues" between the toddler's behavior and play and the parent's or therapist's words can become the vehicle for understanding and resolving the toddler's problems. For example, Jared (in Chapter 7) specified the sources of his symptomatic behavior in play by repeatedly having the dinosaur break down a door and bite the baby inside. His mother realized that he was representing a frightening event that both of them had experienced. This allowed her to see beyond Jared's aggressive behavior to the fear and anxiety that were fueling it. The therapist and Jared's mother put the events and affects expressed in his play into words: "It was so scary when Daddy broke the glass. The glass hit you. Mom's not going to let Daddy do that again." The expression of empathy and clarification in words helped Jared represent his experience at a verbal level and provided him with reassurance that his mother was aware of his fears and intended to act protectively.

Lieberman (1992) points out, however, that it is important not to overestimate the toddler's ability to make use of verbal interventions and recommends that therapists find ways to talk about "big feelings in toddler-size words" (p. 570). The younger the toddler, the more strongly this caveat applies. It is frequently useful for the parent, with the therapist's coaching, to join in the toddler's play as a means of nonverbally dramatizing empathy and protective responses to the child's anxiety. For example, when Jared continued to raise questions and fears about his father's violence in play by having a father figure crash into the family in the middle of a meal, his mother picked up the mother figure and had her push the father figure out of the house, saying, "No, the mom's not going to let the daddy do that."

Representation and Trauma

The toddler's advancing capacity for representing the self in the context of experience carries liabilities when the child encounters stressful or traumatic events. The toddler may construct images of stressful experiences that reflect misunderstandings, confusions of cause and effect, and egocentric perspectives. Jared, even though he had not seen his father for 6 months, implied an ongoing expectation of his father's violent return through his nightly checking to see if all the doors were locked. In the toddler, in contrast to the infant, anxiety can take the form of conscious mental imagery that influences the toddler's view of self and reality. The toddler remembers and thinks about difficult experiences, such as a long separation from a parent, and worries they will occur again. These ideas create anxiety and are often the basis for toddlers' symptomatic behavior.

By early in the second year, children can retain behavioral or "action" memories of events even though they cannot describe the event in words (Bauer, 1996). This implies that they can remember and communicate behaviorally about traumatic events (Fivush, 1997, 1998). Since receptive language development runs a bit ahead of expressive language, it is possible to begin working on the goal of helping a child construct a narrative of trauma midway through the second year by having caregivers put into words what the child is expressing behaviorally.

The capacity for internal representation means that traumatic experiences may affect a toddler's working models, even when the parents are trying hard to provide a sense of security. The implication of this fact in regard to practice is that toddlers' misunderstandings and over generalizations need to be addressed directly in treatment. Because the toddler forms her own impressions and thoughts, guidance-based intervention with the parent alone usually is not sufficient to mitigate the toddler's anxiety. Toddlers need an opportunity to represent their concerns and to have them responded to specifically, which means that in most cases the toddler will be included in sessions with the parent and that therapy will be structured to elicit the toddler's representations of her experience (Davies, 1991). A recent study of intervention with maltreated 3- and 4-year-olds demonstrated that parent–child therapy based on attachment theory was superior to a parent-only intervention focusing on teaching parenting skills. Young children treated in the parent–child therapy model showed more positive self-representations and more positive views of their parent over the course of intervention (Toth, Maughan, Manly, Spagnola, & Cicchetti, 2002). From a developmental perspective, attachment-based treatment of toddlers and preschoolers is particularly timely, because it can improve the parent–child relationship and alter the child's representational models of caregiving and of the self in a positive direction *before* the young child's working models have become stabilized.

Attachment and the Treatment of Toddlers

In the treatment of toddlers and parents, *a primary goal is to strengthen the adaptive features of the attachment* (see Table 8.2). In some cases the focus will be on the parent's own negative or insecure attachment history as it contributes to his or her negative perceptions of the toddler. In less severe cases, the focus may be on the interaction between parental vulnerabilities and the toddler's self-assertion. For example, some parents who have found pleasure in the child as an infant react negatively to the toddler's growing autonomy, experiencing the child's assertion as a struggle for control. Treatment concentrates on reframing the toddler's behavior as developmentally appropriate and exploring alternatives to the establishment of mutually coercive interaction patterns. In other cases, the work focuses on restoring function to a previously adaptive attachment that has been compromised by developmental changes, stress, or trauma. Overall, "the most powerful change agent for young children's development and symptomatology is their relationship with their primary caregiver" (Scheeringa & Zeanah, 2001, p. 811).

TABLE 8.2. Toddler's Developmental Capacities That Can Be Utilized in Intervention

- Ability develops to represent and raise questions about experience through symbolic enactment and play (begins between 15 and 18 months).
- The toddler's strong motivation to know and understand experience makes him interested in pursuing salient issues in treatment.
- Receptive language ability permits the toddler to understand simple explanations of stressful experiences and reassurance (begins at 15–18 months).
- Receptive language ability also enables parents to prepare the child in advance for potentially stressful events, such as brief separations or doctor visits (begins at 15–18 months).
- Expressive language ability permits the toddler to articulate worries, questions, and concerns in simple ways (begins at 20–24 months, and increases rapidly with language development).

PARENT–CHILD THERAPY WITH AN ABUSED TODDLER: A CASE EXAMPLE

When she was 2 years and 8 months old, Kaitlin was physically abused by a 14-year-old female babysitter. Kaitlin's mother found bruises on her back, abrasions and bite marks on her arms and thighs, and blood in her diaper from scratches in her perineal area. Her parents took her to a hospital, and a finding of physical abuse was substantiated. The babysitter confessed that Kaitlin had wanted to play with her while she was watching TV, and that she had bitten Kaitlin hard on the arms and legs, hit her a number of times, and scratched her genital area, causing abrasions with her fingernails.

Kaitlin immediately showed some posttraumatic symptoms, including clinging behavior, anxiety about strangers, frequent waking at night, and frantic crying whenever one of her parents changed her diaper (Scheeringa & Gaensbauer, 2000). Her parents also showed some common reactions to trauma in a young child. They felt sad, helpless, overwhelmed and uncertain how to help her feel better. They were not only angry at the babysitter but also angry at themselves and guilty about having left Kaitlin with an abusive person. These feelings were disabling to them, in the sense that they felt unable to help Kaitlin master the traumatic incident. However, they did not want Kaitlin to be damaged by the trauma and were very motivated to participate in treatment. Prior to embarking on the parent–child therapy, I met with the parents and explained the approach, stating that Kaitlin should be able to use play to demonstrate her ideas about this frightening experience. I normalized her symptomatic behavior as consistent with a young child's reaction to a trauma, and said that their ability to convey understanding of what had happened and to provide reassurance that they would work to protect her in the future would help her put this experience in the past. I suggested that Kaitlin's prognosis was good, since this was a single incident of abuse, occurring in the context of a history of overall good development and secure attachments with her parents. I wanted to give Kaitlin's parents a realistic appraisal of her status, but I also intended to convey hope, because that would mobilize them to work in treatment on her behalf (Scheeringa & Zeanah, 2001).

I saw this family for about 2 months. I had two main objectives: to give Kaitlin a chance to represent her experience and her ongoing worries about it in play; and to help the parents mobilize the strengths in their attachment relationship with Kaitlin, so that she would gain their help in processing the trauma and receive their reassurance that they intended to keep her safe.

We sat in a circle on the floor, and I told Kaitlin that I knew she had been hurt by Jessica (the babysitter) and that her parents and I wanted to help her feel better about it. I said that playing would help us understand her worries. Kaitlin used small dolls to replay the abuse. I said she was showing us what happened. Her affect was sad and anxious, but she seemed driven to play out all the events of that night. After a bigger doll hit a little doll repeatedly, the little doll was taken to a hospital and examined by nurses and doctors. I asked her parents to describe in words what was happening in the play, and Kaitlin's mother retold the story of what happened that night. When Kaitlin presented the same play scenario in the next session, I coached the parents to tell her that they knew what had happened, that they knew Kaitlin had been hurt and scared, and that they knew she was worried that she would be hurt and scared again. They told her that Jessica would never be her babysitter again and that they would make sure that any babysitter they got in the future would not be someone who hurts little girls. They told her that for now the only person they would let take care of her would be her grandmother.

Kaitlin's play in subsequent sessions, as well as her behavior at home, represented questions about how safe she was, especially at night, a time when young children are likely to be more anxious in general, because they are separated from their parents and must give up a sense of control as they drift off to sleep. In sessions, Kaitlin had a "monster" come into the baby's room at night and bite her. At home, she was having trouble going to sleep and was often getting up and going to her parents' bedroom. I pointed out that, even though Kaitlin knew her parents had told her they would not let Jessica come and hurt her again, she still worried about it. In play, Kaitlin's father took an active role by having a father doll kick the monster out of the house. This demonstration seemed to reassure Kaitlin temporarily, but over the next 2 sessions she continued to elaborate questions in play about whether her parents could keep her safe. After the baby was put to bed, Kaitlin had her wake up and fly around the room. She would hit her head against the wall and cry. When Kaitlin's parents used their dolls to stop the baby from being hurt, Kaitlin's baby doll eluded them and kept getting hurt. I made this comment: "Kaitlin, this reminds me of how Jessica hurt you when Mommy and Daddy weren't there. It looks like the baby is showing your worry that Mommy and Daddy won't be able to keep you safe." I turned to her parents and asked them to respond. Her mother said: "We are not going to let Jessica come back to our house. We won't let anybody come into our house at night and hurt you. We'll stop them." After this, Kaitlin's play shifted to more normal caretaking play, with the Daddy doll tucking the baby doll into bed.

Kaitlin's play with the doll who eluded the parents' dolls and kept getting hurt was a clear dramatization of the dilemma of a traumatized toddler. Since young children have relatively few internal resources for mastering trauma on their own, they need external support, particularly from the attachment relationship with their parents. But precisely because toddlers rely much more heavily on the attachment relationship than on themselves to maintain a sense of security, trauma creates a challenge to the attachment relationship. The traumatized toddler implicitly feels that the fact that this frightening and overwhelming event could happen to me must mean that my parent cannot keep me safe and secure. This distressing awareness often leads to behavior that shows the child is questioning the viability of the attachment relationship (Scheeringa & Zeanah, 2001). Kaitlin was able to represent this issue in her play, and that allowed her parents to convey that they understood her worry and that they would act to keep her safe. Near the end of treatment, Kaitlin's parents went out at night a few times, leaving her with her grandmother. This gave her a chance to experience a separation from her parents and to learn experientially that she could be safe while they were away. In the relatively short time of 2 months, Kaitlin's posttraumatic symptoms diminished, which suggested that she had achieved some working-through of the trauma and that she was feeling more secure in her attachment with her parents.

As this case example makes clear, in infancy and early childhood trauma inevitably has a relational component. In the early years, the child depends on her attachment relationships for relief of distress and regulation of affect (Scheeringa, 1999). Kaitlin made a good recovery from a single-incident trauma because her parents were able empathize with and talk about her experience and made strong efforts to restore a sense of protection and to repair an attachment that had previously been a secure one.

Observation Exercises

1. Spend 1 hour observing toddlers and parents in a public place. A park or playground would be best, though a shopping mall or fast-food restaurant would also be interesting sites for observation. Observe for the following:

   a. *Secure base, attachment, and exploration.* If the toddler is in a place where she can play freely, note the balance she establishes between exploration and attachment. Do you see the toddler "checking in" with the parent, either visually or verbally, while she plays? How far does she move away from the parent? What does the parent do to stay in touch with the exploring toddler? What is the toddler's activity level? What evidence do you see that supports the idea that toddlers are intensely interested in learning about their immediate world?

b. *Autonomy.* What examples do you see where the toddler takes the initiative or insists on doing things his own way? How do toddler and parent react when the toddler's assertion of will runs contrary to the parent's wishes or intentions? How do the parent and toddler negotiate conflicts over safety?

2. Spend 30–60 minutes observing in a toddler room in a child care center or preschool.

   a. What individual differences among children do you notice in the areas of motor skills and language ability?
   b. What kinds of play do you observe? Note examples of sensorimotor, imitative, symbolic, and interactive play.
   c. Observe for the "mine" phenomenon, looking for instances of possessiveness or conflicts over toys. How do toddlers respond to such conflicts? How do caregivers respond when a conflict occurs?
   d. Do you see instances of empathy and prosocial behavior?
   e. Do you see instances of the presence or absence of self-control? What forms does self-control take? What appears to precipitate breakdown in the control of impulses?

Interview Exercise

Spend 30–60 minutes interviewing the parent(s) of an older toddler (between 2 and 3 years of age). Ask the parents to reflect on the differences between their child as an infant and toddler.

1. In general, how is she different at age 2, compared with age 6–9 months?
2. How has your relationship with her changed during the past 1–1½ years?
3. What do you recall about her during the 3–4 months immediately after she learned to walk?
4. How has her ability to communicate changed? How has her new ability to understand and use words changed your relationship?
5. Do you find it easier or harder (or perhaps some of each) to parent a toddler, compared to an infant?

CHAPTER 9

Preschool Development

The preschool period, encompassing ages 3–6, is a great transition in development. The child evolves from an egocentric toddler with limited capacity for understanding the self and the world into a child of the middle years, who has much in common with adults, in that she can think logically, maintain self-control, and empathize with others. Cognitively, the preschool child moves gradually from magical thinking to thinking that is more logical, shows understanding of cause and effect, and distinguishes between fantasy and reality. A major effect of these cognitive changes is that by age 6 the child's view of self begins to be more realistic. So, there is a corresponding movement from an egocentric, self-centered view of the world to a decentered, more objective view that understands that many events happen without reference to the self. The preschool child's relationships change as he becomes more autonomous. Relationships with peers become very interesting to the preschooler and have implications for development. In interactions and play with age mates the preschooler gains skill in empathy, perspective taking, negotiation, and cooperation, and begins to experience the pleasures of friendship. Through these interactions, the child begins to measure himself against others, introducing for the first time social comparison as a component of the sense of self.

The capacity for self-regulation and impulse control improves a great deal between 3 and 6, as the child learns interpersonal coping skills and internalizes cognitive controls and unconscious defenses. She still depends on her attachment relationships, but she slowly learns to manage anxiety by using internal resources and gaining support from others, based on generalizing her working models of attachment. In moral development there is a movement from reliance on outside approval or disapproval to a more internalized sense of values. The child gradually develops a conscience, which imposes internal standards for judging her behavior, creates possibilities for deriving self-esteem based on self-approval, and helps consolidate the child's internalization of the values, expectations, and rules of her family and culture.

The preschool child lives to play. This is the age of individual fantasy play and dramatic play with peers. As with the older toddler, play continues to serve the functions of skill development, exploration of reality, and mastery of anxiety. But imaginative play takes center stage in development, becoming an essential vehicle for constructing and understanding the world as well as facilitating cognitive and socioemotional growth (Piaget, 1962). The central role of play in preschool development will be emphasized and illustrated in this chapter, as well as in Chapter 10, which presents a detailed account of play therapy with a preschool child.

PHYSICAL DEVELOPMENT

The preschooler grows steadily but at a slower rate than the infant and toddler. A comparison of 2- and 5-year-olds shows that the 5-year-old is not just taller but more slender, with proportionately longer legs than the toddler. Her head appears proportionately smaller as well. Brain growth, though slower than in infancy, continues at a rapid pace. In particular, synaptic pruning and myelination continue to increase the brain's specialization and efficiency of function. Myelination of circuits in the sensory and motor areas translates behaviorally into improving perceptual abilities and motor skills, as well as better coordination between the two (Todd, Swarzenski, Rossi, & Visconti, 1995). Different functions of the brain are located in the right and left hemispheres, and during the preschool years the increasing integration of these functions is made possible by the myelination of the *corpus callosum*, a structure consisting of neuronal pathways linking the two hemispheres. For example, the left hemisphere is the site of language production and comprehension, while the right hemisphere is the site of emotional understanding. As the two hemispheres are linked, the older preschool child starts to understand not just another's words but also the emotional nuances the words express (Hellige, 1994).

Physical skills continue to develop steadily. Preschoolers can coordinate the movements of their muscles in gross motor activities like climbing, skipping, hopping, and running. They can throw or kick a ball and ride a tricycle. Because they are stronger and more coordinated, preschoolers thrive on physical activity. In the fine motor area, they become more and more adept at guiding their hands with their eyes. Improving hand–eye coordination enables them to cut with scissors, draw shapes such as a circle and a square, and by age 4 draw human figures that are recognizable. A 2-year-old may draw a series of straight or circular lines and label them a person, but without the child's description one would

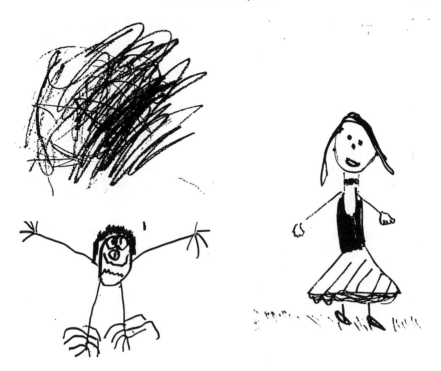

FIGURE 9.1, 9.2, and 9.3. The progression of children's drawing abilities. Figure 9.1 (top left). Age 2 years, 11 months: "Me, my eyeballs, and my body." Figure 9.2 (bottom left). Age 4: "Me." Figure 9.3 (bottom right). Age 5: "Me when I grow up."

not see a person in the drawing. A 4-year-old, by contrast, draws a person as two crossed lines with a circle on top—body, arms, head. She may also add details—fingers, eyes, mouth, hair. A 5-year-old can draw human figures that have more realistic proportions. (See Figures 9.1, 9.2, and 9.3.) Between 4 and 5, fine motor coordination improves enough for the child to be able to handle the fine points of dressing—zippers, buttons, and Velcro straps. Shoelace tying is harder and is usually not mastered until age 6 or 7. Overall, preschoolers take pleasure in the use of their bodies, which work much better than when they were toddlers.

ATTACHMENT

The preschooler continues to depend on the attachment relationship for feelings of security. The preschool child who has a history of secure attachment may show attachment behavior much like a 2-year-old's if he is feeling particularly distressed or anxious, very fatigued, ill, or in pain.

He may run to the parent and cling to her, crying and demanding the parent's attention. More often, however, securely attached preschoolers manage their attachment needs differently from infants and toddlers (Schneider-Rosen, 1990). Because a preschooler can verbalize his wishes, he is increasingly able to negotiate attachment issues with a parent. Bowlby (1969) pointed out that the preschool child's cognitive and verbal skills allow him to enter into a "partnership" with the parent around the goal of maintaining attachment. A familiar example of the child's negotiating ability happens at bedtime. The 4-year-old may say to his father, "I don't want you to go yet. Just read me one more story." His father may respond, "OK, I'll stay a couple more minutes, but then it's time to sleep." Increasing linguistic sophistication allows preschoolers to communicate their needs much more specifically than the toddler can. A child who has been upset by a separation can say, "Mommy, I wanted you and you weren't there!" Being able to communicate directly in words, with the assurance that the parent will understand those words, allows the child to feel more secure and in control.

At the same time, improved memory, sense of time, and understanding of daily routines allows the child to use the parent's explanations to promote feelings of security. The 4-year-old can take in and remember a parent's words: "I'm going to be gone all day. You'll have lunch, take your nap, get up and have a snack, play with your friends, and *then* I'll come and pick you up." Cognitively, the 4-year-old is capable of using events in the routine of the child care center as markers that tell her when to expect her parent to return. She may still miss her parent, but she now has a cognitive means of coping with a separation that the 2-year-old does not yet have. Although the child does not have a choice about the parent's leaving, she now has the ability to gain mastery over separation anxiety by thinking about the parent's absence, by understanding it as part of a plan. Further, the preschooler can draw on internal resources, which include her internal working models of attachment (Bretherton & Munholland, 1999). Instead of needing the physical presence of the parent, she may represent and dramatize attachment seeking through doll play or family play with peers. Working models of secure attachment also give the child confidence in seeking support from other adults and peers.

Studies of Attachment History and Preschool Development

The quality of attachment during the first 3 years has important implications for preschoolers' development. Several longitudinal studies have assessed the effects of secure and insecure attachment patterns on later development. Studies of low-risk middle-class children have found consistency in attachment classification from infancy to age 6. Types of attachment at 12 and 18 months tend to persist through the preschool years, suggesting that parental caregiving styles, working models, and transactional patterns tend to be continuous, and also that internalized working models of attachment and self are being generalized by the child (Thompson, 2000). By contrast, attachment classifications of low-income children are more likely to fluctuate over time, in response to their parents' exposure to multiple risk factors (Vondra, Hommerding, & Shaw, 1999). When risk is low, secure attachment in infancy and toddlerhood predicts adaptive functioning during the preschool years, whereas insecure attachment predicts some difficulties in functioning. A summary of these studies is presented in Table 9.1.

SOCIAL DEVELOPMENT

The preschool years are a bridge between the egocentric toddler and the more socially adept and aware child of the middle years. Preschoolers are learning how to be social, how to take others' perspectives into account. The tasks of social development for the preschooler include learning social skills, prosocial behavior, and values, and learning how to play with peers and how to establish friendships. Preschoolers encounter many situations requiring social competence. New circumstances and developmental change contribute to the need to develop social abilities. Preschoolers are more likely than infants and toddlers to be cared for in large groups. At the same time, the preschool child's growing orientation toward peer relationships and cooperative play with peers motivates him to learn to get along with other children.

Across the preschool years children advance in their strategies for reaching goals in social situations. Young preschoolers may try to get what they want in ways similar to those toddlers employ. A 3-year-old wants the toy another child is playing with and looks for an opportunity to simply take it. By age 4, such physical means are increasingly supplanted by verbal strategies. She may say, "I want to play with that," or, in a more sophisticated approach, "Let's both play with the dishes, OK? I'll make spaghetti." New developments in communication skills and social understanding allow for this change in strategy. The child can express herself more easily now, and she is more able to take another's perspective, which means that she is aware that the other child would resent having the dishes taken away from her.

Prosocial Behavior

Although toddlers act in prosocial ways occasionally, they are most often concerned about their own self-interest and needs. Prosocial increases between 3 and 6. Children learn values about prosocial behavior—

TABLE 9.1. Research on Relationships between Attachment Patterns in Infancy and Functioning of Preschoolers

Preschool children with histories of secure attachment

- *Affect*: emotional openness, more positive affect, full range of affects, good memories of attachment experiences, at age 6 (Main, Kaplan, & Cassidy, 1985; Main & Cassidy, 1988); capacity for modulation of affects and "situationally appropriate" expression of affects (Easterbrooks & Goldberg, 1990).

- *Self-regulation*: ability to cope with anxiety adaptively, either by drawing on internal coping resources or by turning to an adult for help. This capacity for self-regulation, in turn, enables preschoolers to sustain exploration, play, and learning (Maslin-Cole & Spieker, 1990; Vondra, et al., 2001).

- *Generalization of attachment*: readily turn to adult caregivers for support when parents are not available (Sroufe, 1983; Howes & Hamilton, 1992; Howes & Ritchie, 1998).

- *Social relationships*: show more positive affect in peer play and more engagement with peers; show positive expectations of interactions, have more friends, and become more popular with peers (Sroufe, 1989); show good abilities in empathy and understanding others' emotions and intentions (Meins, Fernyhough, Russell, & Clark-Carter, 1998; Greig & Howe, 2001).

- *Sense of self*: confident in solving problems, self-directed, appropriately independent and resourceful; adequate to high self-esteem (Sroufe, 1989).

Preschool children with histories of insecure attachment

- *Affect:* avoidant preschoolers show defensive restrictions on affect and on memories of attachment experiences (Main, Kaplan & Cassidy, 1985); ambivalent children show heightened negative affect, moodiness, and depression (Cassidy & Berlin, 1994; Kochanska, 2001).

- *Self-regulation*: difficulties in affect and behavior regulation, including over- or undercontrol of impulses, lower frustration tolerance, higher levels of anxiety, more negative affect (Easterbrooks & Goldberg, 1990; Vondra et al., 2001)

- *Generalization of attachment*: negative attention seeking, provocative or oppositional behavior toward adults, less comfort seeking from adults, precocious self-reliance, social withdrawal, tendencies to anxiously monitor caregivers' availability at the expense of developing relationships with peers; negative behavior tends to elicit controlling behavior by teachers, which often feels punitive to the child (Bates & Bayles, 1988; Howes & Hamilton, 1992; Howes & Ritchie, 1998).

- *Social relationships*: aggression and negative behavior toward peers; emotional distance, especially in preschoolers with avoidant attachment; exploitative and coercive peer interactions, often with an avoidantly attached child dominating an ambivalently attached child (Troy & Sroufe, 1987; Elicker, Egeland, & Sroufe, 1992); poorer ability in understanding others' intentions and emotions (Fonagy, Redfern, & Charman, 1997; Greig & Howe, 2001).

- *Sense of self*: view of the self as incompetent, based on a history of feeling unable to elicit caretaking from parents; view of the self as not valuable or lovable, which contributes to depression as well as to angry, mistrustful, and oppositional behavior toward caregivers; negative behavior results in rejection by peers, further damaging self-esteem (Greenberg & Speltz, 1988; Sroufe, 1983).

sharing, comforting, helping, controlling aggression—through the ways they have been responded to by parents and others. Parents who model prosocial behavior through their caregiving and provide warmth, nurturance, and clear limits encourage incorporation of prosocial values as part of the child's overall identification with parents. In addition, new cognitive skills such as role taking (the ability to see things from another's perspective), exposure to rules and expectations in the family and preschool settings, and exposure to peer group situations that require cooperation all influence the development of prosocial behavior (Eisenberg & Fabes, 1998).

Peer Relationships

During the preschool years, the child's relationships begin to focus more on peers, although parents remain the central people in the preschooler's life. This shift in orientation can be observed in preschools. A toddler who is dropped off at child care tends to look for a teacher as a substitute attachment figure. A 4-year-old, even though she may have warm relationships with her teachers, looks for her friends. She may see two other children she regularly plays with and asks, "What are you playing?"—or she may propose her own scenario. A 4- or 5-year-old identifies with her peers, intuitively seeing them as the people most like herself. Therefore, she comes to school oriented to telling them what is emotionally important to her—"Look at my new shoes," or, for a child who was scared and excited by fire engine sirens on her street the night before, "Let's say there was a big fire and we're firefighters." She has come to expect responses from her peers, to be noticed and accepted by them.

The increasing valuation placed on the opinions of peers supports the preschooler's cognitive shift toward a more objective and complex view of the world. Egocentrism decreases as cognitive development proceeds. The 5- or 6-year-old is less egocentric because he is more able to take another's perspective. He sees that his point of view is not the only possible one and that the ideas of others must be taken into account. However, the decline of egocentrism is not simply a result of cognitive maturation but rather is influenced transactionally by the child's experiences with peers (Piaget, 1951). The relative equality of power among peers, as compared with the child's relationships with adults, requires the child to take other children's wishes and ideas into account. As peer relationships become more important, beginning at about age 3, the child is increasingly motivated to have enjoyable interactions with peers and to be accepted by them. This motivation fuels the development of skills in perspective taking, negotiation, sharing, and cooperating (Piaget, 1951).

There are positive links between the quality of early relationships with parents and the quality of preschoolers' peer relationships. If a child has had secure and satisfying relationships with parents during the first 3 years, he is likely to be oriented toward peers, to expect that contacts with others will be pleasurable. Toddlers who have experienced a secure base in the attachment relationship explore the environment more confidently, and this includes making contact with other children (Hartup, 1992). Preschoolers with histories of secure attachment have more advanced social abilities, in part because their working models contain positive expectations about relationships and in part because they have developed social skills through interactions with parents (Howes & Ritchie, 1998).

By contrast, insecure working models lead to assumptions that make it more difficult for the preschool to learn social skills in the context of peer interactions. Preschoolers with working models that assume a lack of responsiveness from others may not reach out socially because they are unsure of the response. Those with working models organized around assumptions of interpersonal anger and coercion may seek out or create conflictual situations that confirm their working models. These children may want to interact with peers; however, their efforts to control interactions combine with their impulsiveness and aggression to alienate other children (Rubin, Coplin, Fox, & Calkins, 1995).

In peer interactions, the preschool child learns a great deal about social behavior, building on what she has learned in her family: "Turn taking, sharing, control of aggression, empathy, helping, sex role learning, role taking, strategies of conflict resolution and moral reasoning all develop within the peer group as well as the family and appear to be central to the ability to establish friendships and maintain relationships with others" (Campbell, 1990, p. 142).

It should be emphasized, however, that these skills are in the process of developing during the preschool years. Observations of normal preschool children playing together document frequent conflicts, disagreements, aggressive actions, falling-outs, and disruptions of cooperative play. Triangular dynamics emerge as children vie for one another's attention. Children's feelings are hurt because they are excluded or rebuffed. Egocentrism and possessiveness are common, as children try to force their fantasies on others or refuse to share toys. When conflict erupts, children may become physically aggressive or verbally rejecting (e.g., "You're not my friend!" or "I'm not inviting you to my birthday party!"). Because of the preschooler's wishes to be accepted and valued by peers, however, such conflicts become a laboratory for learning how to resolve conflicts.

The inherent pleasure of fantasy play provides an additional motive for resolving conflict—if the conflict is overcome, play continues (Pelligrini & Jones, 1993). In one of many lovely examples in *Bad Guys Don't Have Birthdays: Fantasy Play at Four*, Vivian Gussen Paley (1988), a preschool and kindergarten teacher in Chicago, describes a conflict between three boys in a passionate disagreement about whether the play will be about Batman or He-Man. Two of the boys have ganged up on the other and are belittling his ideas. The interactional dynamic is complex because, in addition to the attempt to exclude one boy, there is a rivalry for the attention of Mollie, with each side appealing to her to join its fantasy:

> CHRISTOPHER: What are you talkin' about? Mollie's never going to play with you. She's *my* friend.
>
> BARNEY: Are you playing with him or us?
>
> FREDERICK: Say us, say us.

In response, "Mollie purses her lips primly. 'I'm still friends with the whole of everyone. Nighttime, nighttime, everyone goes to bed. The rainbow is outside the window" (Paley, 1988, pp. 17–18). Mollie defuses the conflict by accepting all of them and then adeptly shifting the fantasy to include her favorite character, Rainbow Brite. The three boys, evidently relieved to be out of conflict and back in play, join her idea by agreeing to go to bed. Then they begin discussing the need for guards during the night, and play resumes. Children like Mollie, who have a positive attitude and skills in negotiating conflict, are usually popular among their peers, which in turn supports the development of their social competence (Campbell, 2002).

While preschool children popular with peers are friendly and socially competent, "aggressive and disruptive behavior enhance[s] the likelihood of social rejection, especially among boys" (Hartup, 1992, p. 264). Preschoolers who are negative and aggressive toward others are often avoided and excluded by their peers, fueling a cycle of anger and further rejection. Preschoolers described as "hard to manage" because of behavior problems show higher rates of aggressive pretend play based on violent fantasies, more conflict with peers, and a much stronger tendency to cross over the pretend boundary into actual aggression. Preschoolers whose pretend play emphasizes violent attacks show relatively poor ability to understand the feelings of victims and strong tendencies to identify with aggressors (Dunn & Hughes, 2001). Aggressive preschoolers often misinterpret others' intentions, seeing threat when none is intended, as a projection of their own aggressive feelings. Overall, they show more teasing, bullying, and physical violent actions (Hughes, White, Sharpen, & Dunn, 2000) Impulsive, aggressive behavior in the preschool is one of the most common reasons that preschool children are referred for evaluation. Without prompt and consistent intervention, the aggressive preschooler is likely to remain aggressive because, from his point of view, aggression works. The child who enters middle childhood with poor peer skills faces a big disadvantage, because then peer relationships become even more important as a source of personal competence and self-esteem.

Friendships

Although toddlers show preference for some peers over others, preschool children begin to develop real friendships. Between 4 and 5, children begin to label other children as their friends and in group settings prefer to play with them (Hartup, 1992). For a young preschooler, a friend is someone she likes to play with. Older preschool children often pair up with a close friend in relationships that show other characteristics of friendship, including concern for the other child's feelings, wishes for approval, and displays of affection. These friendships are beginning forays into having a "best friend," which becomes so common during middle childhood. Often children are drawn to each other by similar fantasy interests: "shared pretense is a core feature of their friendships" (Dunn & Hughes, 2001, p. 491). Hartup (1992) notes that because friends spend more time playing together, they have more conflicts, frequently over whose fantasy agenda will control the direction of play. Friends, as opposed to nonfriends, will work on solving these conflicts not just to keep the play going but because of mutual investment in the friendship. Because friends have come to know each other's interests and preferences, they are more adept at keeping play going because they know what to do to reduce conflict (Hartup, 1992, 1996; Dunn & Hughes, 2001).

At the same time, preschoolers with quiet, withdrawn temperaments or histories of insecure attachment may already be showing difficulty in establishing friendships. For example, a fearful or withdrawn child may shrink back from social play and become an outsider in the group. This reinforces his withdrawal and prevents him from learning the pleasures of friendship. Resiliency research has identified having friends as a protective factor and not having friends as a risk factor (Werner, 2000). The ability to make and keep friends depends on having good social skills; in turn, friendships support social development because they give children chances to learn how to interact, negotiate, and solve conflicts in order to keep the friend (Hartup, 1996). Having friends helps children cope with developmental transitions and other stressful situations. For example, children who enter kindergarten with friends or who make friends early in the year and maintain them show better attitudes toward school and better academic performance than those children who have difficulty in making friends (Ladd, 1990, 1999). The preschool period is pivotal in shaping children's later orientation to friendships. Preschool children's experiences with friends create "internal representations of friendship relationships upon which they then draw in subsequent friendships at school" (Dunn, Cutting, & Fisher, 2002, p. 632).

Play and Social Development

The parallel play of toddlers persists into the early preschool years but is gradually replaced by more cooperative play. Two 3-year-olds riding tricycles side by side on the playground enjoy doing the same thing in parallel, but they do not say much to each other or give evidence of sharing a fantasy. By age 4 these children riding tricycles together may be engaged in a more complex and interactive form of play based on a shared idea. For example, they might be playing out a superhero fantasy; rather than simply riding together they are chasing bad guys, and their words and actions create a joint story:

CHILD 1: Batman, they went out by the swings. Let's get 'em.

CHILD 2: No, Robin, they've got laser guns. Let's go back to the Batcave and get our bazookas!

CHILD 1: OK! (*They turn and ride off in another direction.*)

Similarly, the "conversations" of 3-year-olds often sound like joint monologues, but they evolve into dialogues as the children move closer to 4.

Three-year-olds make the transition to cooperative play by watching the play of other children, gradually learning its forms, rituals, and "rules," and then beginning to take roles in it (Paley, 1986). By ages 4 and 5, a great deal of a child's play involves other children as they take roles in a shared scenario. Their conversations often sound like real dialogue, in which the perspective of the other is increasingly taken into account, as they plan and negotiate roles in fantasy play. Here is an example of three 4-year-olds getting started in fantasy play (Paley, 1986, p. 141):

CHRISTOPHER: Come on, Rainbow Brite, I hear a sound in the doll corner. I think it's the good witch.

MOLLIE: OK, Starlite. Margaret, you can be Rainbow's kitty . . . Starlite horsey, come get your food now. Once more now. Time for bed now, horsey. Go to sleep.

CHRISTOPHER: I tricked you Rainbow Brite . . . Lurky is coming! He's coming in the back of us. He might be scaring us!

MOLLIE: Don't worry, Starlite. I put the magic trap under the door. Then we'll give him the poison drink. Don't touch this. It's the poison drink.

CHRISTOPHER: It's poison mud.

MARGARET: Meow, I'm afraid of Lurky.

MOLLIE: I'll keep you safe, little kitty, because Rainbow Brite has powers.

CHRISTOPHER: Yeah, but I got superpower . . . I'm super Starlite! Super Starlite! I never go to sleep to watch for bad guys. I kick at them with my hind legs!

In this brief interchange a number of things occur. One child announces a theme for the play based on characters and scenarios the other two children are familiar with. They quickly assign or take roles and the play begins, with turns in the plot being negotiated on the fly as the drama unfolds. The two principal actors, Mollie and Christopher, have different, gender-influenced ideas about what the story should be about (caretaking vs. danger), but they accept each other's fantasy and Mollie, in particular, finds ways to accommodate Christopher's wishes in order to keep the story going. Implicitly these 4-year-olds are learning and practicing skills in perspective taking, negotiation of differences, problem solving, cooperation, and creating shared fantasy narratives (Dunn & Hughes, 2001).

Culture and Social Development

Although the foregoing discussion emphasizes common processes in social development, the content of children's social understanding varies across cultures, most obviously when the cultures compared have strongly contrasting value orientations. Cross-cultural studies of preschoolers' storytelling and play show how much the young child has already internalized his parents' modeling and lessons regarding the place of the self in social relationships (Haight, 1999). A study comparing narrative themes of middle-class 6-year-olds in the United States and China demonstrated significant cultural differences in their social assumptions. In story completion tasks, Chinese children emphasized observing moral codes, respect for authority, and social connectedness, while American children showed much less concern for correct behavior and authority and a much more autonomous orientation. For example, an American child completed a story about getting separated from her parent in a store by having the child buy some toys with her own money, and then, after looking at a map, finding her way home by herself. By contrast, a Chinese girl imagined the lost child being found by a policeman and taken home. Her mother scolded her, and she felt ashamed and promised to stay close to her mother next time (Wang & Leichtman, 2000).

LANGUAGE DEVELOPMENT

At the beginning of the preschool period at age 3, the rapid acquisition of words between 2 and 3 has resulted in a vocabulary of 1,000 words. Vocabulary continues to increase by about 50 words each month. By age 3, the child has learned the question form. His ability to ask "why" and "what" gives him power over his own learning. The responses of parents and caregivers to his frequent questions increase his vocabulary. The normal 3-year-old's speech is usually clear and easy to understand. By age 4, he is speaking in long sentences (8–10 words) that are grammatically complex and include relative and dependent clauses. By age 7, it is estimated that the child understands about 14,000 words (Rice, 1989).

A 3- to 4-year-old arranges words in the right order according to the syntactical rules of his language. Increasingly, he uses correct grammar, uses present and past verb tenses, and constructs sentences with multiple clauses. Between 3 and 4, children make increasing use of "connecting words," including *and, if, so, because, then,* and *but.* Use of connecting words reflects the preschooler's more complex understanding of reality, because these words denote relationships between things and events, conditional thinking, and causality (Bloom, 1998). Consider a young 4-year-old's running account of playing with a toy car: "When my hotwheels car jumped off the ramp, it was destroyed. But if we have powers, we can fix it. And I *do* have powers!"

Contexts of Language Learning for Preschoolers

Bloom notes that "language is inherently social because it has to be learned from other persons" (Bloom, 1998, p. 332). Young children learn new words and more complex grammar by conversing, by listening to others speaking, and through intentional scaffolding by parents, as when a mother asked her 3-year-old daughter, "What did we see at the store today?" This question encouraged the child to tell a story, using the past tense modeled in the question. The question–answer dialogue continued:

CHILD: We saw alive lobsters.

PARENT: Where were the lobsters?

CHILD: In the water.

PARENT: Yep, they were in a big tank full of water. And what were they doing?

CHILD: They was wiggling their . . . on their heads.

PARENT: You mean their antennas, their feelers.

CHILD: Their feelers.

In this exchange, the parent's questions provided a context that helped the child organize her impressions (Vygotsky, 1978).

However, older toddlers and preschoolers increasingly take charge of their own language acquisition by asking questions and initiating dialogues (Bloom, Margulis, Tinker, & Fujita, 1996). Young children's language development is increasingly influenced by their growing theory of mind understanding: "The persistent desire to convey stems from the child's discovery that other individuals have an emotional and mental life that differs from its own. . . . The child now senses that it has information others lack and vice versa" (Locke, 1993, p. 348). Parental scaffolding and the child's "urge to convey" both shape the quality of the child's ability to express herself in language. Parents who talk with their young children in an "elaborative" style support the development of linguistic, memory, and storytelling abilities. An elaborative style involves asking questions, eliciting details, encouraging evaluation of experience, and helping the child put memories into a broader context. The independent storytelling of older preschoolers who have been exposed to this type of scaffolding shows better narrative skills, better autobiographical memory, and richer, more coherent representation of their experience (Haden, Hayne, & Fivush, 1997).

The capacity to represent experience coherently has a positive impact on preschoolers' self-regulation abilities. Children who can organize their experiences into coherent narratives feel more in control of their affects and have a clearer view of reality. This perspective has implications for child therapy:

> Much of therapy involves attempts by the child and therapist to co-construct, out of children's conflictual and often chaotic experiences, emotionally coherent narratives. Once such narratives are formed . . . children are more capable of regulating their emotions as well as their behavior. (Oppenheim, Nir, Warren, Emde, 1997, p. 284)

Language Ability Shapes Development

By age 4, children have mastered language sufficiently to tell a story using words alone. By contrast, toddlers, because they know fewer words and have not mastered grammar, tend to combine words with actions in order to communicate. Increasingly, during the preschool years, children rely on language over action to express themselves. Their ability to use language has become creative and flexible. Imaginative play also relies more on language.

Children with good language skills are likely to become competent collaborative players (Sawyer, 1997). Older preschoolers have learned that words are useful and powerful. They use words pragmatically and persuasively, and sometimes with an ability to blend words and emotional expression for maximum effect in realizing their goals:

> In a genuinely kind and sweet voice a 4-year-old girl said to her younger brother: "Andy, would you like to play baby? Here's a bottle for you and here's your blanket, honey. I'll tuck you in now." Her brother, this time at least, was persuaded, and lay down on the blanket to be taken care of.

By contrast, preschoolers with language delays often have more difficulty in peer interactions and shared play (Howes, 1992).

Adam, a 3½-year-old, was referred for evaluation by his child care provider, who thought he was either depressed and withdrawn or selectively mute. (In selective mutism, a child has intact language ability but does not speak in situations outside the home.) At school Adam said almost nothing to teachers or peers and did not join in peer play, even though at times he seemed interested in what other children were doing. When I observed him interacting with his mother, he did not appear depressed, nor was he mute. He enjoyed playing and talking with his mother; yet, his expressive language seemed impoverished in vocabulary and under-developed in structure. He spoke in 2- and 3-word "telegraphic" sentences and often omitted connecting and meaning-modifying words. His mother confirmed that the young toddler-level language he showed in my office was representative. This child was not depressed or inhibited but rather lacked the ability to express himself like other 3- and 4-year-olds. Consequently, he was not developing the play and social skills that depend a great deal on adequate verbal skills.

When developmental language learning difficulties are identified in young preschoolers, prompt referral for a language evaluation is essential. Young children with obvious articulation disorders are more likely to be referred for evaluation than children with impoverished language; yet, children with language learning delays are at much greater risk for future difficulties in spoken and written language and reading (Tallal & Benasich, 2002).

Language and the Understanding of Real and Pretend

One of the most salient tasks of the preschooler is to learn to distinguish between fantasy and reality. The development of language supports the development of reality testing. However, between 3 and 4 years of age, the struggle is compounded by the fact that the child is still trying to define and remember the meanings of words. Although the development of language lays the groundwork for an increasingly clear and consensual understanding of reality, at age 3 a child is both wondering if monsters exist and what the word "monster" actually means. It is easy to get confused. Words still have an abstract quality, on the one hand, and they do not mean the same thing to each child, on the other. It is often difficult for young preschoolers to see words as representing a consensual reality; rather, their meanings are more linked to the idiosyncratic reality of each child's experience. This is another reason why play is so important to young preschoolers. By acting out their ideas in play, they can show others what they mean. Action for a 3-year-old is a much more real and reliable mode of self-expression than mere words. However, by 4 and 5 years of age the child's ability to express meaning through language has improved a great deal, and play interactions increasingly rely on words to set the scene and maintain the themes of the play scenario.

> For example, one 4-year-old boy says to another, "Let's say I'm Jim and you're Long John Silver, and we're going to get to the island, but there are crocodiles in the ocean." They kill the crocodiles and reach the island, but one child continues to shoot his gun at the crocodiles. The other child redirects the play, in accordance with his fantasy, by saying, "No, pretend we killed the crocodiles already, and now we're gonna' look for the treasure!" If his playmate now agrees, as he presumably does, language has served to organize and perpetuate the play (Dunn & Cutting, 1999).

Private Speech

Preschoolers talk to themselves a great deal, saying out loud what older children and adults say to themselves in silent thought. "Private speech" accompanies preschoolers' activities and seems to function as self-direction (Berk, 1992). The 4-year-old girl playing by herself with a dollhouse carries out a running commentary that describes what is happening and plans what will happen next: "Now the mommy is going to change the baby's diaper. The baby says, 'Ma-ma, I want my dinner now.' So the mommy goes to the store to get food." Or a 4-year-old boy building with blocks says to himself, "I gotta put the triangle one up here—carefully, so it doesn't fall." Private speech also helps the child exert self-control, as when a child repeats parents' limit-setting words to himself: "Don't run in the house, Amani."

SYMBOLIC COMMUNICATION AND PLAY

Preschool children love to play. Their play is more complex and imaginative than a toddler's, but it is less constrained by rules and adherence to reality than the play of a school-age child. Play takes on a number of functions that support progressive development. Preschoolers' play takes two primary directions, which in practice are often combined. The first involves exploration of reality and especially social roles. By dressing up as adults or as Cinderella or Harry Potter, preschoolers are exploring in fantasy what they may become. The second direction of preschool play involves using play for the mastery of stress and anxiety as well as for the expression of wishes and fears. The 4-year-old boy's superhero play represents an attempt to master anxiety connected with the young child's growing perception that he's a small person in a big world who is incompetent, compared to adults. The process of imagining and carrying out play scenarios supports the development of cognitive skills, such as planning and problem solving, as well as providing the child with opportunities to exercise autonomy and initiative (Piaget, 1962). Play facilitates understanding of emotions and perspective taking: children in dramatic play express strong emotions and must empathize to some degree with each other's ideas and feelings. The negotiation and cooperative planning that occur spontaneously in dramatic play strengthens the child's capacity for self-control. In order to stay within the play scenario, preschoolers will control impulses to act in ways that do not fit the drama they are acting in.

Play Reflects Reality But Is Outside Reality

Winnicott (1971) described play as transitional activity that takes place in a zone between the individual's subjective reality and external reality. The preschool child's play expresses her private fantasies in the public forum of the group of players; yet, the play they create is not bound by the rules of reality. In dramatic play, the imaginable is possible. Bad guys can be killed by laser swords, then rise from the dead to fight again. Princesses are transformed into mothers and then into superheroines. Anger, rudeness, competitive feelings, disappointment, affection, and grandiosity can be expressed in the pretend scenario without eliciting the same responses they might if expressed in reality. Play allows the child to comment on and try to understand reality through a make-believe medium that is under the child's control and therefore more easily manipulated than the actual world (Singer, 1993).

Increasingly, the players acknowledge that they are pretending. While preschoolers sometimes have difficulty distinguishing between fantasy and reality, when they are playing they have no trouble with this distinction. Children know very well when they are intentionally operating within the play frame and when they are not (Woolley, 1997). The imaginative social play of 4- and 5-year-olds almost always begins with the establishment of roles: "I'll be Robin and you be Batgirl, OK?" Preschoolers signal the beginning of play in many ways—by saying "We're playing now" or "Let's say we're on the ice planet" or by a dramatic look or gesture. In the pretend scenario, the child sets his personal identity aside and becomes a character sometimes inspired by adult models, sometimes by figures from the media.

Even though the preschooler changes his identity in play, the play almost always reflects psychological themes and issues that are salient for the preschool child: the imitation of adult behavior; caretaking; practicing of parental, gender, and occupational roles; concerns about body damage and physical vulnerability; and mastery of danger. At times, however, both in peer play and play therapy, the play frame is not strong enough to contain frightening affects, and a child breaks off the play. If one child begins to inject too much aggression into play or becomes a particularly frightening character, another child may step out of the play frame and say, "No, I don't want to play that. It's too scary." Play therapists are also familiar with play disruption when the content of the play produces so much anxiety for the child that he must stop it. This often occurs when a child unconsciously realizes that he is "going too far."

> For example, Gregory, a 4-year-old boy I was seeing in therapy, was having two puppets fight: one was a shark and the other a girl. The shark took the girl's head in its mouth, and Gregory shouted, "He bit her head off!" Then he abruptly put the puppets down and said, "I want to play with the house now." It was unclear to me whether this play disruption was caused by aggressive feelings (toward his younger sister) that felt too strong or by anxiety about body damage. Probably both factors were involved.

Play and Cognitive Development

Play and fantasy create opportunities for the development of cognitive skills during the preschool years. The preschool child uses play to "think" about her experience, considering alternative ways of viewing it and exploring new ways of acting. In symbolic play, the preschooler practices and increases her understanding of cause-and-effect thinking, construction of narrative, and perspective taking (Singer, 1993). Preschoolers with strong imaginative play skills show better understanding of others' emotions as well as superior "theory of mind" abilities. Compared with less capable pretend players, they have better comprehension of the links between mental states, intentions, and actions, which translates into more acute perceptions of relationships and reality in general (Dunn & Cutting, 1999).

By 5 and 6 years of age, children can increasingly describe their experiences in words. This development is not related simply to the accumulation of vocabulary. Rather, it is a result of cognitive abilities supported by and in part developed through playing. Play increases the child's capacity for mental representation by dramatizing in action the child's thoughts and feelings, putting what starts out as an imagined idea into a tangible scenario the child can see in front of her. After a few years of such practice it becomes easier to organize one's thoughts in more purely mental ways, using words rather than action. The ability to mentally organize experience in narrative form promotes clarity of understanding, which in turn has been identified as a protective factor for school-age children who are exposed to stress. Such "representational competence" mitigates the impact of stress and may prevent traumatization, because the child is able to take a more objective and comprehensive view of what has happened. The clear transactional relationship between play and cognitive development suggests that imaginative play and fantasy, rather than simply being regarded as entertainment for the child, should be strongly supported by parents and caregivers during the preschool years (Singer & Singer, 1990).

COGNITIVE DEVELOPMENT

Between 3 and 6 years of age, the preschooler's thought gradually matures to allow for clearer perception of reality. Memory improves in concert with language development. The beginning mastery of language structure and rapidly increasing vocabulary allows for verbal recall of events. The capacity to encode memories in language allows the older preschooler to transcend the "infantile amnesia" associated with early childhood (Simcock & Hayne, 2003). The preschool child, through repeated experiences in conjunction with more extensive language, has developed a larger knowledge base that provides associations and categories for new information. Unlike the toddler, for whom new experiences often seem individual and different from one another, the preschool child generalizes similar experiences. Increasingly, he thinks categorically, using mental representations of previous similar experiences to understand new ones. If a child can link a new experience or piece of information to an existing mental category, he is more likely to remember it. The ability to see similarities coincides with being able to perceive differences and even to think about the process of perception (Deloache, Miller, & Pierroutsakos, 1998). Adults are often surprised by the older preschooler's fresh and sophisticated ideas that reflect his increasing analytical and conceptual abilities, including the realization that "perception informs beliefs" (Wellman & Gelman, 1998, p. 539).

> Consider two examples of a nearly 5-year-old boy reflecting on his experience. As his grandfather was driving him to preschool he piped up from the backseat, "A 'z' is a sideways 'n.' " When they arrived at school he told his grandfather that there was a very big pile of rocks over by the sandboxes. As they walked down the sidewalk at a distance from the play area, he looked puzzled and said "I can't see the pile. It must be gone." His grandfather pointed to the rocks in the distance. The little boy said, "Oh, it doesn't look so big now because we're far away."

In turn, having a larger fund of knowledge allows the preschooler to be a more flexible thinker than the toddler. As a result, preschool children are more adept at assimilating new experiences and unexpected events into their play and thought.

For example, a 3-year-old girl is loading a doll family into a toy plastic van to go on a shopping trip. As she is tipping the top section of the van open so that the doll family will go in more easily, the top unexpectedly comes off, leaving just the floor and seats attached to the wheels. A glimmer of surprise crosses her face; then she says, "They wanted the top off so the sun can shine in. They're going to the beach."

The motivation to assimilate new information is based in turn on the child's increasing perception of the complexities of the world. It is useful to think of a 4- to 5-year-old as a person who is realizing that reality is more complicated than he thought, that causality is mysterious, that there are surprising connections between things, and that there is a great deal he does not know. In response to this awareness, he asks many questions and tries out different versions of reality as he plays. The 4- or 5-year-old's questions about "the big questions" imply surprise, curiosity, and anxiety. He wants to know how God makes rain fall from the sky and what kind of germs make people die. How does a small seed buried in the ground become a bush with tomatoes covering it? A 5-year-old asked his parents, "*How* do you love each other?" Paley (1988) points out that "a relentless connection-making" (p. 12) goes on in the play and dialogue of preschoolers as they attempt to understand reality.

Egocentric Thinking: The Preschooler's Perspective

Jean Piaget (1962) described toddlers and preschoolers (his *preoperational period* encompassing the ages of 2–7) as characterized by egocentric thinking. Egocentrism means that the child sees the world from her own perspective and has difficulty seeing another person's point of view. An aspect of egocentrism is an assumption that everyone thinks and feels the same way as she does. Piaget argued that children during this stage are not able to assume another person's perspective. More recent experimental research suggests that the capacity to see things from another person's point of view is gradually developing during the preschool period. At 4 and 5, children can frequently acknowledge another's ideas, particularly in the context of cooperative play. Researchers on prosocial behavior have demonstrated that, as early as age 2, children can sometimes empathize with the feelings of others (Eisenberg & Fabes, 1998).

A well-known recent Piaget-like theory of mind experiment documents that age 4 may be an important dividing line for perspective taking. In this experiment an adult and a child watch an experimenter put a toy under a box. After the adult leaves the room, the experimenter removes the toy, puts it under a second box, and asks the child, "Where will she look for the toy when she comes back?" Children under 4 point to the second box, where the toy is currently. They focus on the toy's present location and are unable to imagine that the person who does not know the toy has been moved would still think it was under the first box. Increasing numbers of 4- and 5-year-olds understand that the adult will look where the toy was when she left the room, and 6-year-olds universally realize this. This experiment suggests that between 4 and 6 years of age, children are increasingly capable of imagining another's perspective even though it differs from their own (Bartsch & Wellman, 1995). This change in perspective-taking ability also demonstrates the older preschooler's ability to understand that other people can have mistaken perceptions and beliefs. By extension, they are realizing that their own beliefs can be false as well.

This refinement of Piaget's theory illustrates one of the many changes in cognitive ability that occur during the preschool period. Compared with toddlers, older preschoolers show much better ability to sustain attention, to think flexibly, to understand causality, and to distinguish between their thoughts and intentions and those of others (Wellman & Gelman, 1998). Nevertheless, the consistent capacity for nonegocentric thinking does not seem to be fully available to the child until near the end of the preschool period, and it is important for practitioners to keep in mind that the preschooler's capacity for logical thinking and accurate appraisal of reality are limited. We often see in clinical cases that the ability to think in nonegocentric ways is influenced by emotionality, arousal, and stress. A 5-year-old who can show perspective-taking skills in an experimental situation may think egocentrically in a stressful real situation that causes arousal and fear. For example, 5-year-old who is put in time out because he has hit another child is likely to feel unfairly treated. Although he may have some notion that he is being punished for aggressive behavior, his primary response will be egocentric—at an emotional level in the immediate moment he will feel mistreated. Emotionally aroused preschool children also have difficulty sorting out the intentions of others. For example, if another child bumps into a preschooler accidentally, the latter may assume that the act was done on purpose because he was hurt. The ability for perspective taking is present but fragile during the preschool years. In clinical practice, it is important to watch for evidence of distortions and misunderstandings based on egocentric thinking, especially for children who have been exposed to stressful or traumatic events and relationships. The following review emphasizes the constraints of egocentric thinking because, from a clinical perspective, we often find that egocentric perspectives are at the root of young children's symptomatic behavior.

Characteristics of Egocentric Thinking

The following features of egocentric thinking decrease as the child gets older, but they are also subject to the impact of stress.

Understanding of Cause and Effect

The preschooler tends to see a cause-and-effect relationship between things that happen at about the same time. He cannot yet understand that there can be remote or unseen causes. When combined with an egocentric viewpoint, this can lead to serious misunderstandings of reality. For example, a 3-year-old girl whose parents had recently separated said, "Daddy left because we were jumping on the bed that night." In situations of high arousal or strong affect, preschoolers may reverse cause and effect, seeing themselves egocentrically as causative agents. For example, another 4-year-old boy whose parents had divorced explained, "My mommy and daddy got a divorce because they both wanted me to live at their house." It is a short step from thoughts like this to feeling responsible for the parents' separation.

Transductive Reasoning

This is a form of associational thinking in which the child overgeneralizes the results of past experiences. Elkind and Weiner (1978) describe this associational logic as follows:

> A and B occur together
> A is present
> [Therefore] B must be present. (p. 243)

> For example, a preschooler was scared by a loud thunderclap and tornado-warning sirens just as she was entering her child care center. The next day she fearfully refused to get out of the car when they arrived at the center. Her father was perceptive in connecting her present anxiety with what happened the preceding day and reassured her that there would not be a storm. He pointed out that the sky was clear.

It is not always so easy to understand when a child is using transductive reasoning; yet, preschoolers' stubborn or seemingly irrational behavior is frequently caused by this type of thinking.

Personalism

Evident in the previous examples is the preschooler's tendency to personalize events. Rather than being able to think in generalizing or universalizing terms, the preschooler thinks in terms of herself. Paley (1988) writes about a 4-year-old, "Frederick responds to questions about boys and their grandfathers as if they are about himself and *his* grandfather" (p. 12). In the days following the September 11, 2001, attacks, many preschool children who lived far from New York showed anxiety and fearful play, in part because they imagined future attacks destroying their own home and neighborhood.

> On September 13, I was playing in the sandbox with 5-year-old Rebecca, the daughter of friends. Her parents had been conscientious about not allowing her to watch TV and had been careful in what they said to her; nevertheless, her sand play showed that she was aware of the destruction of the World Trade Center and that she had personalized the fears it had engendered. We built a house with wet sand, which she labeled "my house." Then she knocked it down. I asked what happened and she said, "They suicided into it." I did not think she knew what "suicide" meant, but clearly she had heard this word in connection with the destruction of the towers. I said, "Are you thinking your house could get knocked down like those big buildings did?" She said, "Yes." I said, "That was really scary, but it happened very far away and it won't happen to your house."

The preschooler's tendency to personalize has positive implications for storytelling in therapy. The therapist can tell a story about "another kid I knew" that presents the issues a child is struggling with. The story can present an adaptive solution or a more accurate explanation for the child's problem. Preschoolers, as well as somewhat older children, will feel less anxious if the story is about someone else, yet will personalize the story and apply it to themselves.

Animism

The younger preschooler projects her own feelings and characteristics onto inanimate objects, believing that a wave that splashed in her face did it on purpose or that a scratch on the face of a plastic doll must hurt.

Judging Reality by Surface Appearances Rather Than Using Reasoning

Some of Piaget's best-known experiments involved conservation of number and quantity. In one test preschool children were shown 10 vases, each with a single flower in it. The flowers were removed and bunched together. When the flowers are closer together, the preschool child will say there are fewer flowers, whereas a 7-year-old will say that the number of flowers remains the same. For the preschooler appearance alters perception, whereas the 7-year-old uses logic to understand that if none of the flowers has been taken away the same number remains, no matter how they are arranged. In another test, Piaget showed children two identical short, wide glasses filled with equal amounts of water. When he poured the contents of one into a taller, slender glass and asked if one of the glasses had more water in it, preschool children said that there was more in the taller glass. Older children, by contrast, said the amount in each glass was the same because they knew that the actual amount of water had not changed (Piaget & Inhelder, 1969). More recent experimental research documents earlier conservation abilities. However, it is useful to keep in mind the broader implications of Piaget's research: preschool children tend to interpret reality by observing surface qualities, and their capacity for reasoning about changes in reality has not yet developed.

Magical Thinking and the Fusion of Fantasy and Reality

The characteristics of preschool thinking described above cause preschoolers to think in magical terms that compromise accurate perceptions of reality. Although they are working to understand reality, their capacity for reality testing is not well established. They have difficulty in distinguishing between wishes and what really happens; they tend to impose wishes onto reality, often because they want to feel powerful and in control; and they still believe that thoughts and strong feelings can cause things to happen. They tend to believe that dreams can come true. When they have a frightening dream, they often believe it really happened. Since dreams are not under the child's conscious control, he cannot easily see them as imaginary. Rather, they have the power of reality because they seem to the young child to come from outside himself (Estes, Wellman, & Wooley, 1989; Wooley et al., 1999).

MAGICAL THINKING IN A 4-YEAR-OLD: A BRIEF CASE EXAMPLE

To demonstrate the qualities of magical thinking, here is an example from a treatment session with a 4-year-old boy. Brandon had a close relationship with his mother, which was changed by the mother's remarriage. His new stepfather was somewhat distant from him. He felt left out because of his mother's new relationship, and he wanted to regain a more exclusive relationship with his mother by getting rid of his stepfather. He had confided to his mother that he wished his stepfather would go away. But his fantasies of getting rid of his stepfather would provoke counterfantasies involving Brandon's being retaliated against by powerful monsters or robbers. As E. H. Erikson (1963) notes, the preschooler's wish to be powerful competes with feelings of vulnerability based on guilt over aggressive thoughts: "The child indulges in fantasies of being a giant and a tiger, but in his dreams he runs in terror for dear life" (p. 256). Brandon was having scary dreams, which caused him to feel very anxious, because he still believed that dreams might come true. I had told him that I often learned about kids' feelings by hearing about their dreams, and Brandon sometimes described his dreams. In this session, Brandon said, "Let's talk about dreams some more. I have a burning sword that can chop people's necks." I said, "I don't think you've really got a burning sword, but was that in a dream?" "Yeah, I took my sword and chopped everybody on the neck, every robber. But a skeleton knocked the sword out my hand. Then he chased me." I said, "Sometimes when boys have chopping feelings, they get worried that something bad could happen to them because they have those feelings. In your dream, you chopped the robber's neck and then got worried, and the skeleton shows your worry." Brandon said, "I had another dream. A king cobra with a hood came up from a hole at the end of my bed and bit my feet." I said, "That sounds like a scary dream." He said, "In fact there really was a king cobra in my bed because I saw it, and I could feel it biting my feet." He pointed to his heels. "Right now I can feel those bites, they're still hurting." I said, "I'm sure there wasn't a king cobra in your bed and you weren't really bitten, but your dream must have seemed very real." He said, "No, there's a hole in my bed where the snake came out!" I said, "I don't think that's true." He said, "That's right—really I peed in my bed and my pee spot looked like a hole." I said, "Yes, the hole was really your pee spot, but the dream seemed so real that you started to get mixed up and think that the dream really happened."

For Brandon, a real event—waking up to find that he had wet the bed—became the inspiration for a fantasy. This particular fantasy—being bitten by a cobra that crawled up through the "pee spot" hole—may be influenced by guilty feelings about having wet the bed.

Tension between Fantasy and Reality

The preschooler lives with a tension between different ways of thinking about the world. The first way is the egocentric and magical thought of the toddler. In this mode, the child's wishes, fantasies, and dreams influence and sometimes dominate perception. The second way resembles the more mature thought of the school-age child. It is more objective and logical and reflects the child's strong motivation to understand reality. During the preschool years these modes of thinking coexist and alternate. The direction is toward logical thinking, but during this transitional period, when magical thinking remains prominent, the young child's capacity to think logically is frequently compromised by stress, emotionality, disappointments, and compensatory wishes.

Preschoolers demonstrate their wish to hold on to a magical view of the world through their fascination with events that occur miraculously and beings that cannot be seen. Preschool children believe in things they cannot see, like the tooth fairy, and they love to create fantasies about unseen things. These fantasies often reflect their wishes. Paley, in her book *Wally's Stories* (1981), quotes extensively from conversations between five 5-year-olds. For example, she asked children how they knew the tooth fairy was real, and the following discussion ensued (pp. 41–42):

WALLY: The tooth fairy came into my room and woke me up.
TEACHER: What did she look like?

WALLY: She was pretty and had long hair.

TEACHER: Was she old?

WALLY: Not as old as a grand person. As old as you. She put an envelope with money under my pillow.

TEACHER: Tanya says the tooth fairy can't get into her house. Her daddy locks all the doors and windows.

WARREN: She flies through the glass.

WALLY: No, she comes in through the roof.

TEACHER: Where does she get all the money?

WALLY: From the bank.

DEANA: He's right. I *saw* her at the bank. She had purple shoes and red hair.

ANDY: Did she talk to you?

DEANA: She doesn't speak English. I think she talks in Chinese.

EDDIE: Does she, Warren? [Warren is Chinese-American.]

WARREN: Probably she does.

This conversation reveals the preschool child's tendency to interweave fantasy and reality, and presents the tension between the two modes of thinking. The tooth fairy can fly through closed windows, yet she gets her money from the bank. Perhaps Deana did see a woman with red hair and purple shoes who looked exotic enough to be the tooth fairy, and so Deana (at least for the purpose of this discussion) assumed that she was. These children simultaneously show their belief in magic and their attempt to assimilate magic with the concrete reality of everyday experience.

The Influence of Affective Arousal on Preschoolers' Reality Testing

Academic studies show that by age 4 children know the distinction between an imaginary object and a real physical object. For example, 4-year-olds know they can change a pretend scenario by imagining it differently. They realize that "mental images can be manipulated by mental effort" (Wooley, 1995, p. 185). A 4-year-old can imagine herself lifting a heavy boulder—she makes it light with her imagination. This same child knows that she could not lift a real boulder. When asked why she could lift the pretend rock but not a real one, a 4-year-old will readily answer, "because it's make-believe." However, this apparently firm distinction between fantasy and reality can become tenuous when a preschooler is under stress or influenced by fearful affects that cause heightened states of arousal and a decrease in the child's ability to self-regulate. Even in academic experimental studies, if frightening images such as monsters or other images with strong emotional content are introduced, preschoolers' ability to differentiate between fantasy and reality becomes compromised (Samuels & Taylor, 1994).

Context influences preschoolers' reality testing more than older children's. For example, preschoolers are more likely to believe in monsters or witches at bedtime, when it is dark and they are in the position of having to give themselves up to sleep. Every night a 4-year-old girl would leap onto her bed from a distance of a few feet. She explained that if she jumped the witch under the bed would not be able to grab her feet, "because her arms aren't very long." During the day if she was asked if the witch was real, she would say, "Well, not really."

Experimental studies have shown that preschoolers have more difficulty than school-age children in differentiating between memories of actual events and imaginary events or dreams. A 4-year-old is much more likely than an 8-year-old to say that an imagined event really happened (Foley, Harris, & Hermann, 1994). The relationship between fantasy and reality for a preschooler is fluid, and in memory images of what really happened and what the child imagines tend to merge with one another. When an experience has been stressful, young children may add fantasy elements to their memory of it, often in an attempt to gain some psychic mastery over it (Fivush, 1998). This has important implications for the treatment of preschoolers who have experienced disturbing or traumatic events. Traumatized individuals benefit from help in creating a trauma story—an account of what happened—and from the systematic correction of distortions of thinking and perception based on posttraumatic internal imagery and environmental reminders. For young children, a focus on distortions and misunderstandings is particularly important because of their developmentally based tendency to fuse fantasy and reality (Terr, 1991). Preschoolers' behavioral symptoms are sometimes based on such distortions.

TISHA: A BRIEF CASE EXAMPLE

Teachers at 3½-year-old Tisha's child care center where I was a mental health consultant asked me to interview her because she had suddenly become aggressive toward other children and had been trying to paint the mouths of other children with red paint. When I asked if she had any worried or scary feelings, she told me about a physical fight between her estranged parents: "My daddy came over. He fought my mama. My mama fell down and her mouth got bloody. My daddy fell down. His mouth got bloody. I fell down and my mouth got bloody. I fell out of the car on my mouth. It got all bloody." Tisha's mental representation of this frightening scene turned out to contain cognitive distortions. Her mother confirmed that Tisha's father had in fact hit her and bloodied her mouth, and that she had fallen down. That much was an accurate description of what happened, but the rest of Tisha's account was not. Her father had not fallen down, nor had she, nor had she fallen out of a car. The only person bleeding had been her mother. Fear and confusion about what happened became generalized for Tisha, in the form of distorted memories, fears about future vulnerability at school or in the car, anxiety-based aggression at school, and "action memories" of putting red paint on other kids' mouths, a repeated behavior that also reflected her attempt to understand and gain mastery over a terribly frightening event. No one had helped her gain distance from her experience by putting it into words, and Tisha, given her developmentally based limited ability to use language to express affects and to organize experience cognitively, could only act out her anxiety and confusion in behavior that was disturbing and incomprehensible to those who witnessed it. However, when Tisha's actions are viewed in the context of her having witnessed violence, they immediately become meaningful, and not only as symptoms but also as symbolic representations of her experience.

Tisha's teachers set up a conference with Tisha's mother. At her mom's request, I participated in the conference. Her mother said she had not talked with Tisha about this incident, and acknowledged that she herself had been trying to forget what happened. She also said, "I didn't talk to her about it because I thought she was too little to understand." Out of our clearer understanding of Tisha's behavior, we formulated the following interventions: Tisha's mom agreed to talk with her about the violence she had seen, to acknowledge that she understood Tisha's fears, and to reassure her that she would try to prevent such scary things from happening again. She also agreed to tell Tisha that she would keep her safe and that she would not let her fall out of the car. The teachers, with her mom's permission, planned to tell Tisha that they knew she'd been frightened when she saw her mother hurt by her father. They would also state clearly that school was a safe place and that they would always try to keep her safe. The two teachers Tisha seemed most attached to would tell her she could come and be near them if she got worried.

The teachers also planned to be proactive in monitoring Tisha's behavior, watching out for signs of anxiety and being ready to move in to connect with her before she became aggressive. I suggested that when Tisha was aggressive the teachers both set limits and put into words that she was safe and that she didn't need to hurt to feel safe. I suggested they say, "I think you're remembering the scary time when your mommy got hurt. But the scary thing isn't happening now. It already happened. You're safe at school." I provided Tisha's mom with a referral to a domestic violence center where she could learn about legal options. I also asked her to consider a mental health referral to help Tisha process and master a possibly traumatic experience, especially if her symptomatic behaviors at school did not clear up within 3-4 weeks, after the parent and teacher interventions had been tried.

In addition to illustrating an intervention plan to help a preschooler cope with trauma-based fears, this case demonstrates the importance of a strong partnership between day care providers and parents, especially when events at home affect a child's behavior in care. Teachers need to think about the children in their care in terms of the connections between the child's two worlds—the world of home and the world of day care. If caregivers view the child's behavior in this wider context, then they can partner with parents to make the child's experience as secure and continuous as possible (Donahue, Falk, & Provet, 2000). Tisha's teachers had established a strong relationship with her mother, which allowed them to collaborate with her to support Tisha.

REGULATION OF AFFECT AND BEHAVIOR

Increased Self-Control and Inhibition of Impulses

During the preschool years, the child continues to rely on attachment behavior when under stress, but she also makes considerable gains in regulating feelings and impulses on her own. The preschool child increasingly makes use of interpersonal coping skills, internalized defense mechanisms, and even cognitive strategies for dealing with anxiety and distress. Cognitive development makes contributions to the preschool child's ability to exert self-control and inhibit impulses. In part these new cognitive abilities promote feelings of control because they allow the child to understand reality better, so that she is less frequently reactive in the face of experiences that are new or surprising. Factors contributing to increasing capacity to delay or inhibit impulses include the following.

Ability to Imagine and Anticipate Consequences of Behavior

Improving memory and previous social learning enable the child to remember previous consequences and to make choices about future actions on the basis of those memories. A child rejected by peers for destroying their fort by pulling a blanket off the chairs it was draped over sometimes is able to inhibit his impulse the next time because he does not want to be rejected again. It is important to note, however, that having an ability does not mean the preschooler always uses it. The intensity of the preschooler's wishes often causes impulsive actions.

Increasing Categorization of Experience

Increasing categorization of experience permits generalization across similar experiences. For example, a child who has had several babysitters is able to control her apprehension about what the new babysitter will be like.

Inner Speech and Private Speech

The preschool child can talk to herself in order to sort out what is happening and what she plans to do. This gives her a sense of control. She can also remind herself about rules, prohibitions, and expectations, either silently or out loud, in order to guide her behavior.

Increasing Self-Control Based on Awareness of Social Expectations

The child has internalized ideas about acceptable behavior and is beginning to recognize when he has the impulse to break the rules. After age 4 children regularly suppress negative impulses through conscious effort in order to conform to social norms. A child who becomes angry and wants to hit back after another child hits him may stop himself through "effortful control" (Kochanska et al., 2000). Following this inhibition of action he may, of course, express strong emotions by shouting or crying. The intensity of his feeling may reflect both his upset at the other child's violation of the "rules" and the stress involved in inhibiting a strong impulse.

Ability to Displace Real-World Concerns and Anxiety into Fantasy Play

Children use play to compensate for feelings of inadequacy and fears. The 4-year-old, for example, may be anxious about the fact that she is smaller and less competent than adults but compensates by playing adult roles or becoming idealized characters who represent power in her dramatic play. By becoming the powerful queen or heroine, she temporarily diminishes and masters feelings of inadequacy.

Sources of Anxiety for Preschoolers

Some of the sources of anxiety for toddlers—separation fears, problems with self-expression, fear of losing control—cause less pronounced anxiety in preschoolers. Developmental advances have rendered these concerns less stressful. But the preschooler experiences other typical sources of distress and anxiety.

Reactions to Aggressive Feelings

Preschool children are working hard to develop self-control, particularly over aggression but also over wishes to be dependent. When they are unsuccessful at controlling aggression, they may become anxious about the results of their aggressive behavior and about the internal experience of being overwhelmed by anger. The child who is aggressive may already be a fearful child, particularly if he has been treated harshly or exposed to violence; however, the child's egocentric view of his aggressive thoughts and behavior may intensify his anxiety because he assumes that others have similar impulses.

Fear of Being Displaced in the Parents' Affections

Given that many families space their children at 2- to 3-year intervals, the birth of a sibling is a normative event—and a normative source of anxiety—for many preschoolers. During the mother's pregnancy the young child thinks about the baby and worries about being displaced. Volterra (1984) documents the thoughts and behavior of a 2-year-old boy. After this child learned about the coming baby, he became aggressive toward his dolls and younger children. He developed a play scenario in which he, as a policeman, kicked a "bad boy" out of the house. The timing of the baby may temporarily interfere with the preschooler's movement toward autonomy (Teti et al., 1996). In response to anxiety about being less loved, he may show regressive behavior that aims to get his mother to take care of him, as proof that she loves him. When he is at child care or nursery school, he may imagine that his mother and his younger sibling are at home having a wonderful time together. As his sibling gets older he may feel threatened by her developing motor skills and his parents' admiration of them. Finally, he must cope with unacceptable anger toward his mother and the baby, which increases his anxiety. Of course, parents find many ways to help the older child cope, by continuing to support his autonomous functioning, tolerating his temporary regressions, and encouraging his relationship with the baby.

Failures in the Control of Bodily Functions

A preschooler who has mastered urinary and bowel control is upset by lapses in toilet training. The child who wets himself during the day or wets the bed after a period of dryness is distressed by such lapses. Often failures in control indicate reactions to other types of stress—a separation from a parent, the birth of a sibling, or intense arguments between parents. However, parents may increase the child's anxiety by putting pressure on him to stay dry. Brazelton (1992) recommends addressing the primary sources of the child's anxiety rather than focusing on the lapse in toilet training.

Fear and Distress about Being Rejected by Peers

The increasing social orientation of the preschool child means that she is sensitive to how peers perceive her, and by age 5 she may be aware of her reputation and standing in the peer group. To be rejected, teased, or excluded can cause great pain and anger. Because a preschool child thinks egocentrically and still lacks the ability to evaluate the intentions of others, she may hear another child's insult—"You're a stupid poopy-diaper baby"—as if it were true, and react with humiliation and rage. They experience such insults as attacks on their whole person.

Fears Caused by Inadequate Reality Testing and Magical Thinking

The preschooler's ability to distinguish fantasy from reality, especially under conditions of stress, is not reliable. Consequently, young children may become anxious in response to bad dreams, or films or TV programs that show graphic violence or scenes of horror, because they experience the content as if it were reality. Increasing knowledge of the frightening aspects of life can also become a source of anxiety. Learning about death, kidnapping, burglars, or plane crashes can create anxiety because the child personalizes these catastrophes, imagining them as happening to himself or his parents. For example, a 4-year-old whose babysitter told him that he could not stay in the car alone at a shopping center because children were sometimes kidnapped out of cars began to shadow his mother everywhere at home because he was afraid of being kidnapped. The preschooler's dilemma is that his cognitive development is advanced enough to allow him to create images of unseen danger, yet not advanced enough to appraise how realistic his fear is.

Attachment History and Self-Regulation

L. A. Sroufe's longitudinal studies of attachment (1989, 1990) have demonstrated that preschoolers with secure attachment histories continue to turn to adults, such as child care providers and teachers, for support when they are distressed. Their working models lead them to anticipate that they will receive help when they need it. Consequently they seek attention in positive rather than negative ways. Preschoolers with secure attachment histories also show good ability to manage impulses. They are assertive but not aggressive (Bradley, 2000). By contrast, preschoolers with avoidant attachment histories tend not to turn to adults for help in regulating distress. The working models of attachment and self that develop out of the avoidant pattern suggest that others cannot be relied upon for support and that the self is not worthy of being helped. Preschool children with avoidant attachments may turn away from caregivers if they fall and hurt themselves, or huddle in a corner if they are feeling ill. These children also have much higher rates of aggression than children with secure attachments, suggesting both that they feel more hostility and have less ability to regulate aggressive impulses (Sroufe, 1983, 1989; Vondra et al., 2001).

Preschoolers with such difficulties can be helped to move toward more adaptive social relationships if a preschool teacher makes extraordinary efforts to establish an attachment with the child. When a therapist is working with a preschooler with behavioral problems secondary to attachment difficulties, intervention must include not only work with parents but also consultation with the child's day care providers.

Strategies for Self-Regulation and Coping

New self-regulatory capacities emerge during the preschool years that make autonomous self-regulation more and more possible. Nevertheless, we should think of the preschooler as on the way to self-regulation rather than having achieved it. Compared with school-age children, preschoolers are more volatile and less able to maintain consistent self-control. The preschooler increasingly relies on the following self-regulatory strategies.

Play and Fantasy as Displacement of Negative Affects and Impulses

Play increasingly has the function of containing anxiety through displacement. Rather than risk the anxiety that accompanies the direct expression of forbidden aggression, the child displaces aggressive and other negative impulses into play. Paley (1988) catches this idea as she describes the dramatic play of 4-year-olds: "How easy, in play, to disguise the feelings represented by the actions. The more I listen, the more the play seems motivated by that which *cannot* be discussed" (p. 45; emphasis in original).

> In a play therapy example, 5-year-old Andrew had become very rivalrous toward his 2-year-old brother. His brother had recently been praised by their parents for his successful toilet training. Andrew's play became a vehicle for representing his angry perception that his parents appreciated his brother more than himself. Andrew brought a dinosaur he called Chompers to the session. Chompers attacked family dolls, especially a little brother doll, who was punished for unnamed reasons by being thrown across the room and given a potion that would keep him at the age of 1 forever. Chompers's aggression toward the dolls gave Andrew a vicarious outlet for angry feelings toward his parents and his younger brother. His anger was expressed through the play rather than directly and consciously. I commented on his play as representing the difficult feelings children have when they feel their parents favor a sibling. Like Andrew, I used displacement, couching my statements in universalizing terms about the feelings of children in general rather than Andrew in particular.

Internalization of Mutual Regulatory Strategies

During the first 3 years of life, the child and parents have established transactional strategies for regulating affect in the context of the attachment relationship. Although preschool children continue to need help from caregivers to manage emotions, the internalization of dyadic strategies increasingly allows the preschooler to manage anxiety via self-regulation (Bradley, 2000). The preschooler begins to use the social abilities and prosocial attitudes learned in the attachment relationship in peer relations. Children who use these skills to mediate conflicts and disputes with peers feel successful and more in control. They are also popular with other children (Dunn et al., 2002).

Conscious Strategies for Inhibition of Emotional Expression and Arousal

Preschool children have a beginning ability to consciously control their emotional responses. One can see 4- to 5-year-olds, especially boys who are socialized not to cry, working to suppress the urge to cry after being hurt.

> A 4-year-old boy was enjoying roughhousing with his father when he lost his balance and scraped his cheek against the wall. He looked upset, but said, "See you later," and went into his bedroom. Apparently he was ashamed of his impulse to cry and needed to hide it from his father. Alternatively, he may have blamed his father for what happened, and did not want him to know he was angry. In either case, he exerted conscious control over his emotions.

Older preschoolers develop the ability to express "appropriate" feelings and hold "inappropriate" feelings in check. They also begin to show enough control to sustain tasks, at least for a short time, that they would prefer not to do, such as picking up toys (Kochanska, Coy, & Murray, 2001). However, conscious self-regulation is a difficult task for preschoolers. Reliable control over affects does not develop until midway through school age. Preschoolers swing back and forth between self-control and strong expression. The degree of strain they feel is suggested by how excited they become in situations where a full range of emotions can be revealed. This is one reason preschoolers love dramatic play. Play is an arena outside the demands of reality where intense feelings—exuberance, silliness, aggression, disappointment—can be expressed in pretend scenarios that feel affectively real. Child therapists also observe the preschooler's excitement when she realizes that play therapy permits a wide range of emotional expression.

By age 5–6, however, preschoolers become more capable of managing emotions. This general ability has been defined as "emotional competence," an idea that includes being able to express feelings without becoming overwhelmed by them, to recognize the emotional states of others as well as one's own, and to regulate one's own emotions through conscious effort (Saarni, 1999). Emotionally competent preschoolers make a smoother adjustment to school and also become socially competent kindergartners who get along well with peers (Denham et al., 2003). Preschoolers who are less competent in understanding the emotions of other kids have more trouble getting along with peers and are more at risk for social rejection and withdrawal in early elementary school.

Establishment of Psychological Defense Mechanisms

Defenses, as defined by psychoanalytic theory, are unconscious mental operations that serve to protect the child from experiencing anxiety or psychic pain (Freud, 1966). When mobilized in response to internal or external cues of anxiety or danger, defenses help the individual regulate affects and maintain a sense of psychic organization. The motivation for the establishment of defenses in the toddler period comes from awareness of conflicts between the toddler's wishes and his parents'. In order to avoid the anxiety associated with being angry at his parent, the toddler uses the defense of projection, which involves attributing one's negative feelings and impulse to someone else. So the toddler who is angry at her father says, "You're angry at me!" As development proceeds, more sophisticated and adaptive defenses gradually supplant the "primitive" defenses of early childhood. Defenses are one of the normal means of regulating affect and impulse. They only become problematic when they become overgeneralized to situations where they are not appropriate or when they supplant other coping mechanisms such as cognitive and interpersonal skills. Defenses prominently used by preschool children include the following.

Projection. The child attributes his own feelings—especially hostile or aggressive ones—to someone else. A 3- or 4-year-old may accuse a peer he has just pushed as having intended to hurt him.

Displacement. A child who becomes anxious about negative feelings toward a person he cares about directs these feelings toward someone else. Angie, a 3-year-old whose mother was pregnant, became rude and defiant toward one of her child care providers, who was also pregnant. In her own family she was seemingly happy and showed interest in the coming baby. During a brief evaluation this little girl repeatedly played out a scenario in which a baby figure was burned up and then a mother and girl figure held each other close. This child had displaced hostile and ambivalent feelings toward the baby (and her mother) onto another pregnant woman.

Denial. Denial involves saying, believing, or acting as if some painful or anxiety-generating event did not happen. A child may deny to himself that he has violated a parent's rule. Or he may overtly state to another person that he did not violate the rule. This defense, though clearly unrealistic when used just after a teacher or parent has seen him do something wrong, demonstrates the young child's strong need to avoid disapproval. In the therapeutic situation, denial is common if the therapist asks directly about a child's negative behavior. For example, I said to a 5-year-old boy, "Your mom told me you got in a fight with another boy at the park." He replied, "No, I didn't." Another child expressed denial in response to a similar question by completely ignoring it and talking about something else. Denial is a common defense for older children as well, but it is particularly utilized by preschool children. For this reason, it is best to approach anxiety-laden material indirectly, though displacement in fantasy or play.

Regression. This defense involves "turning back to acts, thoughts or feelings which belonged to an earlier stage of development" (Berman, 1979, p. 10). The stereotypical example of regression is when a child whose mother has just had a baby becomes less autonomous, demanding that her mother pick her up, dress her, or feed her. Regression in this example represents anxiety about attachment. The child seeks reassurance that the parent still cares about her, and she communicates this by reverting to attachment-seeking behaviors that had been set aside. Regression can also be used to deny aggressive behavior. For example, a 4-year-old boy who had just wildly thrown dolls and furniture out of the dollhouse in my office began talking "baby talk," apparently in order to suppress the anxiety aroused by his aggressive behavior. Regression is also common at times of developmental transitions. Many children temporarily cope with the stress of beginning kindergarten by becoming more demanding and dependent at home.

MORAL DEVELOPMENT

During the preschool period, the child moves from a moral sense that is based on outside approval to a more internalized sense of right and wrong. At 2 and 3 years of age, children's sense of morality is determined by their wishes for love and approval and their avoidance of disapproval, so they try to avoid behavior that will bring disapproval. Kohlberg (1984) calls this a "punishment and obedience orientation." Although toddlers are aware of parental standards, their internal controls are not well developed and they rely on parents to function as auxiliary consciences (Emde & Buchsbaum, 1990). This is quite different from having an internalized sense of values or conscience. Nevertheless, compliant behavior in toddlers predicts adequate conscience development at age 6 (Kochanska et al., 1995). Preschoolers gradually move from compliance in direct response to parents' requests and commands to "committed compliance," which involves an identification with the parents' perspective and the child's *conscious* sense that she is intentionally doing what the parent wants (Kochanska, 2002).

During the preschool years, progression in cognitive and social development makes possible an internalization of morality. The following discussion presents some characteristics and trends of moral development in children between 3 and 6 years of age.

Distinctions between Intention and Result

Early preschoolers are unable to distinguish between intention and result. (According to our system of law, a crime is worse if someone intended to do it than if it was done accidentally or through negligence, e.g., the distinction between murder and manslaughter.) The young preschool child only looks at the surface of behavior and can't understand motives. Piaget (1948) gave 3-year-olds the following moral problem: One boy was told by his mother not to touch a nice cup. But he was mad at his mother, so he threw it down and broke it on purpose. Another boy was carrying 12 cups on a tray to help his mother get ready for a party. He tripped and all the cups got broken. Piaget asked the children, "Is one of the boys more naughty than the other?" Preschool children regularly answered that the boy who broke 12 cups is naughtier because he broke *more* cups. By contrast, school-age children, who understand the distinction between intention and result, regularly said that the first boy was naughtier because he did it *on purpose.*

Increased Self-Monitoring

The toddler has become aware of parental standards and expectations. During the preschool years, this awareness is increasingly acute. Preschool children are capable of articulating parental expectations. The 5-year-old who instructs her 2-year-old brother to take his plate to the kitchen demonstrates this. As preschoolers consciously internalize standards, they begin to monitor their own behavior. Consequently, they usually know when they have violated a rule or acted aggressively (Turiel, 1998).

The Development of Guilt as a Distinct Emotion

The capacity to feel bad "on the inside" develops during the preschool years. Unlike the toddler, who may feel anxious if he violates a parental rule because he is afraid of punishment, the preschool child begins to understand that he is wrong whether the parent knows or not. This internal awareness of wrong and the painful feeling that accompanies it is the feeling of guilt (Eisenberg, 2000). Kagan (1984) argues that the emergence of guilt is related to cognitive maturation, specifically to the preschooler's awareness that he can choose among alternative actions: "A two-year-old is not capable of recognizing that he could have behaved in a way different from the one he has chosen. But the four-year-old has this ability and so experiences the emotion we call *guilt"* (p. 175). Preschoolers understand that they have choices about how to behave, as well as having a beginning awareness that they are responsible for their actions. Consequently, they can blame themselves when they do not choose to do the "right" thing.

Play as Practice for Morality

As preschoolers begin to think about "good" and "bad," their interactions and fantasy play begin to address explicit questions of what is good behavior and what is not. Because they are trying to figure out these questions on a conscious level, they can easily have their feelings hurt if they think another child is accusing them of being bad. Fantasy play becomes an important vehicle for exploring these questions. In play, one can be Wonderwoman or Batman, whose job is to stop the bad guy, or one can temporarily pretend to be a bad guy *without being bad in reality*.

> A 5-year-old boy who had seen all but the most scary parts of the Harry Potter movies loved to play out heroic scenarios in the role of Harry. But occasionally he chose to enact the role of Draco Malfoy, a mean boy who resents Harry's prominence at their school. As Draco, he would cast spells on the "good" characters Harry Potter and Ron Weasley, freezing them into immobility or turning their bones to jelly. This child had an easy temperament and good self-regulation and was not mean in his interactions with other children. Yet like most preschool children he was aware of mean thoughts and impulses in himself. Playing Draco, he could experience these negative feelings within the safety of pretend. Play gave him a chance to "walk on the wild side" and then return to the good-guy role.

Play also allows children to discharge aggressive impulses in safe ways. For example, two boys have been fighting over a toy and have pushed each other. One threatens to throw the other into the river. The other says, "Like a troll?" and this shifts the focus into play based on the story "Three Billy Goats Gruff." What began as real aggression is displaced into fantasy aggression in which both boys are "safe" and neither has to experience himself as actually bad (Paley, 1986). Through play "antisocial" behavior is transformed into a shared social experience.

Understanding and Following of Rules

Through frequent reminders and limit setting, preschoolers learn the rules of behavior established by parents and caregivers. However, they have trouble understanding the rules of a game. Even when a preschooler grasps the rules cognitively, he tends to see games as vehicles for fantasy. Adults who play simple board games with preschool children find that they often change rules or make them up as they go along. They have little sense of the importance of following the rules for the sake of making the game fair.

> For example, a 5-year-old boy I saw in therapy had learned the rules of checkers and often asked me to play. The game would always begin politely, with several moves that followed the rules. But then he would pick up a checker, raise it high above the board, and shout "Superchecker!" Then Superchecker would fly down and knock all my checkers off the board.

Another issue implied in this story is that preschoolers know that adults are bigger and more competent than themselves. Their frequent tendency to "cheat" and their insistence on winning reflects their attempt to level the playing field by giving themselves advantages over a clearly superior competitor. Young children who become angry at a parent who wins a game sometimes complain bitterly, "It's not fair!" From their perspective as a small person competing against a bigger, more accomplished person, they are right, even when the adult is playing by the "rules." This has implications for parent guidance. If a parent is expecting a 4- to 6-year-old to play by the rules, a therapist can point out that that is expecting too much of a preschool child and might suggest that the child's interest in playing fairly will develop over the next few years.

Social Relationships

The growing importance of social relationships gradually contributes to the development of the conscience. In the early part of the preschool period, the child's egocentrism leads to attempts to get other kids to fit themselves into the particular fantasy she is having. There is often conflict about whose fantasy should dominate; because of this, the collaborative play of preschoolers is unstable. Gradually, however, children come to value relationships over egocentrism. They become more able to negotiate because they can increasingly take the other child's role and empathize with her point of view. They internalize the idea that it is important to be fair to others (Eisenberg & Fabes, 1998).

Transformations in Children's Ability to Accept Responsibility for Their Actions

Young preschoolers have trouble tolerating feeling they have been bad; consequently, they rely a lot on defenses of projection and denial. For example, they may deny that they have hurt another kid, and in fact are likely to blame the victim, saying "He hit me first" or "He was going to hit me." Between 5 and 6 years of age they gradually take more responsibility for their actions. In work with parents, it is often useful to point out that the "lies" preschoolers tell often represent wishes or attempts at self-protection. We can suggest that parents contradict the "lie" without punishing the child for lying.

How Do Moral Controls, Rules, and Values Become Internalized?

A number of processes, both in the environment and within the child, support moral development. These include the following.

Parental Influence

Parents and others repeatedly define expectations and rules for the child. Preschoolers regularly test boundaries, and adults repeatedly clarify what the boundaries are. The child's internal awareness of standards, need for parents' love and approval, and need for regularity and help with self-regulation make her receptive to parents' limit setting. Children with a history of secure attachment are likely to respond to parents' expectations (Kochanska, 2002). If discipline is neither harsh nor absent, the preschool child shows a readiness to take in the parents' rules. Baumrind (1993) notes: "When parents consistently arouse sufficient empathy and guilt in disciplinary encounters to capture the child's attentions, but not sufficient to be disruptively arousing, the child is likely to successively assimilate the parents' moral norms" (p. 1307). At the same time, young children tend to assimilate parental values when the parents' style of discipline is warm, empathic, and well matched with the child's temperament. Empathy and kindness in parents are powerful promoters of conscience development in preschoolers (Kochanska et al., 1995; Kochanska & Murray, 2000).

By contrast, research has linked harsh, authoritarian discipline and physical punishment with poor internalization of controls and values. When a parent is shouting, calling a child names, or threatening to abandon her, the child pays more attention to the parent's intense emotions (and to her own fearful arousal) than to the moral value the parent is asserting. More gentle and rational approaches to discipline keep the child's arousal at a manageable level, with the result that the child is more likely to take in and remember the content of parental expectations (Thompson, 1998). The child who is regularly hurt via spanking or slapping tends to focus on avoiding punishment rather than understanding why a certain behavior is wrong. Physical discipline *impedes* rather than promotes internalization of moral values. Children exposed to frequent physical punishment tend to have poorer internal controls and show more aggression toward peers (Gershoff, 2002). Children whose parents punish them for expressing distress, frustration, or anger develop poorer capacities for regulating feelings and more externalizing behavior problems (Eisenberg, Fabes, Shepard, Guthrie, Murphy, & Reiser, 1999).

Identification

The child who loves and admires his parents comes to identify with them and takes their values into the self. Particularly through identification the child learns "acceptable" ways of expressing autonomy and initiative as well as ways of controlling negative impulses (Kagan, 1984). Toddlers with histories of secure attachments and reciprocal positive feelings are more receptive to the limits their parents set. As preschoolers, they show more evidence of having internalized their parents' expectations and rules, based on positive identifications (Kochanska et al., 1995). On the other hand, the power of identification is so strong that if a parent models dishonest or antisocial behavior, the child will come to feel that he cannot avoid being like his parent even though he may be aware of the parent's violation of social norms (Berg-Nielsen, Vikan, & Dahl, 2002). Such a child may experience confusion and shame over differences between parental and social norms, especially when he enters school.

Increasing Parental Expectations

Parents intuitively recognize the older preschooler's growing capacity to distinguish between intention and result and to empathize with others. In response they increase their attempts to help the child realize the importance of taking the needs and feelings of others into account. In this way, emerging moral abilities based on cognitive development are reinforced by socialization (Kochanska, 2002).

Increasing Empathy

The capacity to empathize continues to develop. The child becomes more able to put herself in another's place and to imagine how it feels to be hurt or teased. Through empathy, the child can understand why she should limit her aggressive impulses toward others (Eisenberg, 2000). Empathy also generates intentional prosocial acts of sympathy and kindness.

> A 5-year-old girl learned that her younger brother had to go the doctor for an immunization she had already received. She observed his apprehension and noted, correctly, "He doesn't want to get a shot." After he went to the doctor, she asked her aunt for paper and markers, and made a card, drawing her brother's face on the front, and having her aunt write on the inside "I hope that shot wasn't too hurting." When he returned, she gave him the card and a cookie.

Increasing Peer Orientation

As peers become more important, it becomes necessary to recognize that others have needs too. Older preschoolers find it quite disturbing if another kid tells them, "I won't be your friend," because friends are becoming so important to them. This encourages them to internalize values about treating others fairly.

Emergence of Moral Reasoning Abilities

By age 4½–5, children become able to explain reasons for moral judgments. When presented with hypothetical stories involving one child teasing or hitting another, older preschoolers will say that it is *wrong* to hit or tease. They can provide a reason for their condemnation: "You shouldn't be mean because it hurts somebody's feelings," or "It's not nice if somebody doesn't share their toys." Such moral reasoning reflects the preschooler's increasing capacities for empathy and perspective taking (Smetana, 1995).

Internalization of the Conscience

The progress of moral development during the preschool years involves a shift from external to internal control. Through the influences and developmental processes described above, the child's control of self moves from outside dependence on parents and other authorities to the inside—to an internal locus of control called the conscience or superego.

THE DEVELOPING SELF

The tension between fantasy and reality in the preschooler's thinking is also reflected in his views of self. The preschool child seems to alternate between grandiose and realistic views of the self. Harter (1998) notes that "young children's inaccurate and inflated self-evaluations should be understood as 'normative distortions' " (p. 589) based on their wishes to be more competent than they actually are. The more grandiose perspective, which is often expressed in fantasy play, serves a protective function, tempering the child's realistic awareness of how much smaller and less capable he is, compared with older children and adults. The compensatory nature of the child's fantasy can be heard in statements of a 5-year-old boy who was anxious about entering kindergarten: "I'm the best basketball player. I already know how to read, even hard books like *Goosebumps*." These inaccurate statements reflected his worry that he would not be able to meet the demands of the "big school."

In spite of normal doubts about the self based on realistic perceptions of inadequacy compared to adults, the preschool child draws on several resources that support the development of feelings of competence and self-esteem. Self-esteem is supported by the child's growing sense of autonomy and coping ability. Preschool children often insist on doing things themselves. They frequently challenge themselves physically. Growing self-awareness allows children to evaluate and value themselves. If they succeed often enough in meeting their goals, they begin to develop an internal locus of control, seeing themselves as competent to make things happen (Harter, 1998). The sense of competence and self-esteem are also supported by the child's historical and continuing relationship with her parents. A child's self-regard is based on a history of secure attachment, parental availability, and emotional support, as well as the child's internalization of her parents' basically positive view of her (Gemelli, 1996).

The preschooler's ability to maintain a positive view of self can be compromised by a number of maladaptive parenting behaviors, including insecure attachment, parental overexpectations that the child repeatedly fails to measure up to, parents' harsh punishment or expression of negative views of the child, and frequent rejection of the child. Such parenting behavior is often the result of intergenerational transmission of insecure and negative attachment patterns, mediated particularly by projective identification, in which the parent projects negative views of the self onto the child (Lieberman & Pawl, 1990). Such projections of the parents' working models of attachment encourage negative or anxious self-representations in the child that interfere with the development of self-love. The child's resulting difficulties with self-esteem confirm Bowlby's (1973) point that the working model of attachment creates the working model of the self as the parent's view of the child becomes internalized. The toddler who has received the parents' support and love, as well as limits, emerges as a preschooler with self-esteem and confidence in his autonomous abilities. The toddler who has been shamed, criticized, negatively characterized, harshly punished, or abused enters the preschool period with a sense of inadequacy, poor self-esteem, and self-doubt (Harter, 1999).

Identification

During the preschool years, identification with parents becomes a primary means of defining the self. Toddlers imitate their parents' behavior, but identification reflects a more global idea: I am like my parent. Between 3 and 4 years of age, the child begins to be aware, both consciously and unconsciously, of similarities between herself and her parents, as well as other important persons in her life. She imitates her mother's behavior and begins to evaluate her own actions in terms of how well they match her mother's (Harter, 1998). She begins to see herself as having psychological qualities like her mother's. Although the child's primary identification may be based on the most obvious similarities, such as gender and physical attributes, identifications occur in many more subtle ways as well and a child in a two-parent family will identify with aspects of both parents. Whether a child develops these more flexible identifications depends on whether sex-stereotyped behavior is reinforced within the family. In families adhering to rigid gender roles, children are likely to be reinforced for identifying with the same-sex parent and discouraged from being like the opposite-sex parent (Elkind & Weiner, 1978). Although children consciously strive to be like their parents, they also *unconsciously* assimilate parental characteristics.

> The son of a thoughtful and rather taciturn father spoke in thoughtful, reasoned tones, constraining his affects, in an eerily perfect imitation of his father. A candid photo of them together showed the father with a quizzical facial expression and the 5-year-old son looking up at his dad with the same look on his face.

An important impetus for identification is the preschooler's growing awareness of the adult's power and competence. Although the child is aware that she cannot do the things her father can do, identifying with him allows her to share vicariously in his power and accomplishments. A strong identification helps allay the anxiety young children feel as they become aware of their relative inadequacies as compared to older children and adults. The child with a positive identification with one or both parents and a history of secure attachment tends to have confidence that she will eventually be able to do things as well as her parent can. Further, strong, positive identifications support moral development, since the child who feels a strong identification with a parent is more likely to assimilate the parent's values and morality. However, if a parent behaves in antisocial, aggressive ways, the preschooler is also at risk for incorporating *those* characteristics into her self-representation.

Gender Identity

During the preschool years, gender identity and sex-role learning become important to the child's definition of self. There are many studies of parental behavior that suggest that sex typing begins at birth. Parents tend to project gender stereotypes onto very young infants, seeing boys as more active and stronger and girls as more fragile and sensitive. Parents respond to girls and boys differently, talking and cuddling more with girls and playing more actively with boys (O'Brien, 1992). Recent studies have refined this view, finding that differential treatment of boys and girls by parents does not occur in all areas of functioning but primarily in response to behavior explicitly resonating gender stereotypes. For example, parents, especially those holding traditional views of gender, may discourage boys from playing with dolls. But in domains of behavior that do not have such specific gender associations, such as sharing or being polite, parents generally have similar expectations for both girls and boys (McHale, Crouter, & Whiteman, 2003).

By the age of 2, toddlers have learned their gender and, through socialization, are beginning to be aware of the characteristics associated with each gender. Once toddlers are aware of their gender, they tend to identify with and imitate the behavior of the same-sex parent. They begin to attend to and assimilate gender-based attributes, as defined by their culture. These understandings gradually become shaped into schemas of "what boys do" and "what girls do" (Liben & Bigler, 2002).

This understanding of gender characteristics specific to the child's culture continues to grow during the preschool years. The dramatic play of 4- and 5-year-olds at times seems to take on exaggerated gender-stereotyped behavior, with girls emphasizing nurturant roles and boys aggressively confronting the dangers of the world.

> As the grandparent of 5-year-old opposite-sex twins, I have had many opportunities to observe and participate in play influenced by gender themes. Fantasy play with them together can be challenging: my granddaughter wants me to help her wrap baby dolls in blankets, while my grandson insists I watch for comets that may hit our spaceship. Sometimes, they will accept my suggestions that the babies can go up in the spaceship.

The formal qualities of play also differ by gender. Boys' play tends to emphasize competition and one-upsmanship, while girls' play tends to be more cooperative, with less emphasis on hierarchy among the players (Sebanc, Pierce, Cheatham, & Gunnar, 2003).

Compared to toddlers, preschool children begin to show a strong preference for play with same-sex peers. In nursery schools and child care centers, 4- and 5-year-old girls enjoy playing together in the doll corner, emphasizing themes of nurturance and caretaking, and becoming brides, whereas boys may act out superhero play involving aggression, magical powers, and overcoming danger. Although boys may join in girls' family play and girls may take roles in boys' superhero play at times, there is a strong tendency during the preschool years for play to be sex stereotyped (O'Brien, 1992). Preschoolers tend to support and admire peers who maintain sex-stereotyped behavior and, to a lesser degree, to criticize or reject those who do not. Boys tend to be more insistent than girls in maintaining gender-stereotyped play themes and avoiding toys associated with girls (Ruble & Martin, 1998). Nevertheless, in the hierarchy of preschoolers' values, moral considerations of fairness take precedence over gender stereotypes. When preschool children are asked whether it is *fair* to exclude children from play on the basis of gender, a strong majority of both boys and girls condemns exclusion (Killen, Pisacane, Lee-Kim, & Ardila-Rey, 2001).

In addition, observations in preschools suggest that girls and boys do play together and that the roles they take sometimes blend stereo-typed masculine and feminine characteristics, with girls combining magi-cal superpowers with caretaking and boys, who usually focus on fighting bad guys, occasionally showing concern about babies. Observational studies in group settings have found that about two-thirds of preschool-ers' play is same-sex and about one-third involves both sexes. The amount of cross-sex play is influenced by the values of teachers. If teach-ers encourage it, there is more cross-sex play (Smith & Cowie, 1991). Overall, in the preschool years, there are strong tendencies toward same-sex play, but there is more fluidity in the amount of cross-sex play and sex-role behavior than in middle childhood, when sex segregation is more rigidly adhered to.

Studies of gender identity suggest that *gender constancy,* the aware-ness that one's gender cannot change, develops during the preschool years (Ruble & Martin, 1998). Younger preschoolers may believe that girls may turn into boys, boys into girls. This is consistent with the pre-schooler's emphasis on imaginative thinking, as well as the awareness that many things about the self do change, including height, weight, strength, and coordination abilities (Harter, 1983b). However, gender constancy is reinforced during the later part of the preschool years by children's internalization of social norms regarding gender. By age 5 nearly all children understand that gender does not change (Szkrybalo & Ruble, 1999).

Sexual Interests and Gender

Preschoolers show heightened interest in sexuality. Parents describe more overt sexual interest and behavior during this period than in either the toddler or school-age periods (Ryan, 2000). Preschoolers show in-creasing interest in their genitals, realizing through experimentation that the genitals are a source of pleasure. Masturbation becomes more fre-quent not just as a means of self-soothing but as a way of getting sexual pleasure. During this period, children sometimes talk about their geni-tals, occasionally play "doctor," and want to see and touch their parents' bodies. It is not unusual to hear from the mother of a preschool boy, "He said he wanted me to take off my shirt so he could touch my breasts," or to hear from a father that his daughter's (or son's) sexual excitement at bath time has led to a request that the father take off his clothes and get in the tub.

Sexual interest is normative during the preschool period, though sex-ual curiosity and behavior are more likely to be seen at home. Sexual behavior does occur in preschool group settings but is less common there because parents tend to teach children that sexuality is a private matter (Larsson & Svedin, 2002). Sexual behavior that is compulsive, coercive, or directly reflective of adult sexual acts is much less common and should be investigated, since it may reflect sexual abuse, witnessing adult sexuality, or exposure to pornography (Hewitt, 1999).

As children imagine themselves growing into adult roles, they think first of their parents—usually the opposite-sex parent—as love partners. For the preschool child the fantasy of the Oedipus complex makes sense: who could be a better partner than the person who has loved and cared for you and whom you feel close to and admire? Who better to feel sexual toward than a person who has held you, caressed you, allowed you to snuggle against his or her body? The notion that the Oedipus complex consists of the child's falling in love with the opposite-sex parent and wanting to get rid of the same-sex parent is an important but only partial description of the wishes of preschoolers. The girl who imagines marrying her father also wants to be just like her mother. Since the preschool child cannot maintain these competing fantasies simultaneously, she may alternate between which parent she demands an exclusive relationship with and which she treats as a rival. Positive identification tempers and alternates with rivalry. Nevertheless many parents observe that between 4 and 5, children go through a period of possessiveness toward the opposite-sex parent and competition with the same-sex parent. Children in families where fathers are absent play out these dynamics with other males in the extended family. In the dramatic play of preschoolers, one can observe triangular, exclusionary themes as children, trying to compensate for their actual status in the family, compete for the more grown-up role. So one boy says to another, "*I'm* the daddy—you have to be the little boy."

There is a curious dichotomy between classic psychoanalytic thinking, which characterizes the preschool period as the Oedipal phase or "infantile genital phase" (Tyson & Tyson, 1991), and academic developmental psychology, which virtually ignores the preschooler's body and sexual interests in favor of studying cognitive and social development. Although we see behaviors that seem to fit classical Oedipal theory—preference for the opposite-sex parent, jealousy toward the same-sex parent, "triangular" play among preschoolers—for most children the Oedipal drama does not cause irresolvable conflict. A more balanced approach would acknowledge that preschoolers are very interested in their genitals and sexuality, but would not argue that the Oedipus complex is the central developmental process of the preschool years. Practitioners familiar with attachment theory tend to see "Oedipal conflicts" as the outcomes of problems of attachment. Children who are intensely possessive toward a parent are most often those who have developed an insecure–resistant/ambivalent attachment or who have experienced disruptions of attachment that have put the security of their attachments into doubt (Erickson, 1993).

Psychoanalytic theory has also emphasized the developmental significance of young children's reactions to anatomic sex differences. Between 2 and 3 years of age, children know that they are girls or boys and that the other sex is somehow different from them. Between 3 and 5, children become aware of the physical differences between the sexes. Preschool children commonly have some worries and questions about sex differences. The awareness of sex differences is a strong challenge to the child's egocentric view that "everyone is like me." Because of the limits of their cognitive abilities, preschoolers may develop wrong and worrisome theories about the reasons for sex differences. Girls, upon seeing boys, wonder if they once had a penis and imagine it was stolen, cut off, or maybe went inside. A 4-year-old girl told me as we discussed sex differences, "I used to have one when I was 1, but somebody took it from me when I was asleep." Boys, seeing girls, imagine they could lose their penis. Psychoanalytic theory presented this issue as a central issue in preschool development. However, I think it makes more sense to see children's theories and concerns about sex differences as a specific example of how preschoolers think, in this case about an issue that is interesting and exciting. Preschoolers work very hard to come up with explanations for what they observe. In part their thinking is a generalization on the accurate view that many things about the body do change. However, their attempt to understand sex differences is also based on a mistaken premise of egocentrism: that all people are the same. Within this premise the theories they develop about sex differences are not so strange.

Racial Identity and the Self

During the preschool years children's cognitive skills in generalization and categorization develop. Children differentiate between girls and boys, younger and older children, and other obvious physical differences between people. By about age 4, children remark on differences based on skin color and begin to identify themselves as members of a particular ethnic group. Racial/ethnic identity becomes an element in the child's emerging sense of self.

Experimental studies asking white and African American preschoolers to indicate a preference between white and black dolls have consistently shown that both groups of children preferred the white dolls. These findings have been interpreted as responses to exposure to racism (Spencer & Horowitz, 1973). However, the preference for white dolls should not be equated with negative self-images in individual African American children, since studies of young African American children have found that their level of self-esteem does not differ from that of white children (Crain, 1996). Instead the preference for white imagery "may reflect young children's identification (of the self) with the (perceived) more valued stimuli" (Spencer & Markstrom-Adams, 1990).

Spencer (1985) found that although African American preschoolers were aware of negative racial stereotypes and may have been directly subjected to racial prejudice, they did not tend to apply these negative views to themselves. Unlike earlier researchers, who assumed that awareness of negative stereotypes must contribute to a negative view of the self, Spencer concluded, "Racial stereotyping in black children should be viewed as objectively held information about the environment and not as a manifestation of personal identity" (1985, p. 220).

APPENDIX 9.1. Summary of Preschool Development, 3–6 Years of Age

Overall Tasks

- Development of play as a vehicle for exploring reality
- Make transition from view of world based on egocentric and magical thinking to a more logical and reality-based view

Attachment

- Attachment continues to provide security when child is under stress (3–6 years)
- Attachment needs are frequently verbalized rather than simply being expressed in action (4–6 years)
- Improving memory and sense of time allow child to cope with separations—the child can understand better when a parent will return (4–6 years)
- Working models of attachment are firmly established and can be generalized to relationships with nonparental caregivers and peers (3–6 years)

Social Development

- Development of social skill through interaction and play with peers; social competence gradually develops through peer interactions involving negotiation about play scenarios, conflicts based on egocentrism and possessiveness, and triangular dynamics involving competition and exclusion (3–6 years)
- Development of verbal approaches to social interaction and conflict resolution (4–6 years)
- Prosocial interaction is elaborated and more frequent, based on increasing identification with adult models and growing skills in empathy and perspective taking (3–6 years)

- Exposure to peer group and prosocial values in preschool settings encourages cooperation, sharing, and problem-solving skills (3–6 years)
- Peers become more important; sustained exposure to peers leads to decreases in egocentrism; the preschooler identifies with peers and is motivated to make interactions with them pleasurable (4–6 years)
- Friendships based on common play interests develop (4–6 years)

Language and Communication

- Vocabulary at age 3 equals about 1,000 words and continues to increase at a rate of about 50 words each month (3–6 years)
- Speech becomes clear and easy to understand in most preschoolers (3–4 years)
- Long, grammatically complex sentences involving 8–10 words and dependent clauses is typical of the speech of preschoolers (4–5 years)
- Out loud self-talk, or private speech, accompanies behavior and play; the child describes and directs his behavior in this way (3–5 years)
- Interactive play increasingly depends on language (4–6 years)
- Language gradually supplants action as the child's primary means of communication (4–6 years)

Symbolic Communication and Play

- Preschooler's play tends to be imaginative, dramatic, and interactive (3–6 years)
- Functions of preschool play: exploration of reality and social roles; mastery of stress; expression of fantasies, wishes, and negative, forbidden, or "impossible" impulses (3–6 years)
- Distinction between real and pretend: this distinction becomes increasingly clear as the preschool period proceeds; play, which children understand is pretend, helps them begin to distinguish between fantasy and reality (4–6 years)
- Play provides opportunities for practicing emerging cognitive skills, including cause-and-effect thinking, construction of narrative, perspective taking, problem solving, and exploring alternative interpretations of reality (4–6 years)

Cognitive Development

- Generalization and thinking in categories increases (3–6 years)
- Improving memory provides a greater knowledge base for categorizing new information; at the same time, a wider range of categories for informa-

tion storage increases the chance the child will remember new information (3–6 years)

- Cause-and-effect thinking: increasing awareness of causality leads the preschooler to look for causal connections between events; however, limitations in the ability to think logically or emotional arousal may lead the preschooler to mix up cause and effect (4–6 years)
- Egocentric thinking persists, causing limitations in accurate understanding of reality; types of egocentric perceptions include the following: inability to assume another's perspective; reversal of cause and effect; attributing the causes of events to the self; transductive reasoning; personalism; animism (3–6 years)
- Magical thinking and the fusion of fantasy and reality are common, especially when affective arousal, as in trauma, influences thinking. In situations where there is need for "hidden" information, such as figuring out how a seed becomes a plant, the preschool child is likely to utilize fantasy as a way of trying to explain reality (3–6 years)

Self-Regulation

- Increasing ability to categorize experience reduces sense of novelty in new situations, resulting in feelings of control and less vulnerability to anxiety (4–6 years)
- Cognitive ability to imagine and anticipate the consequences of behavior contributes to improving impulse control; this ability is increasingly supported by the child's internalization of social expectations (4–6 years)
- Inner speech and private speech are used to sort out experience and provide reminders of rules, prohibitions, and expectations (3–6 years)
- Ability to displace real-world concerns and anxiety into fantasy play and other forms of symbolic expression (3–6 years)
- Internalization of dyadic strategies of regulation: working models of dyadic regulation are generalized to self-regulation (3–6 years)
- Beginnings of conscious inhibition of emotional expression and arousal (4–6 years)
- Psychological defense mechanisms: projection, displacement, denial, regression (3-6 years)

Moral Development

- Gradual internalization of moral values, resulting in the establishment of a conscience or superego by about age 6 (3–6 years)
- Increased self-monitoring: older preschoolers monitor their behavior, applying standards of morality to themselves; however, this is not done consistently (5–6 years)

- Guilt develops as a distinct emotion (4–6 years)
- Rule-governed behavior: with reminders and reinforcement, preschoolers can follow the rules at school or home; however, they have difficulty abiding by the rules of a game, in part because they cannot emotionally tolerate losing, and in part because the fantasies that games evoke seem more important to them than the rules (4–6 years)
- Increasing importance of peer relationships helps children control negative or impulsive behavior because they want to maintain the friendship and approval of peers (4–6 years)
- Moral controls are gradually internalized by age 6 through the following influences: consistent parental monitoring, limit setting, and praising of good behavior; increasing parental expectations as the child's capacity for self-control matures; identification with parental values; increasing capacity for empathy; increasing peer orientation (3–6 years)

Sense of Self

- Self-esteem is supported by child's growing sense of competence, autonomy, and coping abilities (5–6 years)
- Preschool children who have received parental love and support over time tend to have a positive view of self (5–6 years)
- Identification becomes a basis for defining the self; children consciously strive to be like their parents and also unconsciously assimilate parental characteristics (3–6 years)
- Positive identification helps allay the child's anxiety about being small and incompetent relative to adults (4–6 years)
- Gender identity: children demonstrate increasing awareness of gender identity and culturally based sex roles in play and peer relationships (3–6 years)
- Sexual sense of self: during the preschool years sexual interests develop, as manifested in preoccupations with the body, increased masturbation, Oedipal interests, and curiosity and anxiety about sex differences (4–6 years)
- Racial identity: minority children are aware of prejudicial racial stereotypes; the impact of this awareness for self-esteem, however, depends on whether minority children have experienced the positive processes contributing to self-esteem described above (5–6 years)

CHAPTER 10

Practice with Preschoolers

ASSESSMENT

Preschool children are more autonomous than toddlers. They can express themselves in play, art activities, and words. Consequently, assessment approaches that combine parent–child sessions and individual sessions with the child are both possible and useful. In individual sessions a preschool child may be able to represent her concerns in play more freely than with her parent present. As always, assessment must consider all of the developmental domains. Areas particularly useful to observe in the assessment of preschoolers are cognitive processes, play ability, and self-regulation. Children who have difficulties controlling impulses during the preschool years are at risk for problems in social development (Shaw et al., 2003). Cognitive processes should be observed with an eye to possible distortions of experience based on egocentric thinking. Since play supports so many aspects of preschool development, it is important to investigate the child's capacity to use play to create stories, represent ideas about cause and effect, and organize her view of reality. Children who are inhibited in their play may need help to express themselves more freely. Children who are impulsive or have attentional difficulties may benefit from interventions that help them organize their play. The child whose problems with attention, concentration, and impulsivity interfere with play development does not get the practice with organizing the world and thus may be less prepared for more advanced forms of thinking that build on play thinking.

Observation in the Child Care Center as an Assessment Strategy

In addition to play sessions and family interviews, assessment of preschoolers often includes observations of children in child care settings and consultation with child care providers. Over 60% of children 4 and under in the United States are in regular child care (Shonkoff & Phillips, 2000). Mental health referrals of young children often originate from the observations of child care providers who interact with them on a daily basis.

The child care center's importance in the everyday lives of families points to its potential as a site for prevention and early intervention efforts (Collins, Mascia, Kendall, Schock, & Parlakian, 2003). Because child care personnel see so many children, and are therefore familiar with the range of normal expectations for a given age, they often are the first to raise questions about developmental delays. Child care providers are in a position to observe how a child and parent(s) are managing stresses on the contemporary family, because the child's reactive distress usually shows up in behavior at the center. They can observe how the child and parent(s) are handling life transitions, such as the parent's return to work or school, or the disruptive period following separation and divorce. They can see when negative interactions between parent(s) and child are developing, and they can look for signs of abuse or neglect. They can offer emotional support to those parents who are isolated, and they can provide information about child development, discipline, and other parenting issues. Since they often spend 20–40 hours weekly with a particular child who in many cases will have developed an attachment to them, they are also in a strong position to intervene on the child's behalf (Donahue et al., 2000).

Mental health practitioners must broaden the traditional context of agency-based assessment to include observations of children in their home and child care environments. The following case discussion presents an example of child care-based assessment and intervention, in which the clinician's primary role was to help devise an intervention plan carried out by providers and parents.

CHILD CARE CONSULTATION
WITH A PRESCHOOL CHILD: A CASE EXAMPLE

The director of a child care center where I had previously consulted regularly asked me to assess Carlos, a young 3-year-old who had been at the center the previous year and had just returned from a 2-month-long break during the summer. Both parents worked and Carlos was in care approximately 35 hours per week. Carlos's teachers were concerned because of his lack of involvement with peers and seeming mutism. Carlos was a bilingual child who had been exposed to both Spanish and English since birth. During the preceding year, between ages 2 and 3, he had been speaking in school somewhat, and his use of English seemed adequate for his level of development. His play had been more parallel than interactive. Because he was still 2, his teachers had not been concerned. He talked at home and showed no evidence of language delays. His mother, Ana, was from Panama and spoke Spanish to him at home. His father, John, was American and fluent in Spanish, and he alternated between Spanish and English in speaking to Carlos. The parents felt that Carlos's English was as good as his Spanish and did not think his failure to talk at school was related to lack of knowledge of English or anxiety about speaking English. During the 2 months in Panama, he was surrounded by Spanish speakers and primarily spoke in Spanish. Within the first month after coming back to school, his teachers noticed that he was becoming increasingly withdrawn and silent.

My first thoughts were to observe Carlos at the center to try to learn if there were specific factors in the environment that might be inhibiting him from interacting. I also wanted to see how Carlos functioned at home. The descriptions of his talking at home, but not at school, suggested selective mutism. By seeing him at home, I could directly observe his use of language.

Observation at the Child Care Center

When I observed Carlos, I noted that he watched other kids silently but did not interact with them. He stood in a fixed position for surprisingly long periods of several minutes, just watching, with a rather blank look on his face. It was as if his body was mute like his voice. Nevertheless, his eyes showed interest and moved as he watched other kids. Other children tended to pass him by as if he wasn't present. They had already learned not to expect interaction with Carlos. A girl brought a picture of a polar bear to show Carlos. She said something I couldn't hear. Carlos glanced at her, then at the picture, and the slightest whisper of a smile came over his face and disappeared. He did not say anything, and the girl moved away. Seeing that Carlos's eyes carefully followed the activities of other kids helped me imagine that he was not simply detached or alienated. His eyes seemed to express interest and curiosity, despite the apparent withdrawal communicated by his blank facial expression and his almost frozen body posture.

Home Visit

At home Carlos was friendly toward me, though a little shy, and he spoke to me in English. His language skills seemed appropriate for age. He showed me his toys and talked while he drew some pictures of things he was interested in, like dinosaurs. His parents, Ana and John, said he played well with his older brother. During this visit Carlos's mother, Ana, conveyed an eagerness for help and spoke with me openly. Ana told me that she'd really been homesick since her last visit to Panama, during the summer. She had lived in the United States for 4 years, and complained that she still did not feel at home, though she preferred to stay in the United States because of work opportunities for her and her husband that were not available in Panama. She said that Carlos missed their large extended family in Panama. I asked about other stressors currently affecting Carlos, and she could not think of any. She said that she had discussed Carlos's problems at school with her *compadres* in Panama, but reflected that they did not know how to help because they were unfamiliar with life in the United States. I asked if she felt comfortable talking with the child care staff in Carlos's room, and she named one teacher, Lisa, whom she felt was concerned and sympathetic.

Impressions

Carlos had the characteristics of a selectively mute child. Children who are shy or temperamentally slow to warm up are more likely to develop this problem, as are children of immigrants (American Psychiatric Association, 2000). I wondered if Carlos's mother, out of her own discomfort with American culture, may have conveyed to Carlos that the child care center should be an uncomfortable place. In this context, it would have been helpful to observe a drop-off or pickup to see how she interacted with Carlos's caregivers. Even though he was only occasionally resisting going to school, I speculated that he felt insecure being separated from his mother, perhaps because he had internalized some of her discomfort with American culture and her anxiety over separation from her family in Panama.

Since ages 3–4 is a crucial period in social development, when children begin to interact with peers more intensely, I was concerned that Carlos was missing out on learning beginning skills in sharing activities, play, and ideas, and that his inability to enter into peer interactions would over time reinforce and solidify his withdrawn, isolated stance. Consequently, I suggested the following behavior plan in a meeting with his parents and teachers. In this conference, Lisa, the teacher whom Carlos's mother felt closest to, agreed to be a "preferred provider" who would focus on Carlos when possible.

A Home- and School-Based Plan for Carlos

After we discussed my recommendations, I gave everyone a copy of the suggested plan, which is presented below.

1. Increase Carlos's sense of continuity between home and school.

   - *Parents set positive expectations*, telling Carlos that they know he doesn't talk often at school but that they would like him to because it will be more fun for him. Say to him that you know he likes to talk at home and that you think he would like to talk at school.

- *Parents convey enthusiasm/acceptance of school,* so that Carlos feels he has their "permission" to have a good time there.

How to do this:

- Talk about school at home. This should be based on information from teachers rather than asking Carlos what he did at school.
- At drop-off, a brief but enthusiastic conversation should be held between Ana (or John, when he brings Carlos) and Lisa or another teacher. The content should involve something Carlos has done the day before at home. The tone should be warm so that Carlos sees a good feeling between his parent and the teacher.
- At pickup a similar conversation should take place, in which the teacher describes some of the things Carlos did that day. What the teacher says should be informational rather than evaluative of what kind of day he's had. However, if Carlos has spoken more, become involved in a particular activity, or played with another child, this should be pointed out with pleasure and enthusiasm. John or Ana should mirror the teacher's feeling.
- In the end-of-day conversation, the teacher should mention some activities that will be happening the next day. The following morning on the way to school, parent can talk about this in order to help Carlos anticipate his school day.
- For consideration if work schedules permit: (1) Ana or John spends some time at school in the morning, looking at materials, asking Carlos about other kids, engaging him in conversation that elicits his knowledge of school; (2) Ana or John arrives 20 minutes before regular pickup time and spends some time playing with Carlos or watching him play with other kids. (Note: This could be done 2–3 times a week at first, then decreased after a few weeks.) (3) John or Ana go on some field trips with the group. (4) Ana or John comes occasionally to have lunch at school.

- *Peers.* Arrange opportunities for Carlos to play at home with children from his school. At school, teachers say to Carlos: "Your mom told me that Shelby came to your house to play and that you had fun together. You can have fun together here too."

2. Teachers address separation issue directly.

- When Carlos's mind seems to be elsewhere, consider that he may be thinking about and missing his parents. This can be addressed by saying: "Sometimes when kids are quiet, they're thinking about their mom and missing her. Let's do something together so you'll feel better."
- Let him keep a transitional object in his cubby. A family picture is good. If he appears lost, suggest he go and look at the picture. Look at it with him and talk about some specifics about his family.
- Suggest play involving separation themes with a teacher. Using two

houses and dolls, play out directly leaving home, going to school, being picked up, and so on, with Carlos being encouraged to take control of the play.

3. Help Carlos speak and interact with other kids more at school.

- Teachers note and reinforce *each time* Carlos makes a request of a teacher or speaks to another child. Don't interrupt a conversation if one actually happens, but afterward offer positive and specific encouraging statements. For the first 2 weeks, try as much as humanly possible to verbally reinforce Carlos's speaking every time you see it. For example:
  - "That was great, Carlos. You spoke to me and I knew just what you wanted!"
  - "You had fun singing that song with Shelby."
  - "You showed/told Shelby what you wanted and she did it!"

- Teachers look for opportunities to interpret social overtures by other kids to Carlos.
  - "Rosie's showing you a picture of a polar bear. She thought you'd like to see it. Friends like to show each other things."
  - Without forcing, a teacher takes Carlos's hand and leads him over to a table where kids are drawing or working with puzzles. Ask him to sit down at the table, so he can see what they're doing. Then, if another kid offers him a marker, point out: "Kamali wants to share the markers with you. He wants you to color with him."

- When possible teachers arrange pairing him with another kid—for example, walking together on a field trip or going together on an errand with a teacher. Try to build upon natural or accidental pairings. For example, a teacher has been reading to Carlos and another child, then helps them transition into play together.
- Parents express pleasure/happiness when they see Carlos interact with another child at school. For example: "Carlos, I'm so happy that you talked to Andrew. I want you to have friends at school, and talking is a good way to make friends."

Assumptions Underlying the Behavior Plan

The plan was informed by the following ideas:

1. If Carlos senses increased continuity between home and day care via positive interactions between teachers and parents, talking about day care activities at home and vice versa, and having opportunities to see day care peers at home, he will begin to feel more comfortable interacting at day care.

2. If his mother can convey interest in his activities at day care, she will implicitly convey her permission for him to become more involved with caregivers and peers.
3. Frequent positive reinforcement for interacting or speaking at day care will support the development of Carlos's social abilities.
4. At day care, encouraging joint peer attention (Carlos and other kids sharing the same experience) and explicitly interpreting other kids' social cues for Carlos will also support the development of his social abilities.
5. Specificity and detail would help caregivers and parents understand and carry out the plan.

Follow-Up Note

This plan worked well, primarily because his parents and teachers invested in it. Within a month Carlos was speaking regularly to teachers and other children and was playing with a few other children regularly. At the time of the initial evaluation, I proceeded on the assumption that Carlos's difficulties were based on temperament and on an identification with his mother's sense of alienation in this culture. A few months later, Carlos's father contacted me and indicated that he and his wife had been having severe marital conflicts since returning from Panama. This suggested a more compelling explanation for Carlos's increased insecurity and separation anxiety. In spite of this deeper issue, the increased efforts of teachers and parents to help Carlos feel more comfortable with peers supported him in the tasks of social development in the fourth year of life. Their intervention was tailored to this goal and provided the encouragement and frequent reinforcement Carlos needed to find his voice. For this presenting problem an ecological approach was more effective than psychotherapy.

INTERVENTION WITH PRESCHOOLERS: PLAY THERAPY

From a developmental perspective, the aims of therapy with preschoolers often include addressing troubling ideas and feelings based on the child's cognitive limitations and encouraging the child to move toward verbally mediated understanding of his experience. Here are some characteristic objectives in the treatment of preschoolers.

Help the Child Clear Up Misunderstandings

The preschooler's tendency to try to understand reality through fantasy can generate anxiety that leads to symptomatic behavior. For example,

Angie, the child described in Chapter 9 who displaced her anger about her mother's pregnancy into defiant behavior toward her pregnant child care provider, had evidently come to feel that the new baby would take her mother away from her. In a brief parent–child treatment, I coached Angie's mother to talk with her directly about this worry and to reassure her that she would love her and do mommy things with her after the baby was born.

Clarify Overgeneralizations

Preschoolers tend to overgeneralize on the basis of their stressful experiences. While generalization and categorization are normal aspects of cognitive development, generalization of stressful events can disturb the child's ability to assess reality accurately. As a result, children may become anxious in situations that have associational reminders of the stressful or traumatic situation, or even come to associate any anxiety-provoking situation with the traumatic situation. For example, it is common for young children who have witnessed violence to become hypervigilant and expect that violence can occur at any time, even in situations far removed from the original situation. Tisha, the child described in Chapter 9 who was very aggressive with other children at her child care center after witnessing domestic violence, needed explanations from her mother and teachers to understand that she was safe at the child care center and that her teachers would not allow the type of violence she had witnessed to occur there. Her teachers told her that they knew what she had witnessed and that they would not allow grown-ups to hurt anyone at the center. These interventions validated Tisha's perceptions and feelings but identified her overgeneralization as invalid.

Help the Child Move
to Verbally Mediated Understanding of Experience

Talking with a child about her experience by organizing it into verbal narratives that specify cause-and-effect relationships and distinguish between past and present allows her to gain a sense of control and cognitive competence. As a normal part of development, young children and parents co-construct narratives about the child's experience. This process contributes to the child's capacity for self-regulation by increasing her ability to understand and evaluate experience (Haden, Haine, & Fivush, 1997). In child therapy, representing experience in play narratives and words similarly promotes regulation of affect and behavior (Slade, 1994). Verbalizing feelings allows the child to get some distance from strong impulses and affects so that she does not have to act on them immediately. Being able to substitute thinking for acting promotes a sense of mastery and self-control. As the child gains some verbally mediated mastery over anxiety-producing internal feelings and impulses or stressful past situations, she is likely to become less symptomatic. This objective is particularly important in therapy of children who have difficulty controlling impulses. Since preschoolers are not able to represent all their feelings verbally, the therapist needs to encourage the process of verbalization and verbally mediated thinking by putting into words what the child symbolizes in play. This accomplishes several things:

- The child feels she is not alone with her problems; as the therapist puts thoughts and feelings into words, she feels that someone else understands.
- Her experience is given shape and meaning, enabling her to have a clearer sense of reality and of the distinctions between past and present.
- She gains a means of thinking about her experience and gradually can begin to talk about it herself; she is developing representational competence.
- Her experiences and affects are linked together in a way that makes sense.

USING PLAY IN THE TREATMENT OF PRESCHOOLERS

Since preschoolers readily utilize pretend play to represent experience, play can be the social worker's entry point for a dialogue—involving both action and words—about the child's difficulties. This displacement of real experiences into play creates a safe vehicle for mastering stress or confusion. In part, play provides a means of dramatizing one's concerns beyond mere words; in another way, play provides protection: play is about fantasy characters, not about the self. Practitioners should pay attention to the story and themes represented in preschoolers' play. It is useful to assume that the child's play is telling a story that reflects his concerns.

Preschool children understand the distinction between real and pretend. They are also able to step out of play temporarily, much like the movie director who yells "Cut!" and tells the actors what she wants them to do and then shouts "Action!" to resume the drama. Therapists can make use of the preschooler's ability to distinguish between the play frame and the reality frame. The therapist can at times stop the play briefly and comment on its content and then resume play. Even though a child may not welcome such breaks in the play, they feel normal to her.

Most preschool children, once they have begun to feel some trust in a therapist, prefer that the therapist play with them, as opposed to passively observing their play. A smaller number of children prefer that the therapist stay outside the play, and this must be respected. During the preschool period, players take roles and act them out, which means a preschool child will expect the therapist to become an actor in his play scenario. The therapist must be willing to become a player. As a participant-observer in the play, the therapist can learn how the child constructs his experience and is in a unique position to make interventions, both within the flow of play and by stepping out of the play to comment on it (Chethik, 2000).

In the case that follows, we examine the use of play therapy with a 4-year-old girl whose development was interfered with by medical treatment for a cancerous brain tumor. We look at the preschooler's ability to use play to communicate concerns she is not yet able to express in words, as well as the therapeutic potential of play interpretation. Before presenting the case, I will discuss the problem of developmental interference, with particular reference to the interaction between extended medical treatment and the preschooler's developmental tasks.

MEDICAL TREATMENT
AS A DEVELOPMENTAL INTERFERENCE

As medical treatment for childhood cancer has improved, larger numbers of children are surviving malignancies that previously were almost always fatal. Paradoxically, successful medical treatment may produce negative developmental side effects. The prolonged and invasive treatment common to cancer therapy protocols may constitute an interference to subsequent development in young cancer survivors (Rowland, 1989). Children treated during the toddler and preschool years are particularly vulnerable to developmental interference (Mulhern, Wasserman, Friedman, & Fairclough, 1989). This is consistent with the general findings of developmental research suggesting that the younger the child, the fewer internal resources he has for coping with stress.

Cancer treatment typically involves the onslaught of a number of stressors, including hospitalization, anxiety about dying, pain from spinal taps, bone marrow aspirations and other procedures, nausea and weakness as side effects of chemotherapy, bodily changes such as hair loss, loss of familiar routines, disruption of friendships, and in some cases separation from parents. Some cancers have more severe short- and long-term developmental effects. For example, brain tumors—the second most common type of childhood cancer—generally require surgery, radiation, and chemotherapy; this necessary, intensive treatment, however, often leads to cognitive deficits in attention, memory, cognitive processing speed, visual–motor integration, and in the long run to lower IQ and nonverbal learning disabilities (Armstrong, Blumberg, & Tolendano, 1999).

Rutter (1981) noted that the capacity of preschool children to cope with future stresses was reduced by the stress of multiple hospitalizations. Coping styles developed in response to hospitalizations tended to persist even if they were not adaptive from the perspective of the tasks of future development. Many preschoolers develop a precocious maturity, becoming unexpectedly compliant with treatment; however, this precocity may become generalized and show up later as inhibitions and behavioral rigidities that interfere with development (Rowland, 1989).

Compared to the school-age child, the preschooler's internal mechanisms for coping with stress are not yet well developed. The more sophisticated defenses characteristic of the school-age child—repression, rationalization, denial in fantasy—are not yet in place. Lacking adequate coping strategies, the preschooler is more likely to become overwhelmed during stressful procedures and may either shut down emotionally or lose control and dissolve into tantrums (Chen, Zeltzer, Craske, & Katz, 2000). Prolonged invasive medical treatment is likely to interfere with a number of developmental tasks of the preschool child, including the development of an autonomous self, beginning peer relationships, elaboration of play and fantasy, and control of one's body in terms of regulation of body functions, physical activity, and mobility. At a time when these developmental issues are in ascendancy and therefore subject to disturbance, cancer treatment and hospitalization cause the preschooler to experience a loss of autonomy and self-control, increased dependency, isolation from peers, restrictions on freedom to play, restrictions on physical activity and mobility, and physical vulnerability because of invasive procedures and the side effects of chemotherapy (Chang, 1990).

During the preschool period the ability to play imaginatively is a major adaptive mechanism for the mastery of stress as well as the primary pathway for exploration that facilitates learning and socioemotional development. Play supports the development of autonomy and initiative. Cancer treatment disrupts the child's ability to play actively and strenuously, and has inhibiting effects on her ability to fantasize (Erikson & Steiner, 2001). Recent research suggests that a more global "repressive adaptive style" in which children restrict affect and behavior is common in survivors of childhood cancer (Phipps & Srivastava, 1997). When young cancer survivors return to school, they may be inhibited in expressing feelings and take passive roles in peer interactions (Sexson & Madan-Swain, 1993).

Such inhibited behavior can be understood from the perspective of attachment. Although still reliant on the attachment relationship when under stress, the preschool child is moving toward a sense of the self as autonomous, self-reliant, and purposeful. This movement is supported by an internalized secure base of positive working models of attachment (Main et al., 1985). When a preschool child experiences prolonged stress due to illness and medical treatment and must revert to dependency on parents and other caregivers, her developmental progression toward autonomy may be compromised. Behavioral and affective inhibition can be based on other factors, including temperament and a history of insecure attachment; however, even a preschooler with a history of secure attachment and adequate development can be thrown off track by exposure to severe stressors and may adopt an inhibited style that emphasizes security at the expense of exploration and autonomy (Lieberman & Pawl, 1990). This pattern is particularly likely to develop when parents fearfully overprotect the child after treatment is completed (Scheeringa & Zeanah, 2001). An inhibited child does not compel attention as dramatically as a child whose behavior is impulsive or out of control. However, serious inhibitions during the preschool years may have a negative impact on the child's ability to interact with the world and thus foreclose many normal developmental opportunities, including openness to learning in middle childhood.

The likelihood of developmental interference is increased by the preschooler's cognitive characteristics, including egocentrism and prelogical, magical thinking, which does not distinguish clearly between intention and result or between cause and effect, especially when stressors are operating. Consequently, a preschooler may develop distorted notions about the causes of her illness, including mistaken associations between the onset of the illness and coincidental external events, and is likely to regard invasive and painful medical procedures either as sadistic abuse or as punishment for misdeeds. Further, the preschooler has limited ability to understand abstract explanations of medical issues that she may overhear in the hospital and is prone to impose idiosyncratic constructions on them (Bergmann & Freud, 1965).

PLAY THERAPY WITH A PRESCHOOL CHILD: A CASE EXAMPLE

The case of Katy is an example of a developmental arrest caused by a preschooler's reactions to a serious illness following an early history of excellent development in the context of a stable and loving family (Davies, 1992). Although the cancer treatment was sometimes traumatic and at other times quite stressful for this 3- to 4-year-old girl, her previous excellent developmental progress and remarkably supportive parents combined to protect her from more severe effects of the treatment. Katy was buffered by other protective factors, including middle-class status, her parents' high levels of education, and family and friends who supported the family in many ways, including providing care for her younger brother. Nevertheless, she did show evidence, at age 4, of developmental arrest in the social and affective areas.

Medical History

Up to the onset of her medical symptoms at age 3, Katy was a vivacious, outgoing child who played vigorously and had a good sense of humor. Near her third birthday, her parents noticed that Katy seemed to become moody and that she "stopped playing." Over the next 3 months she became more and more somber and less and less active. She complained of feeling weak and began to have headaches. However, her pediatrician could not find any evidence of illness. When she refused to get out of bed because her head hurt, her parents took her to the emergency room, where she was diagnosed with a malignant brain tumor.

The tumor was removed in an 8-hour surgery. Katy was in considerable pain for 10 days following surgery. Over the next 7 weeks of hospitalization she had several minor surgeries, including the placement of a shunt to drain fluid from the surgical site, two repairs of the incision, and the placement of a Broviac catheter in her chest wall. (A Broviac is a catheter tube that is inserted into the vena cava, the large vein near the heart. It is used for the administration of chemotherapy. The toxic cancer medications would have severely damaged Katy's veins if dripped into her arms; by using the vena cava, where the volume of blood is much higher than in the arm veins, the medications were diluted more quickly and did not cause vascular damage.) All together, she underwent general anesthesia six times. One repair of the incision was done without anesthesia and seems to have been traumatic: Katy became hysterical and had to be held down, and the doctor yelled at her to stop crying as she restitched the wound. She also received cranial radiation, which caused her to lose her hair.

Over the next 15 months, Katy was hospitalized 10 times for 2-day periods for chemotherapy. As she realized that the chemotherapy made her feel terribly ill, she began to resist it and had to be coaxed by her parents. She told her parents that she thought the chemotherapy might make her die. Most of the time, however, she seemed to submit passively. There were also many other invasive procedures, ranging from extremely uncomfortable and at times painful spinal taps to needle pokes for IV (intravenous) intubation and blood draws. Her parents reported that Katy was forced in the hospital to do things she didn't want to do—to have IV needles changed, to be awakened at night to go to the bathroom, and in general to adapt to the hospital routines. Another consequence of her illness was that she had to be kept away from other children when she was out of the hospital. The chemotherapy had compromised her immune system so that an ordinarily mild illness such as measles would be life-threatening to Katy.

Her parents and the medical staff, however, had explained what was happening to her, and her parents had been remarkably supportive and consistent with her in spite of the tremendous stress her illness imposed on them. One of her parents had been with her at all times when she was hospitalized. Katy, for her part, had been cooperative or stoic in response to all but the most surprising or painful procedures. By the standard of overt distress, which is commonly seen in the literature as a measure of coping (Blount, Davis, Powers, & Roberts, 1991), Katy seemed to have tolerated her medical experiences well. She had used an array of coping mechanisms, including the support of her parents and the medical staff, complying with medical procedures, and defense strategies such as denial and blocking of affects.

Assessment Impressions

I began seeing Katy when she was 4 years and 8 months old. At that point her cancer treatment was completed, and medically she was doing well. Her parents were aware that her cancer could recur and also that she would be at risk for developing leukemia later on. They referred her because she had become such a serious, quiet, inhibited child, quite different from the vivacious 2-year-old they remembered. They were concerned that she had reactions to her hospitalizations and fears of death that she could not talk about. She often hinted that she remembered stressful medical procedures but avoided her parents' attempts to talk with her about them. Like other young children who have experienced stressful medical interventions, she apparently attempted to cope with conscious negative memories by suppressing them (Chen et al., 2000). She was extremely cautious physically and no longer threw herself into play. She refused to do "risky" play like swinging, jumping, or climbing. Katy told me she thought she'd gotten cancer because she fell off the jungle gym when she was 3. She was enrolled in part-time day care but was standoffish with other children and played mostly by herself, probably because she had missed out on learning to play with other children over the previous year and a half, and also because she was still afraid of catching a disease from another child. She also seemed arrested in her ability to play. At home, at day care, and in the early treatment sessions, her play had a constrained, tentative, and obsessional quality and lacked the rich fantasy themes typical of a 4-year-old. These were indicators that her experience with cancer treatment was interfering with her development. My impression on meeting Katy, however, was that she had a full range of affect and fantasy available to herself but that she kept them under wraps. She was nearly silent in sessions. Nevertheless, I felt engaged with her and believed that beneath her inhibitions and affective constriction she might be imaginative and articulate.

A Developmental Treatment Approach

The treatment goals were as follows:

• To help her recover the ability to play. This would open up for her an age-appropriate pathway for developmental progress and the mastery of stress.
• To help her gain some mastery over the traumatic aspects of cancer treatment by playing out in an active way those experiences she had previously had to submit to passively. An essential part of this goal would be to give Katy a chance to present a range of affects—especially anger and negativism—that she had suppressed during her medical treatment.
• To help her differentiate her experience with cancer from her present experience. This would involve helping her see cancer treatment as a past experience, not a lens for viewing the present.

Katy's symptoms did not meet the criteria for a diagnosis of posttraumatic stress disorder. However, I suspected that her cancer treatment had been traumatizing and that her defensive avoidance of spoken memories and feelings about her treatment might mask other symptoms (Erikson & Steiner, 2000). Traumatization during medical treatment is associated with poorer long-term adaptation for child cancer survivors (Barakat, Kazak, Gallager, Meeske, & Stuber, 2000). Further, Katy's parents' description of her as quieter, more inhibited and self-contained, less active physically, and less social raised the possibility that her reactions to cancer treatment had interfered significantly with the precancer trajectory of her development and might crystallize into more serious difficulties with anxiety and depression when she entered middle childhood (Pynoos, Steinberg, & Piacentini, 1999).

The therapeutic approach in this case was a focal psychotherapy to help a child master a developmental interference (Chethik, 2000). The treatment modality was individual play therapy and parent guidance. (The parent work will not be described because it was minimal. The case is atypical in this respect. Ordinarily, parents also need a chance to work through the traumatic impact of their child's life-threatening illness. Katy's parents had done a remarkable job in helping Katy cope with her illness and in coping with it themselves. From the beginning of her illness, they had demonstrated resiliency by actively evaluating treatment options and forging an alliance with the medical team [McCubbin,

Balling, Possin, Frierdich, & Byrne, 2002]. They had already made extensive use of outside supports, including a family intervention during Katy's illness.)

The play of preschoolers in the therapeutic situation is best seen as the child's representation of significant aspects of her experience and as a commentary on what her experience has meant to her. Starting from this assumption, the practitioner attempts to understand the meaning of the play and then to provide interpretive commentary that helps the child take a new perspective on her experience, with the aim of reducing developmental interferences. At the outset, the therapist makes statements about the problem for which the child has been referred. I told Katy, "Your mom and dad wanted you to see me because they think you might have some worries and scary feelings about cancer and the hospital. My job is to help girls with their worries, and your mom and dad thought I might be able to help you." If this problem statement is salient for the child, play representing the child's experience of the problem begins to emerge, often in the first session. For Katy, this took the form of her laying out 20 or so rectangular blocks and then placing small dolls lying down on each of them. I watched her and said, "This is too big to be a family; there are so many beds, I wonder if it's a hospital." Katy looked me in the eye and said, "Yes." Through this process the play becomes focused, organized, and meaningful. The child preconsciously understands that the therapist sees play as a representation of experience and begins to use it to express what has been difficult for her. In order to help focus the treatment I had a toy doctor's kit and some medical paraphernalia—surgeon's mask and cap, IV tubing and tape, and the like—available for Katy's use. I never directed her to play with these materials but pointed out that she could use them to show me her worries, just as she could use the more standard child therapy toys.

Course of Treatment

Katy's early play was inhibited and constrained. She chose to draw and play board games, speaking little, and avoided developing any fantasies in her play. I was content to give Katy some time to acclimate to the therapeutic situation. Feeling forced and controlled had been inevitable features of her medical treatment. I felt that it was particularly important that Katy not feel forced in this relationship. I saw the early sessions as an opportunity to establish a friendly and supportive relationship with Katy. Her drawings were mostly of rainbows and hearts. As she drew, we spoke about the bright colors she liked to use, and I commented that she seemed interested in practicing getting her rainbows just right. We also played Candyland, a simple board game appropriate for preschoolers, since it is based on chance and does not require the use of strategy, which is generally beyond the cognitive level of preschoolers (Schaefer & Reid, 1986). Katy took pleasure in winning the game, though she seemed to be working to keep her affects in check. This was consistent with the affective restraint that had been an adaptive coping device when she was in the hospital. My main intervention during these early sessions was to mirror her excitement and pleasure in a slightly exaggerated manner in order to model the possibility of a wider range of affect.

After Katy became more comfortable showing pleasurable feelings, I began to model negatively toned feelings. For example, in the third session, I offered her Play-Doh. Play-Doh is a good material for eliciting affects of anger and frustration. Children like to pound on it and work it vigorously. As Katy pounded on Play-Doh with her fist, small breakthroughs of affect began to occur. When a piece dropped on the floor and Katy looked displeased, I amplified her facial affect by saying, "That stupid Play-Doh! It fell on the floor!" Katy was pleased and repeatedly dropped the Play-Doh, while I continued to express irritation. My aim was to demonstrate to Katy that negative affects could also be safely expressed within the therapeutic situation.

The first significant play commentary Katy made on her hospital experience appeared in the third session, after we had played with the Play-Doh. In the course of playing catch, Katy began hitting me on the head repeatedly with a foam ball. Given that Katy had had many hurtful things done to her head, I did not think this was random or merely diffusely aggressive behavior. I told her that of course it didn't hurt to be hit with the soft foam ball but that I would pretend to be hurt. I complained a lot about being hurt, and she continued to hit me with the ball with a grim expression on her face. I also pretended to be mad, which she thought very funny. When she took up this play in the next session, I focused it around her medical treatment. I told her I would pretend to be a kid at the doctor's office who was getting hurt by what the doctor was doing. As she hit me with the ball, I said, "Doctor, that hurts. I don't like you to hurt me. I'm getting mad at you for hurting me." After a bit I stepped out of the play and said, "I'm showing how kids get very angry when the doctor hurts them." At this point, Katy got a girl doll, took off its clothes, and began taping an IV tube to its chest. I spoke for the doll and asked if what the doctor was doing would hurt. Katy, as the doctor, gave a small, enigmatic smile and mumbled incomprehensibly. (This, it appeared, was her representation of the doctor—someone who did hurtful things, all the while smiling and mumbling, but not being responsive to her feelings or questions.)

Following this direct representation of medical procedures, Katy's play became more symbolic but still affectively salient. She developed a game of throwing markers on the floor and telling me, "Pick 'em up!" This was repeated many times. I asked her how I was supposed to feel about having to pick the markers up all the time, and she said, "You don't like it." I echoed this feeling each time she threw them on the floor. I commented that she was helping me understand how it felt to be forced to do something you don't want to do. I said her mom had told me she'd been forced to do a lot of things when she was in the hospital. Over the next few sessions, she elaborated the game. We would both pretend to go to sleep in our chairs. While I remained asleep, she would get up and throw markers and crayons all over the floor. Then she would turn over the play chairs with a big thump, which would be my signal to wake up and pick everything up. Within the play, I said, "I hate to be woken up. I don't like to be forced to pick all this stuff up." Katy said, "You have to." I commented that a kid in the hospital wouldn't like it when the nurse woke her up and forced her to have a shot or made her get up and go to the bathroom.

This hospital play scenario was fully elaborated in a session 2 months into the treatment. As usual, Katy threw markers on the floor and turned the chairs over. While I was sleepily picking things up, I complained that I hated being awakened in the middle of the night and that I wanted to be home in my own bed. I didn't want to be in this stupid hospital. She said, "Now you have to get up and pee." I said, "I'm not going to, and I'm not going to take my medicine either!" Katy looked very grim and said, "You can't say that." I said, "I don't care! I hate this hospital!" She hit me on the shoulder, looking very stern. I said, "Why am I in this hospital?" She said, "You have cancer." I said, "I hate cancer and I hate chemotherapy, because it makes me feel so awful. I'm not having any more chemotherapy or radiation!" She said, "You have to have surgery." I said, "No!" She hit me again and said, "You already had your surgery." I said, "Yes, and it hurt so much after I woke up." She said, "Now you're going to get a Broviac." I said, "What's a Broviac?" She said, "It's just a little tube that goes into your chest." I said, "I'm not getting any Broviac!" She hit me again and said, "Yes you are, and you're going to get an IV and a shot too." I made several comments at the end of this hour—that she had helped me know how it felt to be in the hospital and shown me many of the things that she hadn't liked, that she had helped me feel how scary it could be for a kid, how mad a kid could get about having all kinds of hurting and scary things done to her, how a kid hated to be forced, and how confusing it felt when doctors, who were supposed to be helping, sometimes did things that hurt a kid.

In the sessions immediately following, Katy began to take the role of the patient. For example, she took the cushions off my office chairs and lay down on them. She instructed me to get some puppets who should wake her up. The puppets told her it was time to wake up, and she woke up with a vengeful look and began pummeling the puppets until they were knocked off my hands and flung across the room. When I had the puppets say, "Wake up. It's time to take your temperature and go to the bathroom," Katy bit the puppets and threw them against the wall. Then she made a bed out of blocks and put a girl figure on the bed. She built up the sides of the bed and placed other figures there, standing over the girl. I commented that the girl looked as though she was in the hospital, and Katy confirmed this. Then, in a representation of the pain she experienced in the hospital, the figures standing over the girl pushed blocks on top of her. I said, "I think you're remembering about doctors and nurses looking down at you. What happened to the girl showed me how confusing it could be to have doctors hurt you when they were supposed to be taking care of you."

Over the next several sessions, Katy's play shifted from hospital themes to themes of protection and safety. She crawled under a chair and refused to talk to me. She brought her hand out from under the chair and motioned that I was to chase it with my hand. My hand chased hers but was never able to catch it. Then she began grabbing my intruding hand and throwing it out from under the chair, and looked very pleased with her ability to repulse me. I commented that it looked like she was in a very safe spot under the chair and that it must feel good to be in a safe spot. She probably felt in the hospital that there weren't any safe spots. She couldn't get away from having people do things that scared her and hurt her, and she must have wished then for a safe spot. I said, "In our game, you're the one in control. When my hand comes in, yours is too fast and always gets away. Or else your hand is too strong and throws mine out. I bet you wished that you could have thrown those doctors and nurses away from your bed in the hospital."

By now the therapy was in its third month, and Katy's parents were reporting that she was much more social at school, that she was less inhibited, and that she was expressing negative or angry feelings much more openly. She was becoming very bossy to her brother and had some angry outbursts toward her mother. Her mother had been taken aback, because this was so unlike Katy. Her parents were pleased, however, because Katy was expressing a wider range of feelings.

The last month and a half of treatment focused on themes of mastery and putting her illness in perspective. I have selected 3 hours during this final phase that seem not only to summarize these issues but also to underscore the strong progressive developmental forces in Katy, which were becoming more available to her.

In the first of these hours, Katy pushed a chair over to the window, got up on it, and looked out at a nearby park. She pointed out a playground. Then she began jumping off the chair. At first she held my hand each time, then began jumping off on her own. I said, "This reminds me of how you used to be afraid of jumping or falling, because you had the mix-up that falling off the jungle gym made you get cancer. Now, I see that you can jump without being too scared." Katy did not respond verbally but went into the closet and pulled the door shut. She pretended to be a kitten locked in the closet, and it was my job to let her out. Several times when I opened the door, she had a very somber expression and I commented that the kitty was looking sad. About the fifth time I opened the door, she had a very happy expression and pranced around the room, flapping her arms, pretending to fly. This scenario was repeated about four times. Then, when I opened the door, her expression was threatening and she poked at me with a coat hanger. Next she huddled up in the corner, hiding her head. Finally, the flying girl came out again. I commented that her happy play reminded me about how she felt before she got cancer. But then she got sick and felt awful and scared and sad and just wanted to huddle up and hide from people who might hurt her. Sometimes she was also very angry but was afraid to let people know she was mad. I said, "Now that you're feeling much better, it seems like you can be a happy, flying girl again who can do lots of things. Maybe you're not so worried now about getting sick again."

A few days before the second significant hour in the final phase, Katy had had her 6-month CT scan and it had been normal. Katy spent much of the hour showing me tricks she could do. She jumped off the chair in a number of different ways: first off the seat, then higher from the arm, then backward off the seat. She did somersaults and pretended to be a ballet dancer. I admired all the things she could do and complimented her abilities and her initiative. She also spent a good deal of time carefully building a house out of Lincoln Logs. I was pleased to see this kind of play because it is a normal type of skill-building play for a 5-year-old. A shift from play referring to trauma to such developmentally appropriate and conflict-free play is one of the signs that a child is becoming free from preoccupation with trauma-based anxiety.

At the beginning of the third significant hour, which occurred a few sessions before treatment was concluded, I began by saying, "Your mom told me that your CT scan showed you don't have any more cancer." Katy said, "Yes," and immediately became the kitty. She had me pull the two office chairs together to make a bed. The kitty climbed on to the bed, yawned, stretched luxuriously, and went to sleep. She smiled in her sleep, and I commented that the kitty looked like she was having nice dreams. Then the kitty climbed down and frolicked around on the floor. I said, "The kitty looks like she's feeling very good. I bet she's happy now because she doesn't have to go to the vet all the time or stay in the kitty hospital." The kitty answered by rolling around on the floor, stretching, and going to sleep. Then kitty woke up, looked very alert, and began bringing me things in her teeth: a plastic dinosaur, a little plastic table, a piece of string. I said, "The kitty's very good at picking things up with her teeth." Then I decided to reintroduce the medical theme into the play,

saying, "I don't know if you can carry that big doctor's kit in your teeth—
it might be too heavy." Katy grinned at this challenge and picked it up in
her teeth and carried it over to me. Then she opened the kit and immediately took on an angry expression. She dumped everything out and scat-
tered it across the floor. I said, "The kitty doesn't like all that doctor's
stuff. Maybe it reminds her of the vets and the kitty hospital." She took a
surgeon's cap and mask and stuffed them in a drawer and slammed it
shut. I said, "The kitty hates all that doctor's stuff. She doesn't even want
to see it." Then she initiated a game of chasing a ball and bringing it back
to me. Once, while chasing the ball, she came across the doctor's kit and
flung it across the room. I said, "The kitty doesn't like that doctor stuff
because it reminds her of when she was in the hospital and people did
things that hurt her. But it's very good that the kitty is healthy now
because it means she won't have to stay in the hospital. She'll still have to
go to the doctor for checkups and tests, but that won't be like staying in
the hospital." Katy handed me a toy syringe and motioned for me to give
her a shot. I did and said, "That shot was to keep you from getting sick. It
didn't seem to hurt too much." She handed me the stethoscope, and I listened to her heart and said, "It sounds very good." The kitty yawned and
stretched contentedly. I summarized this play by saying, "I know that
you're just like the kitty—you're very happy to be feeling good again."

During the remaining few hours before termination, the medical
themes were absent from Katy's play. However, more generalized issues
of anxiety about being hurt and feeling safe were brought up, particularly
in response to the pressure of termination. For example, Katy spent a lot
of time standing on the arm of the chair looking out the window and she
wanted me to be close to her. She repeatedly pretended to lose her balance and had to grab onto me to keep from falling. I said, "This reminds
me how you used to be afraid of falling because you thought that had
caused your cancer. But that's not true. Falling down didn't cause it." I
also said, "Since you've been seeing me, you've been feeling lots better,
lots happier, and you can do more fun things, like play games with other
kids and even climb to the top of the jungle gym. Maybe you're worried
that when you stop seeing me, you'll start falling again. But that's not
going to happen because you've been practicing and you've gotten very
good at climbing and jumping and at keeping yourself safe. And now
you don't need to get extra worried about falls and bumps because you
know that even though they might hurt they're not going to make you
sick."

Discussion

At the end of this 5-month-long therapy Katy was far more expressive,
showed a fuller range of affects, was much less anxious about her physi-

cal safety, was more active physically, and was more social. The intervention helped her give up her internal preoccupation with and anxiety
about her medical experiences. There are other factors besides therapy
that contributed to her resumption of an apparently normal developmental trajectory. These included her relief that she was feeling better physically, her opportunity in the day care center to become a "regular kid"
interacting with other kids, and her parents' ability to support her assertiveness and expressiveness.

Play therapy enabled Katy to represent in play her subjective account
of cancer treatment. Her play presented a story of a young child who felt
frightened, helpless, and rageful, was confused by the pain of treatment
that was supposed to help, and viewed herself as a victim of sadism and
perhaps as deserving punishment for being bad. This affectively rich play
representation was very different from her self-presentation while hospitalized, when for the most part she was subdued, compliant, and cooperative. Out of necessity, Katy had developed the ability to modulate and
contain anxious reactions to all but the most painful or frightening procedures. Her precocious defenses and her ability to accept the support of
her empathic and competent parents made it appear that she was coping
well with her difficult medical treatment. However, as the story of her
play suggests, it is important to distinguish between immediate coping
and actual mastery.

Katy's play in therapy suggested that her coping capacity represented a self-protective process developed in a series of psychic emergen-
cies, not psychological mastery of the experiences. After her medical
treatment ended, the need to understand, master, and integrate her experience with cancer still remained. Paradoxically, her defenses had become
organized around the need to suppress activity and affect; consequently,
the normal means a preschooler uses to master and understand experience—play and fantasy—had become inhibited and were less available to
Katy as vehicles for mastery. For this reason, *restoring the ability to play
became an essential goal of the early stage of therapy.*

Katy's continuing reliance on the emergency-based defenses was
having more pervasive effects on her development because she tended to
overgeneralize them to nonemergency situations. The inhibitive strategies she developed during hospitalizations—compliance, overcontrol of
affects, emotional withdrawal—became maladaptive when applied to
normal tasks of preschool development such as entering into peer relations and developing the capacity for initiative through imagination and
physical activity.

By abstracting the main trends of the therapy, we can see how Katy
gradually mastered these developmental interferences. At first Katy was
inhibited in affect, fantasy, and activity level. After I indicated interest in
her hospital experiences and encouraged the expression of affect, Katy

progressively found ways to represent the negative feelings associated with cancer treatment. In the hospital play, Katy first attempted mastery through role reversal, putting me in the position of the hurt, frightened, angry child. Such role reversal was typical of preschoolers' tendency to represent anxious or traumatic experiences in compensatory ways. They try to deny and master real-life experiences of anxiety and helplessness by taking the roles of powerful, magical figures. By taking the role of the sick child, I had the opportunity to put Katy's unspoken story into words and to empathize with her experience. Essentially, Katy "taught" me how it felt to be helpless, scared, and impotently angry, and I responded by acting out and articulating those feelings in order to convey understanding of what she had been through. Once a play dialogue had been built up, with Katy in the powerful role and myself taking the weak role, I began to conceptualize her experience of medical treatment, define its limits, and differentiate it from present reality.

An important shift occurred when Katy gave up the medical play and established her "safe spot" under the chair. By controlling and repelling my play intrusions into her safe spot, Katy was mastering the repeated intrusions during her hospitalizations. I emphasized her ability to gain control. During the last phase of treatment two themes coexisted. One was oriented to the present and involved testing her physical abilities by jumping off the chair and doing somersaults. I acknowledged Katy's physical competence and used her physical activity as an opportunity to contradict her earlier belief that physical daring had been the cause of her cancer. Occurring in the context of therapy, Katy's physical activity represented her struggle to master fears of body damage. (During this period, her parents reported that she had resumed climbing on the jungle gym and was swinging again.) The second theme was play that "summarized" her experience with cancer and placed it in the context of her life. This was expressed through the kitty character, who seemed to go through cycles of intense anxiety and anger followed by relief and contentment. I interpreted this play to help her construct a view of her illness as a painful and frightening past experience that she would remember but was separate from her current life.

As she was able to represent the story of her cancer treatment and have it confirmed and then interpretively differentiated from her current experience by a therapist to whom she had become attached, Katy was gradually able to gain a significant degree of mastery over a series of extremely stressful experiences and to resume an adaptive developmental trajectory. The preschool child—because of her egocentric perspective, limited internalized coping mechanisms, and limited abilities in understanding and communicating verbally—may especially benefit from *play* interventions that help promote mastery of developmental interferences.

Observation Exercise

Spend 1 hour or more observing in a preschool or child care center. Focus on the following:

1. *Dramatic play.* Choose a group of children who are playing together. What are the themes and plots of the play? What roles do children choose or assign one another? Is the play gender-segregated or not? How do the children deal with disruptions of the play scenario caused by conflicts over whose fantasy will prevail? What reflections of the mass media do you see in the play?

2. *Peer relationships.* Choose two or three children who are playing together, either in dramatic play, building play, or other activities. Can you discern elements of friendship in the way they relate to one another? How do they resolve conflicts that arise? To what extent are other children allowed to enter or excluded from the play activity?

3. *Relationships with adults.* How much do children interact with their teachers versus other children? Do you see attachment-seeking behavior? How do children cope with separation when their parents drop them off at the center? Do you see different styles of relating to teachers—such friendly interaction, clinging, or withdrawal?

4. *Self-control.* Observe for potentially stressful situations—separation from parents, conflict with another child, having to wait to get the teacher's attention, and the like. What strategies for self-regulation do you observe? Do you see instances of aggression? What seems to have precipitated aggressive behavior? Do you see instances of prosocial behavior?

CHAPTER 11

Middle Childhood Development

The school-age child seems calmer, somewhat more serious, and less spontaneous than the preschooler. The preschooler handles the need to learn about the "real world" by assimilating reality into fantasies driven by her wishes and needs. In middle childhood, extending from age 6 to the onset of puberty between 10 and 12, the child gradually comes to see the world as a place with its own laws and customs, which she must learn about and assimilate herself into. The child shifts from seeing herself as at the center of the world to realizing that the world is complex and that she must find her place in it.

The preschooler creates himself through his imagination; while imagination and play remain important to the school-age child, he increasingly establishes his sense of self through a long apprenticeship of gaining skills. This theme is most clearly symbolized by the progressively more complex skills learned in school, but the themes of "learning how to" and "getting good at" increasingly inform the child's efforts in other activities, such as sports and hobbies. School-age children learn that success is based on practice, which helps explain their intensity and persistence as they work on building skills.

A 10-year-old neighbor boy was shooting baskets in my driveway, over and over, when it began to rain. During a 10-minute period, it rained harder and harder, but he still kept shooting. My wife came home and said, "Hey, Liam, don't you know it's raining?" He said, "I've been through this before. All I have to do is keep focused."

This boy's behavior, although funny because he was standing out in the rain, illustrates many of the capacities of school-age children: sustained concentration, belief in practice, and keeping a purpose in mind in spite of distractions.

Middle childhood, also referred to as the "latency" period in psycho-analytic theory, is characterized by the child's capacity to maintain states of self-control, calm, pliability, and educability (Sarnoff, 1976). Good self-regulation is essential to the developmental tasks of school age, which involve the child's developing a sense of her capacity to work, to learn skills through practice, and to develop feelings of competence and self-esteem based on how she compares with peers.

What is happening within the school-age child that supports the development of calm, educability, and self-control? The following over-lapping advances in development occur during the middle years:

• *Improved self-regulation.* The child can use many cognitive strate-gies to assert conscious control over impulses. Unconscious defense mechanisms are regularly utilized to control impulses and fears.

• *Internalization of the conscience and related advances in moral develop-ment.* The child now has an inner sense of right and wrong; so, that she approves of herself when she does something right or resists a bad impulse and feels guilty when she does something wrong. This internal-ized conscience helps the child control negative or antisocial impulses. The child gradually accepts personal responsibility for her behavior, with correspondingly less reliance on projection and displacement of blame (Zahn-Waxler & Kochanska, 1990; Kochanska, 1994). Moral controls are also supported by identification with parents' and peer group's values, by a growing sense of fairness and awareness of the social value of adher-ing to rules, and by a growing capacity to see things from another's point of view.

• *Advances in reality testing and cognitive development.* Egocentrism diminishes, with the child increasingly able to take the "decentered" view of the observer, seeing events more objectively and in context, with less reference to the self. Basic reality-testing capacity is now established: the child makes increasingly clear distinctions between fantasy and reality, thought and action, his thoughts and feelings and those of others. Atten-tion span, concentration, and the ability to focus on a task all improve. Learning can now be based on observational ability, logic, and cause-and-effect reasoning.

• *Increased ability to substitute thinking, words, and fantasy for impulsive action.* Increasingly during middle childhood the child becomes capable of substituting thinking for doing and of using reflection and fantasy as a means of rehearsing actions.

• *Increasing peer orientation.* The child moves into the social world of peers. The child's self-esteem and view of self are increasingly based on recognition and acceptance by the peer group and by the child's inner assessment of how she is doing compared to peers. Desire to fit into the peer group becomes a powerful motive for following rules and maintain-ing self-control.

PHYSICAL DEVELOPMENT

The child's rate of growth during middle childhood is steady and occurs at a slower rate than during early childhood. At age 6 children weigh an average of 48–49 pounds and are an average of 42 inches tall. By age 11, they have reached about 58 inches in height and weigh about 80 pounds. These figures are based on the 50th percentile for height and weight, and there are considerable variations around this mean. Boys are on average slightly larger than girls until about age 11, when the girl's earlier growth spurt begins. Since this growth spurt is linked to puberty, which occurs approximately a year earlier for girls, girls begin to develop secondary sex characteristics during the last part of middle childhood, whereas boys retain the prepubescent body shape until about age 12 or 13 (Elkind, 1994).

In the past 20 years, pediatricians have become concerned about the rapidly increasing incidence of obesity in school-age children in the United States and other industrialized societies (Miller, Gold, & Silverstein, 2003). Obesity is defined as being 20% over one's expected body weight for height and age. By the late 1990s 20% of American children met the criteria for obesity (Wilson, Becker, & Heffernan, 2003). Although obesity is linked to genetic predispositions, cultural change has influenced children to eat more and be less active physically. Increased television watching, less physical exercise, food advertising directed at children, and larger portions in fast-food restaurants have been implicated in the increasing rate of childhood obesity. Obese children are at risk for early health problems, including hypertension and diabetes, and, since obesity tends to persist, for serious health problems in the long term. They are also more at risk for social rejection and consequent low self-esteem. Rejection by peers is a particular risk to development in middle childhood because of the value children place on how other kids view them (Morgan, Tanofsky-Kraff, Wifley, & Yanovski, 2002) .

Gross motor skills—running, climbing, kicking, throwing—are well developed at the beginning of middle childhood and continue to improve throughout the period. Individual differences in gross motor coordination become important because in middle childhood athletic ability becomes a measure of competence, in the eyes of both the individual child and his peers. Children put considerable energy into becoming proficient at team and individual sports. Children with poor gross motor skills are often teased and suffer social rejection (Smyth & Anderson, 2000).

Fine motor skills are also perfected during this period. Hand–eye coordination necessary for writing and drawing improves during the early years of middle childhood, and by third or fourth grade children are often skilled at writing rapidly. Children with delayed or awkward fine motor skills may have academic problems during the early elementary years as they struggle to write or copy mathematics problems. Fine motor difficulties require careful assessment, since poor handwriting or copying ability can be part of a pattern of neurological dysfunction based on learning disabilities, (Hooper, Swartz, Wakely, deKruif, & Montgomery, 2002).

Since new levels of cognitive functioning, including reasoning ability, develop in middle childhood, it is important to note that brain development undergoes significant changes during the early part of this period. Some areas of the brain are growing more nerve pathways, while others are eliminating unused synapses and increasing the number of others in the interest of developing more specialized functions (Nelson, 2000b). The frontal lobe of the cerebral cortex develops more rapidly between 5 and 8 years of age. This is the area of the brain associated with consciousness and thinking processes involving language (Janowsky & Carper, 1996). In the prefrontal cortex, synaptic pruning and myelination occur at an increased rate during early middle childhood, considerably later than in other brain regions, and these changes coincide with the emergence of higher cognitive functions associated with the prefrontal cortex—working memory, planning, and inhibitory control (Johnson, 1998).

THE TRANSITION FROM PRESCHOOL TO MIDDLE CHILDHOOD

Although most theories of development regard the years of middle childhood as a distinct period, it is useful to think of the years from 5 to 7 or 8 as a *transitional phase* during which the abilities of the middle years are developing rapidly but may not be consistently present (White, 1996). The first- or second-grade child often seems to straddle the preschool period and middle childhood, at times advancing in cognitive skills and real-world abilities, at other times relying on egocentric thinking and imagination. It is therefore important to describe this transitional period in order to appreciate the tasks and stresses that 6- and 7-year-olds encounter.

The period from years 5 to 7 or 8 historically has been defined as a turning point in development across cultures, as a time when the child becomes capable of reasoning, learning, and perceiving reality accurately. Cognitive and emotional maturation allow the child to function autonomously and to learn new skills that prepare her for adulthood. Familial and social expectations of the child also change. Formal schooling begins at age 5 or 6 in many societies; in cultures without formal education, apprenticeship for adult work skills and social roles begins at this age (Rogoff, 1998).

Entering School

When the child enters school, she experiences separation from parents in a more structured environment than preschool. She must adapt to elementary school routines and learning activities that place demands on her cognitive abilities and adapt to new people in authority. The transition is also psychological. The child knows she will have to function more autonomously. She may be intuitively aware of the demands school places on her to marshal new cognitive abilities, which during this phase are on the way, but perhaps not fully developed. From the perspective of the 5- or 6-year-old, entry into school may seem like an awesome task. Relationships with adults change, from more supportive preschool teachers (significantly, they are also called "caregivers") to kindergarten teachers who focus more narrowly on the child's cognitive skill development and provide less one-on-one interaction (Rimm-Kaufman & Pianta, 2000). Adequate self-regulation developed during the early years predicts the child's ability to maintain the self-control and concentration needed for school work (Howse, Calkins, Anastopoulos, Keane, & Shelton, 2003). The capacity to make and maintain friendships has been found to be a protective factor in the transition to school and is associated with positive attitudes toward school (Ladd, Kochenderfer, & Coleman, 1996). Making friends in kindergarten provides feelings of security during the transition, and, at the same time, paves the way for growing primacy of peer relationships across middle childhood. Good friendships in the early grades may be particularly important in supporting school adjustment for boys. While friendships are important for girls as well, they have the additional support of experiencing their relationships with teachers more positively than boys do (Ramey, Lanzi, Phillips, & Ramey, 1998). Girls identify with their female teachers and use them as models of how to behave and how to approach academic tasks. There are comparatively fewer male teachers in the early grades, so boys usually lack immediate role models whose presence encourages positive attitudes toward learning. Whether the lack of male teachers becomes a risk factor for a successful transition to school depends, of course, on the balance of other risk and protective factors (Valeski and Stipek, 2001).

School Entry, Preschool Experience, and Class Status

The benefits of high-quality preschool or Head Start experience for future school performance have been documented in longitudinal studies (Ramey & Ramey, 1998). Children who have had good preschool experiences make better adjustments to elementary school. This is significant because children who start out better tend to do better over the long run: "Individual differences in children's school outcomes, especially achievement, remain remarkably stable after the first few years in school" (Rimm-Kaufman & Pianta, 2000, p. 494; Eccles et al., 1998). Poor children exposed to multiple poverty-related risk factors gain the most, as measured by subsequent literacy skills, academic achievement, and high school graduation rates (Weikart & Schweinhart, 1992).

A national survey of over 3,500 kindergarten teachers provides evidence that the transition difficulties are real for many children entering school. One-sixth of children entering kindergarten were perceived by their teachers as having serious difficulties adjusting to the expectations of the school environment. The findings reflected social stratification in American society, with teachers in middle-class school districts reporting few problems with school transition. In many poor districts, teachers perceived 50% of entering kindergartners as having *serious* transition problems. (Rimm-Kaufman, Pianta, & Cox, 2000).

DISADVANTAGED CHILDREN IN KINDERGARTEN: A TEACHER'S STORY

When I began volunteering as a teacher's helper two-thirds of the way through the year in a public school in a poor community, I noticed a great variety among the 25 kindergartners in their abilities to follow directions, perform academic tasks, and maintain behavioral control. When I asked their teacher to give her impressions of the children and the challenges of teaching, she said, "The thing I have the hardest time with is where my kids are, compared with the district's new standards of where they're supposed to be at the end of the year. I have maybe 7 or 8 out of 25 who will definitely be ready for first grade. Most of them have made a lot of progress learning the classroom routine and basically what's expected when you're in school, but I wish I could have them for another year, now that they're getting used to school. Almost none of them went to any kind of preschool. You can see the results—most of them at the beginning of the year couldn't recognize letters and numbers, let alone write them. The Head Start program here has such a long waiting list that only a few of them could get in. And those are some of the kids who are at grade level academically. My kids *all* come from poor families, and they have so many challenges in their *lives*, it's really hard for them to focus on learning to write letters. Three of them are living in foster homes; two have a parent in prison; Angelita's mom died last summer; most kids are in single-parent families and their moms are *stressed*; some have dictated stories to me about punching fights between their parents; several kids are living with their grandmothers and I don't know where their parents are; three I suspect, are mildly retarded or have language delays and I'm sending them to be tested—and I know that would have been picked up if they'd been in Head Start. It's quite a list, isn't it?"

Current national policy is moving toward cutting funding of preschool preparation for disadvantaged children, even though current funding allows only 60% of eligible children to enroll in Head Start (Children's Defense Fund, 2002, 2003). The Bush administration, while emphasizing school accountability regarding students' performance at the elementary and secondary levels, as of June 2004 continues to support funding cuts in Head Start and child care subsidies (Mezey, 2004).

Parents' Responses to the Transition

Beginning school is a developmental transition for parents as well, symbolizing for many parents their child's capacity for being on her own and creating for some parents a sense of loss of the close relationship of early childhood. Parents' attitudes and circumstances can have a strong impact on the child's transition into school. If a parent is encouraging and positive, the child is likely to enter school more confidently. If a parent is anxious or stressed, the child may pick up on these feelings and become anxious about school. The quality of connection established between parents and school in the transition seems to have important effects on the child's trajectory of relative success or failure in school. Strong parent–school relationships provide shared expectations and support for the child to do her best. By contrast, when parents feel alienated or disengaged from their child's school experience, the child feels a lack of support. Her home and school environments feel fragmented and discontinuous, and risk for lower performance increases (Pianta & Kraft-Sayre, 1999).

Children's Responses to the Transition

Once in school, children intuitively realize that fantasy and play are not adequate vehicles for mastering the developmental tasks of middle childhood. They become aware that they will be evaluated by the skills they develop. They realize they must learn to read and write and become proficient at organized games and sports. For the 5- to 7-year-old, meeting these demands of reality, however defined by his culture, often seems daunting. He is becoming aware of the abilities he is expected to develop but is also aware that he does not yet possess them. He observes the superior skills of adults and older children and wonders how he will be able to learn them. Most children use this concern as a source of motivation and work hard at learning academic skills. First graders often appear serious and absorbed when they are trying to learn a mathematics concept or sound out a passage in reading. On the other hand, the strain of stretching their cognitive abilities and adapting to the requirements of learning helps explain their high level of activity on the playground and the emotional volatility at home that is common in 6-year-olds.

THE STRESS OF STARTING SCHOOL: A BRIEF CASE EXAMPLE

Tanisha, a 6-year-old I saw in play therapy, expressed her anxiety about starting first grade by reversing roles with me. During several sessions before school began, I became the student and she was my teacher who carefully looked over my writing of the alphabet. She corrected my "mistakes" and was stern and bossy. She sent me to the principal's office so that he could examine my papers. In play she was presenting her apprehensions that she would not be successful and that her teacher would not think her work was good. However, within a month of starting school, Tanisha began playing a kind, supportive teacher—a reflection of her first-grade teacher—who gave stars on many of my papers and allowed me "extra time" to finish my work. This new content suggested she was realizing that the demands of school would not be beyond her ability and that she could succeed. As therapy proceeded, I always knew when this bright and conscientious child was struggling to master an academic task, because the role play involving the stern teacher and the student who made many mistakes would resurface. Parenthetically, adjustment to school was not Tanisha's primary issue. Her mother, whom she had not lived with for much of her life, was dying of AIDS, and treatment focused on her reactions to loss and her anger and disappointment that her mother had been largely absent from her life. This example, however, suggests that practitioners need to be alert to the developmental hurdles a child is coping with and be ready to tailor interventions to help the child master current developmental tasks.

Other children may temporarily shrink back from the reality expectations of early middle childhood by trying to hold onto the wishful and omnipotent orientation of the preschooler. This can mean different things. For some children, it may reflect temporary anxiety about performance. For other children, holding onto a younger child's orientation may be a sign of lags in development.

SIGNS OF DEVELOPMENTAL LAG: A BRIEF CASE EXAMPLE

Jason, age 6, refused to do schoolwork in first grade and constantly tried to get other children to play with him while class was going on. This child was developmentally somewhat immature. His fine motor coordination was not well developed, and he resisted trying to write letters because their shaky appearance made him feel inferior. In play sessions, he created elaborate scenarios of teams of dinosaurs fighting on another planet. When I attempted to inject a reality orientation into this play by asking if the dinosaurs went to school (a foolish question), he said, "We don't have schools on this planet!" Jason's behavioral regression and attempt to hold onto a fantasy orientation reflected his intuitive awareness that he was less ready for school than other children in his class. When clear limits, in the form of a behavioral plan, were put in place, his behavior gradually conformed more to classroom expectations. Over the course of the year, his cognitive skills seemed to mature and he mastered the academic expectations of first grade. The spurt in cognitive maturity that many children show at age 6 did not occur for Jason until he was nearly 7.

This example underlines *the importance of recognizing individual differences in the rate of development.*

During this transitional phase, children also struggle with the implications of having a conscience. An internal conscience requires the child to monitor and set limits on her own behavior. It also punishes the child with negative feelings—guilt, shame, anxiety—when she violates her own internalized sanctions. The task of coming to terms with the presence of rules on the inside is frustrating and anxiety-producing for 6- and 7-year-olds. They still have strong volatile impulses, yet an internal voice warns and corrects them. When the conscience is newly internalized, children can be particularly hard on themselves and reactive to feelings of guilt and self-blame. They are especially sensitive to being scolded because the adult's reprimand awakens the internal voice of conscience and makes them feel doubly punished. Because young school-age children are working hard to establish internal rules, they are quite sensitive to violations of rules by others. They may point out that other children, especially younger siblings, are behaving badly. They may also monitor their parent's behavior. At times they may act impulsively, as if trying to deny the existence of the conscience, only to be painfully reminded of its presence when they feel guilty afterward. A 6-year-old girl captured the dilemma of feeling controlled by a internal voice when she screamed to her mother, "I hate my conscience!"

ATTACHMENT

During the middle years, the child's reliance on attachment to parents continues to decrease. The school-age child has many more strategies for emotional regulation than does the younger child. Consequently, he handles on his own many situations that would have elicited attachment behavior when he was younger. School-age children are more capable of autonomously coping with novel situations, separations, and mild circumstances of threat or danger. Attachment needs are also increasingly transferred to peer relationships as friends begin to provide some of the emotional security and satisfaction that have been present in the parent–child relationship.

Children still show attachment behavior, in terms of wanting physical closeness, toward parents in many situations. Although 9-year-olds, for example, are capable of putting themselves to bed, most prefer to have a bedtime ritual with parents that affirms their ongoing attachment. In situations of stress, such as serious illness or injury, traumatic experience, or loss of a loved one, school-age children register their need for protection and security by activating attachment behavior. Moreover, attachment behavior increases during the transition to middle childhood, particularly in response to entry into school.

ATTACHMENT BEHAVIOR IN RESPONSE TO STRESS: A BRIEF CASE EXAMPLE

Six-year-old Abby was referred by her single mother midway through her kindergarten year. Although Abby had a history of solid development, she began to show symptoms of separation anxiety when she began kindergarten. This coincided with her mother's taking a job requiring an hour's commute each way, which meant that Abby spent about 11 hours each day in school and child care. Abby's reactions to this new schedule and the emotional demands of formal schooling included anger at her mother when she was picked up at the end of the day, shadowing of her mom and clinginess at home, and coming into her mother's bed each night. She also had retrieved her transitional object—a tattered blanket—and would wrap herself in it when she got home every day. Abby's mother said that prior to entering school these symptoms had not been in evidence. Abby's teacher said she was doing very well in school.

In a play session Abby chose big and small opossum puppets. (I had bought these to help children express concerns about attachment and separation: the baby opossum could be Velcro-attached to the parent's back.) Abby played out a repeated scenario. The mother and child opossums would be together with their tails entwined hanging from the doorknob. Then the mother would leave, and a skunk puppet would come and try to eat the baby, but the mother would come back and rescue her. Similarly, a baby turtle would swim away from her mother and be eaten by a shark. The mother turtle would come and punch the shark in the stomach, and the shark would burp the baby up and they would be reunited. Abby got a lot of pleasure out this play, and I pointed out that the babies liked to be with their mothers and they even worried about bad things happening when their mothers were gone. I said also, "Even girls can worry when their moms are gone for a long time." Abby agreed this was true.

Abby was a resilient child who was stressed by the new cognitive demands of school tasks, by the intensity of her schedule, and by long daily separations from her mom. She had to function at a high level during a long day with several changes of environment. She seemed to hold things together at school and child care, but when her mom picked her up she showed intense attachment behavior and regressive behavior, including dependence on her security blanket and coming into her mom's bed.

In a short-term intervention I framed Abby's difficulties as reflecting anxiety about separation. Her mother and I came up with a plan that emphasized her attachment to her mother: Abby's mother designated a special time for them to play together three times each week; she made an album of photos of herself with Abby for Abby to take to child care, with the instruction that Abby could look at the pictures if she got lonely; she began putting Abby's feelings about missing her into words. Additionally, we held some joint sessions with Abby and her mom to talk directly about her separation reactions. In these sessions Abby's mom told her that she knew it had been harder this year because the days were longer and they were apart for much longer times. As we talked about these issues, Abby would not say much but would cuddle up on the couch next to her mom. In one of these sessions, her mother commented that Abby had enjoyed swimming lessons last year but this year had complained almost every time she went to swimming class. She said, "I think it's because she was in a small, heated pool last year, and now she's graduated to a big unheated one." We asked Abby about this, and she said it was true. I was struck by the aptness of this change as a metaphor for the transition to middle childhood. I said that maybe that was the way this whole year had felt—that starting kindergarten and being away from her mom all day was like jumping into a big cold pool and it made her upset and worried. I said that now that her mom understood what worried Abby, she could help her feel better.

Attachment History and School-Age Development

Attachment history in infancy and toddlerhood continues to be a predictor of adjustment in middle childhood (Weinfield, Ogawa, & Egeland, 2002). The child's internalized working models of self, others, and relationships are carried forward, affecting self-confidence, independence, and peer relationships (Grossman et al., 1999). The longitudinal studies of Sroufe and his colleagues, which have been described in previous chapters, show that school-age children with histories of secure attachment are "less dependent, less often isolated and less often the passive recipient of aggression" than children judged insecurely attached in the early years (Sroufe & Jacobvitz, 1989, p. 197). They are also more self-confident in meeting the tasks of middle childhood, which require increasing ability to function independently. Quality of attachment during the first 2 years continues to differentiate between children through the end of middle childhood, especially when they are not exposed to multiple risk factors. A recent study of Sroufe's original infants demonstrated significant continuity between their Ainsworth attachment classifications, and classifications at age 20, using the Adult Attachment Interview (Waters, Merrick, Treboux, Crowell, & Albersheim, 2000).

SOCIAL DEVELOPMENT

The tasks of social development are more complex for school-age children as compared with younger children. The school-age child enters the larger world, symbolized by elementary school, and must learn its values, rules, and routines. He must learn "appropriate" behavior in this larger context through interactions with adult authorities as well as with peers. In middle childhood, even though parents remain central, other adults and peers take on increasing importance.

Social Perspective Taking

During the school-age years, children become increasingly sophisticated in understanding the perspectives of others. The preschool child tends to see the situations of others egocentrically and tries to assimilate another person's viewpoint into her own viewpoint. Beginning at age 6, the child becomes more able to see and acknowledge another person's different point of view. Over the next several years the child gradually realizes that there can be multiple ways of viewing a situation and can imagine how her own ideas appear to another person.

By ages 10–12, a child can hold opposing or different viewpoints in mind at the same time (Harter, 1999). For example, an 11-year-old girl in a divorce adjustment group described her feelings about her mother's upcoming remarriage: "Sometimes I wish she wasn't getting married again. He is nice and everything, but it's going to feel strange with him living with us. I asked my dad, and he said he didn't care if she got remarried. I think he doesn't like it. But maybe it will be a good thing, because I see that my mom's a lot happier now. I want her to be happy." This child understood the perspectives of others as she reflected on her own. She also demonstrated a related capacity that develops during late middle childhood—the ability to tolerate emotional ambivalence. The capacity to acknowledge having two feelings simultaneously has a developmental progression. Preschool children take an all-or-nothing perspective: they say that a person cannot feel happy and sad at the same time. They cannot yet take a balanced perspective on others in terms of seeing another person's "good" and "bad" qualities. The ability to understand ambivalence and to see others as well as the self as a mix of characteristics develops during the school-age years and is clearly present at about age 10 (Harter, 1998).

Because of their perspective-taking skills and repeated exposure to social cues and rules, school-age children are more adept than younger children at sizing up the feelings, wishes, and expectations of others and the social demands of a situation. For example, an 8-year-old at a religious service may be restless or bored, but he knows he cannot express these feelings except in a whisper. Further, he knows he must wait until the service is over before he can be active. By contrast, a 4-year-old may say in a normal voice during the service, "Daddy, when is it going to be over?" The 4-year-old has trouble containing her restlessness. As her own needs become imperative, she has less ability to behave in socially appropriate ways.

As perspective taking improves, so does the child's ability to see below the surface of behavior and to attribute psychological qualities and motives to others. Up to age 8, children tend to describe others in terms of their behavior and physical characteristics. After 8, because of improving ability to analyze and synthesize information, they begin to describe others in terms of internal psychological characteristics. A 7-year-old may say, for example, "Andy runs around too much and yells too much," whereas a 10-year-old describing the same child might say, "Andy is really hyper and silly, and is always trying to get you to pay attention to him." This ability has analogues in the perception of social situations. Children become more able to infer other people's intentions and the psychological resonances of communication. For example, a preschool child may be confused by an adult's sarcastic remark because she cannot understand its psychological intent, whereas an older school-age child has a strong emotional response because she understands the hostile intent of the statement (Dews et al., 1996).

Prosocial Behavior

The capacity for prosocial and altruistic behavior is not firmly present until middle childhood. Prosocial behavior requires the ability to take the other person's point of view, to be able to deduce the feelings of others, and to temporarily set aside one's own needs and desires. Prosocial behavior is supported by the internalization of moral standards, by the cognitive changes that create increased objectivity and decreased egocentrism, and by exposure during the preschool years to situations requiring the development of social skills. Prosocial and altruistic behavior increases with age, particularly when children are exposed to adult models of altruism. School-age children are more likely to notice when another child needs help and more likely to provide it (Eisenberg & Fabes, 1998).

Gender and Prosocial Behavior

Numerous studies have shown that girls show more prosocial behavior and empathy for others than do boys. Across middle childhood, compared with boys, girls' behavior becomes increasingly prosocial and their moral reasoning demonstrates somewhat more capacity for role taking and empathy (Eisenberg & Fabes, 1998). Girls tend to identify with caregiving roles, receive more support for conflict-resolving behavior, and are socialized to be attuned to the emotions of others (McHale et al., 2003).

However, the findings that girls show more prosocial behavior than boys are not entirely consistent across studies, and many studies find very small or insignificant differences. Given this mixed picture, it is important not to make extreme contrasts that suggest girls are caring and helpful and boys are not. In observational studies of school-age children's actual prosocial behavior, the differences are small. Cultural values about gender influence general perceptions of difference: "Sex differences in self- and other-reported prosocial behavior may reflect people's conception of what boys and girls are *supposed* to be like rather than how they actually behave" (Eisenberg & Fabes, 1998, p. 754).

Friendships

School-age children's close friendships are based on mutual liking, sharing of interests, and gender. Same-sex friendships become the norm as gender identification becomes more firmly established and children take in culturally based gender expectations. The same tendency toward choosing as friends people who are similar to oneself leads to increasing same-race friendships as children get older (Hartup, 1992). Across middle childhood, children's friendships deepen and their ideas about what a friend is evolve. For a 6- to 8-year-old, the idea of a friend is organized around concrete activities: "Jenna is my friend because we like to play with our dolls together." Older children begin to think of friendships as relationships that involve common values, commitment, loyalty, mutual support, and responsibility (Rubin, Bukowski, & Parker, 1998). An 11-year-old boy said, "James is my best friend. He treats me nice and he helps me. Like my mama said I couldn't go out of the house without picking up my stuff, and James helped me so we could go soon. I help him too if he needs it."

Friends serve a number of functions. Since friendships are more egalitarian than are relationships with adults, they provide the child with a sense of identification with another person who is like themselves. Rather than comparing themselves with adults, whose abilities are generally far beyond the school-age child's, they can more comfortably compare themselves with friends. They also may gain some relief from guilt or shame by seeing that their friends are not always successful at living up to the dictates of conscience. By observing their friends, they are relieved from the need to be perfect and can become more self-accepting (Gemelli, 1996).

Stable friendships during the early years of school provide support for the transition into middle childhood, and later for the transition to middle school (Ladd, 1990, 1999; Wentzel, 1999). Older school-age children with close friends are able to confide in and gain support from them at times of family disruption, such as separation and divorce. Attachments to friends serve some of the same functions of attachment to parents by helping the child feel secure and understood (Dunn, Davies, O'Connor, & Sturgess, 2001).

Working things out with friends also provides practice in resolving conflicts. Although children who are good friends have frequent conflicts, they are also motivated to resolve conflicts in order to preserve the friendship. Consequently, friends are more likely to disengage from a conflict than to attempt to win through coercion (Laursen, Hartup, & Koplas, 1996). By contrast, children who are extremely shy, aggressive, or coercive of others tend to have fewer friends and more unstable friend-ships, which deprives them of some of the "developmental advantages" of learning social skills through relationships with friends (Hartup, 1992). Children who are rejected by peers make poorer adjustment to school. When antisocial school-age children do have friends, they mutually rein-force antisocial behavior, supporting each other in defining themselves against social norms. The choice of antisocial friends has been linked to histories of coercive parent–child relations during the early years (Dishion, Patterson, & Griesler, 1994).

Peer Group, Social Reputation, and Self-Esteem

Social reputation becomes important during the middle years, as children begin to reflect on their status in the group. School-age children are increasingly aware of how others see them. It is very common for school-age children to comment on one another's performance in school: "I'm on math level 16, and you're just on level 12?" School-age children inter-nally acknowledge the validity of peer evaluations, if they are accurate, and tend to incorporate them into their self-evaluations (Altermatt, Pomerantz, Ruble, Frey, & Greulich, 2002). A child who is sought out by peers *knows* he is popular and gains in self-esteem from that knowledge. Because social status becomes a defining part of the sense of self during the middle years, children with lower social reputations commonly expe-rience anxiety about themselves and suffer low self-esteem. In the social world of older school-age children, kids who are socially withdrawn, aggressive and impulsive, or have unusual self-presentations and man-nerisms, as in Asperger's syndrome or autism, are increasingly seen as socially deviant and are increasingly likely to be actively disliked and rebuffed by peers (Rubin et al., 1998; Dodge et al., 2003).

TEMPERAMENT AND PEER RELATIONS: A BRIEF CASE EXAMPLE

Eric, a 9-year-old, seemed, according to his parents' history, to fit Kagan's (1989) temperament category of the behaviorally inhibited child. Children of this temperamental type are seen as shy or "slow to warm up." They show "high sensitivity to stimulation, gradual adaptation to change, and a tendency to withdraw under stress" (Lieberman, 1993, p. 120). Behav-iorally inhibited young children are at risk for problems of social with-drawal in middle childhood, and are more at risk for anxiety disorders (Rubin et al., 2003).

Eric's presenting problem was school refusal. He frequently got stom-achaches and headaches in the morning before school and tried to talk his parents into believing he was sick. Eric's teacher noted that he was neither a popular nor an unpopular kid but that he did not seem to know how to reach out to other kids. She said that his quiet demeanor caused him to be ignored by other boys in the class. Eric was a thoughtful and bright child, and he directly told me, "I don't want to go to school because I don't have friends there. Last year I had friends in my class, but this year none of them are in my class." He said that a lot of the boys act tough and mean and that he didn't like that. He was repelled by their aggressive behavior, even though they did not pick on him. He also said that they all hung out together and chose each other when teams were being picked. He said, "I'm not that good at football because I really don't like it, so they choose me last." I asked how that felt, and he said, "Kinda bad."

Eric was a self-sufficient and sensitive child who had many interests. He was not depressed. He had enough personal "dignity" to avoid the fate of many withdrawn children—being teased and bullied. But he was not assertive in trying to make friends, and when a peer did something he did not like his only strategy was to withdraw. Eric's difficulties in finding sympathetic peers were exacerbating his temperamental shyness and causing him to lose self-esteem.

The consequences of social withdrawal for children like Eric increase as they get older because rejection by peers becomes more active. By late school age "socially withdrawn children, unlike normal children, may begin to attribute their interactive failures to internal stable causes" (Rubin et al., 2003, p. 385) and are at increasing risk for depression (Asendorpf, 1993).

Children with significant chronic health problems may also feel isolated in the peer group, with potential effects on self-esteem. School-age children are more aware than younger children that their illness makes them different from peers. For example, a child with hemophilia, a hereditary disease affecting only males, must avoid bumping into things because this may cause uncontrolled bleeding under the skin. This means that he must be very careful in play and not engage in contact sports. In this culture, a big part of a school-age boy's self-esteem depends on his athletic ability. This avenue of self-esteem is largely closed off to kids with hemophilia. Severe asthma can also limit children's ability to participate in sports. Children with poorly controlled diabetes or sickle-cell anemia may require frequent hospitalizations and be absent from school often. At the same time, kids who have an obvious disability or who cannot participate in regular activities may be stigmatized by other children, with negative effects on self-esteem (Marshak, Seligman, & Prezant, 1999; Peterson, Reach, & Grabe, 2003).

Influence of the Group

School-age children define themselves as group members, not just as individual friends. Groups in middle childhood are organized around gender and sex roles, ethnic/racial identification, common interests, and social status. Within these groups, there are hierarchies of popularity and dominance. For example, in the group of boys that plays football at recess, the best players are likely to be given the most respect by others. Children are very aware of the social groups.

> A bright and precociously reflective 10-year-old girl described the groups in her class as she talked about her concerns about not fitting in: "There are three groups. There are the snobby popular girls. I don't want to be with them because they're mean to the kids that aren't popular. They're always telling lies and saying nasty things about the kids that aren't in their group. Then there are the dweebs. They're the ones the snobby girls are mean to. Then there are some kids like me who aren't in either group. I'm not a dweeb, so they don't tease me, but sometimes I think if I have a friend who's a dweeb, the snobby girls will think I am one. I feel guilty when I stay away from a dweeb who really is nice, just because I'm afraid of being treated mean by the snobs. I don't want to be one of the snobs because all they do is talk about clothes and how much money their families have and act mean to other kids except their own group."

This child's statement expresses the concern children have about being accepted in a group, as well as clearly describing the *status hierarchies that emerge in middle childhood*. Older school-age children are very concerned about their popularity. They worry about losing status. In part, this worry is realistic. As children move toward early adolescence, peer group relations become more unstable and children sometimes find themselves demoted to a less popular status (Rubin et al., 1998). Concerns about status may be particularly strong for older school-age girls, and they express these concerns in different ways than boys. Although very few girls physically attack other children, recent research suggests that "relational aggression" is common in girls' peer groups (Crick, Casas, & Nelson, 2002). Those girls who accept the pressure to compete for status and power use relational aggression, which involves manipulativeness, exclusion, back-stabbing, malicious gossip, and verbal put-downs, in an attempt to compromise the social position of their target. The girl quoted above was struggling, with great integrity, to avoid being pulled into this pattern.

Once in a group or clique, children are to a fair degree influenced by group norms, and peer pressure becomes a strong force. However, much peer pressure reflects adult values that children have internalized (Hartup, 1992). Children with internalized prosocial values resist the ideas of other children who suggest antisocial behavior. Nor are they likely to be pulled into antisocial peer groups. By contrast, "antisocial norms are most likely to be pressed on children who are already disposed to be antisocial and aggressive" (Hartup, 1992, p. 275). Research findings do suggest that parents are wise to be concerned when the school-age child consistently associates with aggressive, antisocial friends. By early adolescence deviant peer associations clearly influence delinquent behavior (Dishion, Andrews, & Crosby, 1995).

Aggression, Bullying, and Victimization

Physical aggression is fairly common in preschoolers, especially boys. During middle childhood direct physical aggression diminishes greatly. For preschoolers, aggressive behavior often has an impersonal, instrumental quality: the child pushes another child who has a toy or piece of territory he wants. The superior verbal and social skills of school-age children allow them to ask, cajole, or, at times, threaten in order to get what they want. For the majority of school-age children who are not typically aggressive, a physical attack on another child is unusual and is likely to reflect a personal animosity, a hostile intent, or a reaction to the other child's provocation (Coie & Dodge, 1998). Since school-age children more easily distinguish between unintentional and intentional acts, they are more likely to forgive accidents, yet also more likely to retaliate if they recognize the other's hostile intent.

However, the frequent aggressive behavior of a small number of children contrasts with these general trends in middle childhood. These children are bullies, who, instead of giving up physical aggression, come to rely on violent acts, threats, and coercion as primary ways of exerting control over peers and maintaining status (Olweus, 1993). Bullying is responsible for much of the physical aggression observed in school-age children. It begins to emerge in some children by age 5 or 6, but is most common in later middle childhood and early adolescence (Smith & Brain, 2000). Male bullies use both physical and emotional strategies in attacking victims, while girl bullies tend to rely on relational aggression. Children who bully have often been subjected to punitive, coercive parenting and physical abuse, suggesting that their treatment of victims is modeled on how they have been treated (Snyder & Patterson, 1995). Research suggests that the same children, about 10% of school children, are bullied repeatedly. If victimization persists these children, often unpopular kids already suffering rejection from nonbullying peers, may become depressed as well as increasingly isolated. Some children attempt to break out of the victim role by becoming bullies themselves (Hanish & Guerra, 2003).

Although most children are neither victims nor bullies, they may witness bullying regularly. Many are disturbed by the cruelty they see but do not know how to combat it.

> A 10-year-old boy told me, "There's this kid named Jimmy who picks on Ryan every day. Ryan is kind of short, and he's hyper and kind of dorky. Yesterday, Jimmy came up behind Ryan in the hall and pushed him down for no reason, and the day before he took his lunch bag and stuck it in the trash. One time, he pulled down Ryan's pants. That was really bad." I asked what he felt when he saw these things happen, and he said, "I hate it. But I don't try and stop Jimmy. Nobody does. I think because we don't want him to do the same stuff to us."

School-age children tend to believe, with justification, that much bullying occurs "under the radar" of adult observation. In part because they believe this, victimized children often do not ask for help from school personnel. Antibullying curricula are only somewhat helpful, and current approaches to school intervention against bullying emphasize active monitoring by adults and the development of peer support systems (Naylor, Cowie, & del Rey, 2001).

LANGUAGE AND COMMUNICATION

By age 7 the child has a basic grasp of the syntactical and grammatical structures of her native language. Compared to the preschool child who was learning basic language concepts and rules, the school-age child is learning variations of the rules and more difficult constructions such as the passive voice. Vocabulary continues to increase, though not as rapidly as during the preschool years. By age 10, the average child has a receptive vocabulary of 40,000 words (Anglin, 1993). Although there is a range of language ability across individual children, school-age children generally possess sufficient facility with language to express what they are thinking and to tell coherent narratives having a beginning, middle, and end. However, these gains do not mean that it becomes easy for school-age children to talk about emotionally charged topics. It is one thing to describe the ordinary events of the day and another to reveal distressing or conflictual *feelings*. Consequently, play and other types of symbolic representation continue to be essential forms of communication in intervention with school-age children.

Language and Cognitive Development

Language sophistication depends on cognitive development. When children acquire the ability to reverse their thought, they are able to understand transformations in syntax. For example, in order to understand the meaning of a sentence written in the passive voice, "She was liked by her teacher," the child must be able to translate it into the active voice, "Her teacher liked her" (Elkind & Weiner, 1978). The ability to make such changes automatically depends on the capacity for reversibility, which develops between 6 and 8. In a similar way, the ability to perceive nuances and to make comparisons, which develops during this period, allows the child to understand more subtle comparative words. By age 10 children have developed good morphological skills that allow them to understand new words by looking at the morphemes that make them up. For example, a 10-year-old can deduce the meaning of a word or phrase she is not familiar with, such as "reflecting pool," by analyzing its component parts (Anglin, 1993).

Between 8 and 10, children develop an appreciation for wordplay and jokes that depend on double meanings. They can understand and enjoy asking riddles such as "Why is a library so tall?" (because it has so many stories) or the mildly dirty joke "Hey, did you read the book called *Under the Bleachers* by Seymour Butts?" Figures of speech that would puzzle a 4-year-old can be understood by 7- or 8-year-olds. I was playing cards with a 7-year-old who said, "I might have a trick up my sleeve." Playing dumb, I said, "But you're wearing a short-sleeve shirt, so how could you?" He responded, "That's not what it means. It's not really in my sleeve. It's in my mind." School-age children can also begin to appreciate metaphor, simile, and the condensed imagery of *haiku* poetry. An 8-year-old girl, Carol Moore, wrote this *haiku*:

> "Waves slap on the shore
> And make noises like houses crumbling
> Many houses falling down." (in R. Lewis, 1966, p. 114)

Language ability is also influenced by the child's language environment. Children whose parents have over time talked to them and encouraged them to put feelings and ideas into words and particularly into narratives are more likely to have good language skills. In turn, these children share ideas with peers and improve their language skills further. Children whose parents have read to them regularly during the preschool years develop better literacy skills in elementary school (Reese & Cox, 1999).

The cognitive shift toward decentered perspective taking means that school-age children can use language to communicate in new ways. While a preschool child has trouble identifying another's perspective, the school-age child knows that others see things differently than she does. The practice she has had negotiating with peers during the preschool period, combined with cognitive advances and increasing peer orientation, has prepared her for communication that takes another child's ideas into account. Older school-age children are more sophisticated in perspective taking and can shape what they say to fit their perception of the other's viewpoint. For example, a 10-year-old boy who collects superhero comic books communicates in a specialized language when talking to another collector. When he talks to an adult who does not know much about these comics, he can realize this and provide more explanation (Sonnenschein, 1988).

Language and Self-Regulation

The maturing of language and cognitive abilities during middle childhood has important implications for self-regulation. As the school-age child becomes increasingly adept at putting internal states into words—

worry, frustration, anger, and other feelings—he becomes more able to delay acting on his feelings. The diminishing use of physical aggression is related to the child's growing verbal skills, which he uses to assert himself. At the same time verbal aggression tends to increase, in the form of teasing, insults, and gossip (Rubin et al., 1998). The child learns that speaking his mind can be an effective way of gaining perspective on private thoughts, both through his own self-reflection and through the feedback he gets from others. When parents encourage verbal expression, they convey that words can be used to understand the world or resolve conflict. This promotes the use of verbalization as a means of regulating affect and impulse. By contrast, in families where verbal interaction is discouraged, interpersonal empathy is devalued, or secrecy is enforced, the school-age child does not feel permitted to put private thoughts into words. In dysfunctional families where sexual abuse occurs, for example, the child is compelled to be silent and often has no outlet except private fantasy for coping with the trauma of abuse (Fivush, 1998).

Language Issues for Immigrant Children

Immigrant and refugee children face learning challenges based on lack of facility in English. In 2002 it was estimated that there are over 4.5 million children attending U.S. schools whose first language is not English (National Association for Bilingual Education, 2002). These children must learn English in order to function in school. Often they start out behind and have trouble learning English quickly enough to master academic concepts presented in single-language classrooms. They are not simply learning a second language but also a second culture. They are socialized in their first culture by their parents and in the second by teachers and others. They may also be subtly or directly pressed to maintain their first language by their parents. Frequently they must function as translators for parents, and, in a role reversal that can produce anxiety and resentment, the child may become the parent's guide for navigating the new culture (Crawford-Brown & Rattray, 2001). Risks to academic achievement of immigrant children are heightened when parents have a low level of education and poor English language skills, which means they are not able to help children with homework or help them navigate the school system (Zhou, 1997).

Recent research on language acquisition has rejected older ideas that bilingualism impedes cognitive development. Children are able to learn a second language without compromising their cognitive abilities (Bialystok, 2001). Some recent studies have found superior cognitive skills in bilingual children, especially those who have learned multiple languages from infancy (Bialystok, 2001). For immigrant children, however, the degree of support a child receives, on the one hand, for learning the second language and, on the other, for retaining her first language

affects whether she will be competent bilingually and biculturally or conflicted about language and identity. If an "English-only" approach is
taken by schools, she will feel that her native language and culture are
devalued. But if her parents do not encourage biculturalism, she may feel
conflicted about learning English and the culture underlying it. Such conflicts may represent an intergenerational rift in the family regarding children's assimilation into American culture, with negative effects on children's self-esteem and academic aspirations (Fong, 2003). Immigrant
children and children whose families speak languages other than English
are more often referred for assessment of learning and psychiatric disorders; however, "Many of the behaviors considered problematic by teachers are, in reality, characteristics of students who are in the process of second language acquisition" (Canino & Spurlock, 2000, p. 29).

PLAY AND FANTASY

As the middle years proceed, the fantasy play so prominent during the
preschool period declines. It is often said that play is the work of the preschooler. For the school-age child, a work orientation emphasizing intellectual mastery and physical competence gradually supplants play as a
compelling interest (Erikson, 1963). Children who continue to insist that
play is their reason for being are increasingly seen as immature. In part
this shift in orientation is forced on the child by external reality: she must
learn to work in order to master school tasks, which require her increasingly to be organized, logical, and unplayful. But new cognitive capabilities increase her internal motivation to learn new skills. These rapid cognitive advances offer the child the possibility of understanding the world
through systematic, logical thinking, replacing the preschooler's tendency to try to understand through imaginative thinking. Play remains
important to the school-age child, but fantasy play is gradually supplanted by the organized and ritualized play of games and sports (Rubin
et al., 1998). At the same time, children may continue fantasy play by
themselves and with best friends. Play of all kinds continues provides
children with a break from the demands of reality. For this reason alone,
play remains very important to school-age children because so much of
their time in school is spent working on intellectual tasks.

Games with Rules

By age 4, preschool children can learn how to play simple board games.
They can count, take turns, and understand that winning depends on
reaching the last square first. However, preschool children do not enjoy
structured games as much as fantasy play. Games with rules constrain

their egocentric imagination, and they have not yet developed far enough cognitively to be intellectually interested in the structure and logic of a game. They often cannot accept losing and may quit or cheat to avoid losing or react with intense disappointment if they lose. By 6 or 7, however, children can learn somewhat more complicated games, play by the rules more gracefully, take some pleasure in following the twists and turns of the game, and enjoy exercising their skills. They still may be intensely competitive, intent on winning, and disappointed in losing. However, even though games are competitive, they are explicitly social and cooperative, since the players must follow a set of rules for the game to go on. Young school-age children often have difficulty learning their roles in complex games like baseball, and mistakes based on excitement and impulsiveness are common. A few years ago I went to my 7-year-old niece's T-ball game. When a ball was hit to the center of the infield, *all* four infielders ran toward it. The shortstop picked up the ball and threw it to first base, but the first baseman was not on the base to catch it because he had run toward the ball. As children reach 10–12 years of age, they begin to enjoy games that involve strategy rather than chance (Bandmaster & Senders, 1988). Games also symbolize the child's developing peer orientation and become one of the important vehicles he uses to assess his status among peers. Skillful children are respected by peers. Children who frequently ignore rules, blow up in the middle of a game, or otherwise "spoil the game" risk rejection by peers.

The structure of the games of middle childhood mirrors many of the general developmental tasks of this period. Organized playground games such as kickball, soccer, basketball, hopscotch, and jump rope implicitly socialize children to take turns, improve their skills, focus on planning and goals, exert sufficient control over emotions to allow the game to proceed, and follow the rules (Piaget & Inhelder, 1969). Learning to play games with complicated scenarios and rules requires self-discipline and concentration.

Even the spontaneous fantasy play of school-age children frequently becomes ritualized and rule-governed. For example, 10-year-old boys in play with action figures often devise elaborate systems of rules for combat. School-age children often create structure around physical activities, turning rough-and-tumble play into games with rules (Pelligrini & Smith, 1998).

For example, at a family picnic a group of cousins, girls and boys, ranging in age from 8 to 12 were taking turns swinging out on a rope and dropping into a river. Gradually, they began suggesting specific ways of doing this, and a competition evolved, with more and more elaborate tasks being proposed. They had to turn around on the rope and face the bank before dropping into the water; or skim the water with their feet before letting go; or grasp their knees after letting go, to cannonball into the water. Implicitly, they seemed impelled to introduce structure, competition, and consensually defined skills into what had begun as spontaneous play.

Hobbies as Play

Typical school-age activities such as hobbies and collecting depict the evolution of play. Children collect dolls, comic books, sports cards, action figures, rocks, soda cans, or colored glass beads, to name a few. Commercial interests appeal to and exploit school-age children's passion for collecting by continuously creating new collectible objects, often as spin-offs from popular children's movies. Sometimes children assemble collections of disparate objects that have personal meaning and keep them in a special box (McGreevy, 1990). Other hobbies involve craft projects, plastic models, or making things out of scrap materials. Girls tend to spend more time with hobbies, as they have conventionally been defined (McHale, Crouter, & Tucker, 2001). However, many older school-age boys avidly follow sports and make a hobby of learning statistics and legends about athletes, especially those they identify with. Anna Freud (1965, p. 84) suggested that hobbies are "halfway between work and play" because they involve mental skills of organizing and categorizing objects or the ability to build or assemble things, yet also are vehicles for the expression of fantasy. Studies of the relationship between how school-age children spend their free time and developmental success in adolescence suggest that "structured activities such as hobbies and sports are the most development-enhancing ways for children to spend their time" (McHale et al., 2001, p. 1774). These findings are consistent with Werner's (1993) argument that participation in structured extracurricular pursuits and hobbies promotes resiliency by helping children feel "solace in adversity and a reason to feel proud" (p. 49).

Fantasy

The movement from social dramatic play to organized games tells only part of the story of the evolution of play. In middle childhood, a kind of mental play, internal fantasy, increases as play with peers becomes more ritualized. Fantasy continues to fulfill the functions that dramatic play did for the preschooler: pleasure, imagined fulfillment of wishes, exploration of reality, imagining oneself in more advanced roles, rehearsal of actions and plans, and understanding the emotions and perspectives of others through identification and role playing (Seja & Russ, 1999). These fantasy activities contribute to children's abilities in creative thinking and adaptive coping (Russ, Robins, & Christiano, 1999). In psychoanalytic theory, internal fantasy is seen as a substitute for action and is therefore associated with the capacity for controlling behavior. Fantasy provides the school-age child with an outlet for expressing wishes that are not possible to achieve in reality, as well as negative thoughts and feelings that would invite punishment or criticism if expressed in action.

School-age children often keep their fantasies private from adults. Their involvement with fantasy is most often registered by their interest in movies, TV programs, and popular books, such as the Harry Potter series. Fantasy is also evident in the kinds of play they do alone or with best friends. Two 10-year-old boys had seen the film *Desperado*, a story of revenge featuring extreme violence. When they were playing together they sometimes acted out scenes from the film and sometimes drew elaborate pictures of the main character mowing down 20 adversaries. The appeal of such play is that it supports the school-age child's wish to be competent and powerful, even in the face of extreme odds. These two boys were not aggressive in their behavior toward each other or other children. Their wishes to be powerful and dominating were contained in fantasy. In general, however, the content of children's fantasy becomes more realistic and social as they move through middle childhood (Sarnoff, 1976). Instead of daydreaming about being a superhero, like a 6-year-old, a 9-year-old imagines himself being a hero on his sports team.

COGNITIVE DEVELOPMENT

By age 7 the child is moving away from egocentric thinking and is using logic. The child becomes aware that intuition based on an awareness of surface appearances is not always correct (Smith & Cowie, 1991). Piaget's famous experiments with mass and volume illustrate this shift in thinking. Piaget and Inhelder (1969) described middle childhood, specifically 7–12 years of age, as the phase of *concrete operations*. Unlike toddlers and preschoolers, who solve problems by manipulating objects physically, the school-age child learns about reality by manipulating the objects of his perception *mentally*. The essence of the move from Piaget's sensorimotor stage to the stage of concrete operations, then, is *a shift from action to thought*. During the preschool period, the child has slowly developed the ability to represent experience mentally, a process that goes hand in hand with the development of language. Mastery of language, which proceeds rapidly across the preschool period, provides the school-age child with a vehicle for organizing experience mentally.

Concrete operations involve basic reasoning processes but are distinguished from formal operations—abstract, hypothetical thinking—that develop in adolescence by the fact that the child can only use them to think about objects that are visible in front of her rather than purely mental phenomena. In the conservation experiment with water in different containers, for example, the school-age child looks at concrete reality and thinks about what she observes, reasoning that since no water was added the amount of water is the same (Kagan, 1984). She realizes that the shape of the containers makes the amount of water look different, and she is aware that if the steps in the procedure were reversed the amount of water would be the same. Her thinking involves *reversibility*, which Piaget posits as a hallmark of concrete operations. Instead of being tied to her immediate impressions, a child can systematically think back over what she has perceived. For example, by age 8, she can learn a reverse procedure to check a math problem: if $10 - 6 = 4$, then I can check my answer by adding, $4 + 6 = 10$. In the conservation experiment an 8-year-old is likely to explain that the water could be poured back into the first container where it would look exactly as it did at first, using reversible thinking to prove that the amount is the same (Piaget & Inhelder, 1969). Reversibility increases the child's ability to think more flexibly, and is an example of a more general trend in school-age development, the increasing ability to look at reality from multiple perspectives and to solve problems using multiple strategies (Siegler, 1996).

The ability to flexibly perform mental operations based on logic and reasoning, however, requires another developmental advance— "decentration." To think logically, the child must be able to distinguish between the subjective and the objective. Piaget argued that the shift from egocentric to decentered thought between the ages of 6 and 7 heralds and makes possible the development of higher-level cognitive functions. When the child begins to see reality from the decentered as opposed to the egocentric perspective, he is freer to use the more analytical and logical perspective implied in concrete mental operations (Piaget, 1952b). The ability to decenter also allows for a clearer understanding of causality. Unlike the more egocentric preschooler, the school-age child can separate his fantasies from the actual causes of events. A 9-year-old, for example, may be sad and angry about his parents' separation, but he is less likely than a preschooler to believe something he did caused the separation. In middle childhood impressionistic, intuitive thinking remains important, but thinking characterized by reasoning and analysis now is also available.

Recent developmental theory challenges Piaget's view that stagewise maturation is the primary determinant of the course of cognitive development. When children are asked to think about their everyday experience, as opposed to being tested with experiments that implicitly are unfamiliar contexts for thinking, they often appear more advanced than Piaget's research suggests. Recent research on children's reasoning suggests that "children will exhibit different levels of cognitive skills and abilities as a function of their level of knowledge in different domains"

(DeLoache et al., 1998, p. 801). For example, young school-age children can develop expertise at chess and, because of their knowledge, demonstrate much better problem solving and strategy skills *in chess* than adults who are chess novices. However, these skills tend to be domain-specific to chess playing rather than generalizing to other types of problem solving (Schneider, Gruber, Gold, & Opwis, 1993).

Cognitive Advances in the Transition to Middle Childhood

The maturing of the prefrontal cortex, which becomes evident between 6 and 7, correlates with a number of changes in perceptual and cognitive abilities that appear at about age 7 (Luciana & Nelson, 1998). Along with the more general shift toward decentration and improved perspective taking, the abilities listed below provide the foundation for concrete mental operations.

Spatial Orientation and Understanding of Space

The child knows her own right from left at age 6 but has difficulty saying which is the right or left side of a person sitting opposite her. By ages 7–8, she is able to do this. Beginning around age 6, the organization of children's drawings begins to reflect their improving understanding of spatial relationships, relative size of objects, and relative distance (Dennis, 1992). A 4- to 5-year-old's picture of her mother and herself, for example, may show two figures about the same size who, because they are placed in the middle of the page, appear to be floating in air. Next to the human figures is a house that is smaller than they are, drawn without any hint of depth and distance perspective to clarify why a house would be smaller than people. A 6- to 7-year old's drawing, however, shows a more realistic understanding of space: there is a ground line at the bottom of the picture, usually signaled by green grass or brown dirt; the human figures stand on the ground and more accurately represent the relative sizes of a mother and child; the relative size of the birds flying overhead and their distance from the figures in the foreground is shown by sets of two small curved lines joined in the middle to represent wings. Between 6 and 10, understanding of space increases; by age 10 children's drawings begin to reflect a use of linear perspective, so that the spatial organization of their pictures is consistent with what the eye sees (Case, 1998).

Time Orientation

Older preschool children know the days of the week, but children are not able to learn to tell time or understand how the calendar is organized until about 7. This becomes possible because of advances in the understanding of numbers. By about age 7 the child understands that numbers represent sequence of time and that time can be divided into minutes and hours (Case, 1998). This clearer sense of how time is organized allows school-age children to think ahead and to plan their actions more efficiently than a preschooler can.

Seriation

In one of Piaget's tasks, children were asked to arrange 10 sticks of uneven lengths in an order from shortest to longest. Preschool children typically could not accomplish this. They might get a few of the sticks in the correct order, but then seemed to get mixed up and arrange the rest in a random order. By contrast, 7-year-olds grasp the concept of a series governed by some ordering principle and are able to arrange the sticks correctly. This ability to apply a concept of size, weight, length, or some other quantifiable characteristic to a group of objects is one of the building blocks of mathematical understanding (Bisanz & LeFevre, 1990).

Visual Organizational Ability

The child becomes "less and less bound by the organization or lack of organization of visual materials he looks at. Increasingly, he is able mentally to reorganize materials into patterns that are more interesting or satisfying" (Elkind, 1994, p. 123). The school-age child can look beyond surface perceptions to imagine new patterns, whereas the preschooler has difficulty doing this. Elkind and Weiss (1967) demonstrated this change in the ability to organize visual materials by asking children to name pictures of objects that were pasted on a page in a "disordered array." The objects were placed at odd angles and showed no organized pattern of alignment in relation to one another. When preschool children were asked to name the 15 objects, they seemed to become confused by the lack of organization of the objects. They named some objects twice and did not name others. Younger school-age children, ages 6–8, had no trouble naming all the objects, because they mentally organized the disarrayed objects, using a systematic strategy of scanning the objects from right to left or up to down.

A more homely real-life example of the child's visual organizational ability is demonstrated by the job of cleaning up her room. While many children do not like to pick up their rooms, an 8-year-old can generally do it without assistance because she can bring order out of chaos mentally, thinking about where things go. By contrast, a 5-year-old is likely to feel overwhelmed by toys strewn across the floor because she is not yet able to construct an image of the room with everything in its place. Consequently, the younger child will need an adult to help her organize the task.

Part–Whole Discrimination: Ability to Move between Details and Overall Perceptions and to Perceive Multiple Variables

Preschool children may focus on specific aspects of a picture or on the whole picture but have trouble moving back and forth between the two levels of perception: "When young children are asked to compare complex figures, such as two houses that are alike except for the number of windows, they say the two are the same if they find only one similarity, without any further exploration for possible discrepancies. Children of seven or eight explore both houses systematically before deciding whether the two are alike or different" (Elkind, 1994, p. 123). The child is now able to perceive two or more aspects of a problem at once. The ability to move back and forth between parts and wholes, between details and larger organizing ideas, is the basis of categorization and classification. Children's ability to think about problems using multiple perspectives gradually increases as they move through middle childhood.

Auditory Processing

School-age children, compared with preschoolers, are more able to process information given orally. They are more adept at using verbal cues to understand a problem. This ability is based on their more sophisticated grasp of language and their improving capacity for strictly mental representation. It has clear implications for school performance, since teachers frequently give directions and define problems using words alone.

These changes in cognition and perception that emerge during the early part of middle childhood are of critical importance because they are needed for the learning tasks children confront in elementary school. The elementary school curriculum assumes by second and third grade that children possess these abilities. Those children who do not, for whatever reason, are at a tremendous disadvantage and are at risk socially and emotionally (Eccles et al., 1998). A third-grade boy who had average overall intelligence but serious learning disorders that put him far behind his peers told me, "I'm the dumbest kid in my class." As is typical of younger school-age children, this boy was not able to take a balanced view of his weaknesses and strengths. His evaluation of himself in absolutist terms, characteristic of his level of development, contributed further to his low self-esteem.

Attention

Attention involves the ability to select what we perceive and focus on, and to screen out other stimuli. "Paying attention" also implies that we will process and perhaps remember what we attend to, as opposed to surrounding events that do not have our attention. At the same time, attentional ability has limits, both developmental and absolute. Younger children are more distractible and have shorter attention spans, and anyone can lose focus because of strong distracting stimuli or internal feelings of disinterest (Flavell & Miller, 1998). Flavell, Green, & Flavell (1995) provide a useful metaphor for contrasting the attentional abilities of preschoolers and school-age children: a 4-year-old's attention is more diffuse, like light from a lamp shining in all directions, while an 8-year-old can direct her attention, like the focused beam of a flashlight.

There is a dramatic increase in the components of attention during middle childhood, including selective focus, attention span, and systematic planning about what to attend to. These gains occur both as a result of new cognitive skills based on brain maturation, and reinforcement by school expectations and routines. By age 8, children can consciously will themselves to maintain attention. This is particularly obvious, for example, when a child is working on a page of math homework he would prefer not to do, yet keeps at it until he has completed it (Flavell et al., 1995). Although the hyperactivity symptoms of a child with ADHD draw the most attention, his relative inability to organize and maintain attention contribute most seriously to his academic deficits (Barkley, 2003).

Memory

Memory improves with cognitive development. During the preschool years memory grows with language development. Memories that are encoded verbally are more firmly registered. During the school-age years, improving memory is related to the child's increased speed and more sophisticated strategies for processing information. In early childhood, by contrast, children process information more slowly, which means that they tend to " 'lose' more information before it can be encoded" in the short-term memory store (Schneider & Bjorklund, 1998, p, 470). *By the end of the middle years, the child's ability to categorize memories and deliberately recall information is nearly as efficient as an adult's* (Schneider & Bjorklund, 1998). School-age children remember more than preschoolers do because they intuitively apply rules for recalling information. After age 7, children also become conscious of memory strategies and can intentionally invoke them. They have learned to sort information by time, place, category, and other cues, all of which serve to organize memories and thus facilitate recall. As the ability to think in categories improves, so does memory, because categories allow for more effective storage of information. Memory capability also increases because the child's knowledge base is growing ever larger. In processing information, the school-age child, who has a bigger knowledge base than the preschooler, does not have to attend to the parts of a message she already knows. This in turn increases processing speed for the parts of the message that are unfamiliar, with the result that these parts are more likely to be remembered (Kail & Salthouse, 1994).

A related recent concept about memory efficiency is called "fuzzy trace theory," which argues that if a child perceives an event he is already knowledgeable about or which fits into existing categories, he does not need to remember the details. It is sufficient, and more efficient, to remember the *gist* or essence of what occurred (Reyna & Brainerd, 1995). Preschoolers tend to have trouble extracting the gist of a memory. School-age children are much more able to pull out the essence of what happened (Marx & Henderson, 1996).

Improved memory ability allows the child to keep a sequence of steps in mind, which means he can follow stepwise instructions common in academic tasks (Case, 1985). These developing memory abilities are reinforced by school tasks, which encourage children to intentionally remember information. Motivated by school tasks, older school-age children create conscious strategies for remembering—repeating information to themselves, or creating mental cues, categories, or images that help them remember (Schneider, 2002).

> An 8-year-old girl who was learning the multiplication tables told me, "I kept having trouble with the nines, but then my aunt told me a trick— you can always tell what the next one is going to be by adding 10 and subtracting 1, like 6 times 9 is 54, so you know that 7 times 9 is going to be 63."

The Executive Function

This child's statement about memory provides a specific example of a more general process that emerges in middle childhood: the executive function, or metacognition, the ability to think about how one is thinking and, by extension, to use such analysis to solve problems (Flavell, 2000). Kagan (1984) contrasts the differences in cognitive abilities of preschool and school-age children by pointing out that school-age children make more use of "executive processes," by which he means *skills in approaching and thinking about problems*. These cognitive skills enhance ability to solve problems. Table 11.1 summarizes Kagan's discussion of the executive processes and elaborates their impact on problem solving.

The executive function provides conscious supervisory awareness that oversees thinking about problem solving. The ability to maintain a monitoring perspective on one's thought processes allows for more flexible thinking, detection of errors in thinking, and the generation of alternative solutions to problems. Hughes states, "Executive functions are crucial in situations that involve novelty, trouble-shooting, multiple-constraints, and ambiguity" (Hughes, 2002, p. 69). Executive functions

TABLE 11.1. Executive Processes and Problem Solving in Middle Childhood

- *Ability to articulate a problem and generate ideas about what actions can be taken to solve it.*
- *Knowing cognitive strategies that will help in problem solving.* For example, a school-age child who is told to remember a set of pictures will spend time studying them because she knows the extra attention will help her remember them; by contrast, a 4-year-old will not look at the pictures for as long as the school-age child does, apparently because she does not yet understand that a longer study will improve memory.
- *Knowing when to activate cognitive rules and strategies to solve problems.* Essentially, school-age children ask themselves, "What do I need to think about to figure out this problem?"
- *A more flexible approach to problem solving.* A preschool child is more likely to persist in solving a problem in the same way, even if he is not succeeding, while a 9- or 10-year-old is more likely "to discard inefficient solutions that are not working and to search systematically for better alternatives" (Kagan, 1984, p. 231).
- *Longer attention span, ability to resist distractions, and better control of anxiety.* More solid self-regulation, including especially the ability to inhibit frustration and wishes to give up, allows school-age children to keep focused on problem solving even when the problem is hard to solve.
- *Ability to continuously monitor performance.* The child can pay attention to how he is working on a task and evaluate whether he is on the right track.
- *Faith in her ability to think about problems.* A younger child stops trying if she cannot figure out a problem, whereas a school-age child knows from experience that thinking can work.
- *Awareness of shortcomings in thinking.* Older school-age children are usually aware when a solution they have arrived at is inadequate. Unlike preschoolers, who are less concerned about mistakes or ideals of performance, school-age children have internalized standards of performance that cause them to search for the best solution to a problem.

Note: Data abstracted from Kagan (1984).

are somewhat in evidence during the preschool years, but they emerge most clearly in middle childhood (Luciana & Nelson, 1998). The following example illustrates the executive function at work in a rather precocious child.

Hilary and Henry, 6-year-old twins, were sitting on the kitchen floor at their grandmother's, cracking almonds with nutcrackers. Henry cracked a nut and found an almond with two segments instead of one and exclaimed, "I got twins!" Hilary very much wanted to find "twins" herself. She gradually became frustrated as she cracked several more almonds and found only singles. Her dissatisfaction with this hit-or-miss method impelled her to try other ways to find twins. She stopped cracking and told her grandmother, "We need to make a scale because I think twins are heavier." Her grandmother made a scale by suspending two plastic cups from strings at the ends of a coat hanger. Hilary began "weighing" pairs of almonds until she found one that was clearly heavier. She cracked it and found twins! Then she had another idea: "If I shake the almonds, I think the twins will rattle more." She tried this method and it also worked.

This child's creative and flexible thinking demonstrates the emergence of the executive processes. Hilary's grandmother's supportiveness also clarifies that the development of executive processes is shaped by adults' scaffolding (Neitzel & Stright, 2003).

Deficits in executive processes have been implicated in disorders with a strong neuropsychological component, such as autism and ADHD (Ozonoff & Jensen, 1999; Perner, Kain, & Barchfield, 2002). The cognitive processes of children with normal intelligence who have autism or ADHD highlight the deficits in executive functioning. Autistic children, even those in the "high-functioning" category, have significant deficits in their abilities to think about thinking, to self-monitor, and to think flexibly (Russell & Hill, 2001). Children with ADHD show other difficulties in executive function. They have problems inhibiting impulses and easily diverge into off-task behavior, which compromises their academic progress (Adams & Snowling, 2001). Compared with normal children, they "lack strategic flexibility [in thinking], display poor planning and working memory, and are poor at monitoring their own behavior (Hughes & Graham, 2002, p. 135).

SELF-REGULATION

Cognitive processes increase self-regulation as middle childhood proceeds. The ability to think about experience logically and coherently reduces the child's anxiety. The school-age child understands the world and himself better than the preschooler does. He can more precisely appraise stressful situations and take coping actions that are appropriate (Saarni, 1999). Because his reality testing is more accurate, he is less vulnerable than the preschooler to fears of the unknown. The school-age child's improving capacities for sustained attention and goal-directedness implicitly permit him to maintain self-control. At the same time, psychological defense mechanisms become more sophisticated as means of protecting the child from anxiety. As the repertoire of defenses expands, the defenses themselves become more efficient.

Anxiety during Middle Childhood

School-age children respond with anxiety to some of the same situations that were troublesome in early childhood: separation, worry about losing control, fear of body damage, and confusion about reality. However, for children who have histories of secure attachment, live in safe circumstances, and have not been traumatized, these earlier sources of anxiety are not so pressing as for the younger child. They also have more ability to handle these sources of anxiety. Their cognitive abilities make it easier for them to sort out whether a situation is really dangerous. They have had enough experience in the world to appraise situations and the intentions and emotions of others more accurately (Saarni, 1999). For example, a 3-year-old who is threatened by another child may become terribly anxious because he cannot separate the threatening words from the actuality of being hurt. By contrast, a 10-year-old has learned that threats and the actions described in threats are frequently two different things. So, when a peer casually says, "I'm going to kick your butt," he can appraise the threat by evaluating the context in which it occurs. He may conclude, without much conscious thought, "This is my friend. He likes to push people around with words, but he doesn't get in fights. What he really meant was that he didn't like it that I took the rebound away from him. I don't have to worry about this." On the other hand, if the other child's tone is angry or if he is known to act with physical aggression, the child will appraise the threat differently and get ready to protect himself.

The anxieties of the school-age child match the developmental tasks of middle childhood. She is particularly concerned about being rejected or excluded or seen as inadequate by peers, and, in part, evaluates her abilities based on the feedback she receives from peers. Consequently she is very aware of her performance—in academics, social relations, or athletics—compared with that of peers. The school-age child has a firm self-representation and can look at herself from an outside perspective. When her performance falls short of her self-image, she may become anxious. This anxiety may be increased by the conscience's moral self-criticisms. However, the older school-age child with a well-established and securely-held sense of her abilities is less likely to be made anxious by criticism from peers (Pomerantz & Saxon, 2001).

Strategies for Self-Regulation and Coping

Several components of self-regulation come together in middle childhood. These emerging self-regulatory abilities contribute to the evident calmness, self-control, and ability to sustain attention that we see in normal school-age children. When school-age children are faced with external or internal stressors, they are likely to take an active coping stance, drawing on their own self-regulatory strategies or seeking help from others. They are motivated to exert control over stressors and avoid passive acceptance (Saarni, 1999). The consolidation of effective self-regulatory strategies in middle childhood serves the child well when he encounters stressors common in the transition to early adolescence and middle school (Rudolph, Lambert, Clark, & Kurlakowsky, 2001).

Representational Competence

The cognitive and linguistic advances during middle childhood promote an increasing ability to mentally organize and make sense of experience. The capacity to think about stressful experiences reduces anxiety. Representational competence also has an interpersonal, communicative dimension in the middle years. The child can tell the story of his experience with clarity, including a description of how he felt (Frijda & Mesquita, 1994). The school-age child can gain relief from anxiety because he is able to describe what happened.

> An 8-year-old boy who got lost in the woods near his house came home and told his father, "I went to a new part of the woods—not where the path goes—and I got lost. I looked around, and I couldn't see any houses. There was a hill, a little one, and I went up to the top of it, but I still couldn't see where I was. I was really scared. Then I saw this old barbed wire. It was just on the ground. I followed along it, and after a little while I could see the townhouses near the other parking lot. Then I knew where I was, and I ran home." This boy was agitated when he came home, but he visibly calmed down after he told his story and his father listened to it. He was able to reduce his fear by communicating what happened to him.

Cognitive Control of Emotional Arousal

The school-age child is less at the mercy of strong emotions than the preschooler, because he can use mental strategies to inhibit the expression of his feelings. If he perceives it is in his best interest to suppress or hide how he is feeling, he can do so more easily than a preschooler. An 8-year-old who is being scolded by an adult may be angry, but may hide his feelings because he is aware that getting angry will increase his punishment (Saarni, 1997). If he experiences a disappointment, he can rationalize distress, saying, for example, "This isn't so bad. I'll get over it." He can combine rationalization with denial: "It's not that important to be the team captain as long as I get to play."

Social learning theorists define self-control as a special aspect of self-regulation that involves the ability to remain focused on a goal in the face of stress or interference (Patterson, 1982b). Increasingly, school-age children make this a conscious process and use cognitive strategies to maintain a focus. This behavior is also based on the child's belief that he can take action to alter events rather than simply relying on chance (Eccles et al., 1998).

> An 8-year-old who is up to bat maintains his concentration on the pitcher in spite of being razzed by the opposing players, who are yelling, "Hey batter, you can't hit, you'll miss it by a mile." This child hears the heckling and understands its intent is to ruin his concentration. He

controls his affective responses and also may use internal talk ("Just watch the pitcher. Be ready to swing if it's a good one.") in order to stay ready to hit the ball.

Use of Emotions as "Internal Monitoring and Guidance Systems"

Emotions themselves are the indicators of how a person is feeling and therefore contribute to self-regulation. Like attachment, "emotional security" is a set goal in humans—we strive to maintain felt security or psychic equilibrium (Cummings & Davies, 1996, p. 125). A range of emotional responses, not simply anxiety, can signal the need to make efforts to restore a feeling of security. The school-age child differentiates among her emotions and knows more clearly than the preschooler what they mean (Bradley, 2000). She is therefore less likely to be overwhelmed by strong emotions in a stressful situation.

Ability to Remain Focused on Goal-Directed Actions Even When External Support Is Not Being Provided

While preschool children are distracted by both external stimuli and their own thoughts, school-age children can resist distraction and sustain their attention. This ability is based on increases in attentional ability, the cognitive skill of being able to imagine the sequence of steps needed to achieve a goal, and on the sense of oneself as autonomous (Eisenberg et al., 1996). Preschoolers, by contrast, often need the support of others to maintain goal-directed behavior (Case, 1998).

Ability to Delay Gratification Based on Cognitive Evaluation

Harter (1983b), summarizing studies where children were offered a bigger reward if they were able to wait and a smaller one if they were not, states, "A steady decrease in the choice of the less desirable reward was obtained across kindergarten through sixth grade, indicating that children were increasingly able to delay gratification in anticipation of the more desirable reward" (p. 348). As children proceed through middle childhood, they become less impulsive and more thoughtful in their decision making.

Ability to Understand the Concept of Planning and to Make Conscious Plans

By age 8, children can think through several steps in a plan of action. Conscious planning helps the school-age child remain focused on a goal and allows her to resist distractions and frustration when things do not go according to plan (Harter, 1999).

Growing Ability to View Tasks Incrementally

Compared to preschoolers, school-age children are much more able to understand that their skills will improve gradually through practice and repetition. Consequently, they are more able to take an incremental approach, realizing from previous experience that practice and "trying again" will allow them to achieve goals that initially are difficult (Borkowski & Muthukrishna, 1995).

Use of Social Comparison

In middle childhood, children assess their performance by comparing themselves with peers. This is different from the comparisons preschoolers make. The comparisons of preschoolers in the transition to middle childhood are more concerned with making sure they are being treated fairly or getting the same privileges as are given to peers. Older school-age children compare themselves with peers in order to assess how they stack up. The desire to compare favorably with their peers serves to inhibit school-age children from acting in ways defined as "deviant" by the peer group, thus stimulating self-regulatory actions.

Influence of Internalized Feelings of Self-Pride and Self-Shame on Behavior

The school-age child realizes he may feel badly afterward if he does something that deviates from his internalized values. He is also aware that he will feel good about himself if he accomplishes a goal he approves of (Bandura, 1994).

Capacity to Tolerate Conflicting Feelings

This ability corresponds with the cognitive capacity to see alternative interpretations to a problem. At ages 9 or 10, children acknowledge that they can feel more than one emotion at the same time. The child can accept that there may be negative and positive aspects to a situation. This ability to tolerate ambivalence allows the child to contain her feelings rather than acting in response to them.

Increasingly Effective Defense Mechanisms

A greater range of psychological defenses becomes available. These "higher-level" defenses are more effective in helping the child cope with anxiety and, compared to the more "primitive" defenses, they interfere less with the child's overall functioning. Table 11.2 defines the defenses that develop during middle childhood.

TABLE 11.2. Defenses in Middle Childhood

- *Repression.* Involves the elimination, or "forgetting," of unacceptable feelings, impulses, or thoughts from conscious awareness.
- *Sublimation.* Avoiding direct awareness of aggressive impulses and sexual curiosity through "neutralized" activities, such as games, collecting, projects, creativity, and (in general) interest in things outside the self.
- *Reaction formation.* Turning an impulse or wish into its opposite. An example is the transformation of the preschooler's intense interest and curiosity about sex differences to the school-age child's tendency toward sex segregation—"Boys are stupid. We're not letting any of them in our club."
- *Displacement in fantasy.* Impulses that would be negative, aggressive, intrusive, or antisocial if acted out are experienced "at a distance" through fantasy. Displacement in fantasy can involve either the child's own fantasizing or her enjoyment of TV shows and movies where impulsive, aggressive behavior is depicted.
- *Isolation.* Involves repressing the affect connected with a thought so that the thought has a "neutral" quality. Very frequently school-age children can describe a stressful event in a matter-of-fact tone but have trouble answering when asked how they *felt* about it. This is isolation at work.
- *Doing and undoing.* Expression of a negative impulse, followed immediately by its opposite. A child who is angry with her parent—either directly or privately—undoes the impulse by being oversolicitous, apologetic, or spontaneously saying, "I love you, Mom."
- *Turning against the self.* Involves punishing the self for having a forbidden impulse. In response to anger toward a parent, for example, the child feels guilty and "beats himself up" by condemning himself.

Based on A. Freud (1966) and Berman (1979).

Automatic use of defenses, as well as conscious suppression and self-distraction, helps account for the school-age child's ability to avoid distressing feelings. Parents sometimes worry that a school-age child is not showing the emotions she "should" feel. For example, the school-age child whose parent has recently died may appear to be unaffected because she is using the defense of isolation. She may also immerse herself in action to avoid thoughts about the loss, or resist and avoid talking about the parent's death in order to avoid painful feelings. School-age children can only tolerate the pain of grieving for brief periods, and these defenses help them manage and reduce the intensity of painful feelings (Webb, 2002). (This is not to say that school-age children do not grieve but rather that they may grieve in spurts over time or express their grief behaviorally through increased attachment behavior or sleep disturbances.) Such defenses parallel the school-age child's general tendencies to be present-oriented rather than thinking much about the past and to focus attention on concrete experience at hand.

Self-Regulation and Culture

Different cultures and subcultures have contrasting values regarding the display of emotions. Children learn these display rules during the toddler and preschool years, and by school age implicitly know what kinds of emotional expression are expected or permitted in particular situations and relationships. They have internalized rules and schemas that guide them in expressing feelings, covering them up, or transforming them in some way, depending on the social situation (Saarni, 1999). Self-regulation must be understood in this context. For example, Chinese children also learn an expressive style that emphasizes restraint of emotional expression and calm demeanor. In Chinese culture "impulsiveness," or poor self-regulation, might be defined as being boisterous in the presence of adults (Bond, 1993). American culture, by contrast, does not require as much deference and restraint, and children know that many adults accept expressions of excitement.

Within American culture, however, different groups have contrasting rules for emotional display, which in a climate of racism may be misinterpreted. For example, school-age African American children may talk more loudly and excitedly when in a group than white children do. This is consistent with the rules of emotional display many African American children have learned. However, their behavior may be equated with a lack of control or impulsiveness by a white teacher or clinician who has been socialized to be more restrained in displays of emotion. This misinterpretation of a cultural difference, perhaps intensified by prejudice, may turn into a judgment about mental health (Canino & Spurlock, 2000).

Self-Regulation and Coping in Dangerous Environments

The school-age child, more than younger children, comes into direct contact with his community. He may ride the bus or walk to school. On the streets in poor urban neighborhoods he may be exposed to threats and danger, and in consequence may develop coping strategies that would not be appropriate in safer neighborhoods. It is important to assess whether a child's fears and anxiety are realistic in order to understand whether his self-regulatory strategies are adaptive. If a child lives in a dangerous neighborhood where he is threatened or exposed to violence and where people he knows have been victimized by crime, it is appropriate to be afraid. A child in this situation, rather than having a separation anxiety disorder, is, from an attachment perspective, behaving appropriately when she insists on staying near her parent. Alternatively, a school-age child who has been exposed to violence in his neighborhood may adopt an alert, aggressive stance as a means of self-protection, and may gang together with peers as a means of mutual protection.

MORAL DEVELOPMENT

During middle childhood moral abilities expand and are refined. The decline of egocentric thinking supports moral development. By ages 7–8, the ability to take a decentered perspective allows the child to balance self-interest with the social norm of following the rules. Rather than thinking only about herself, the school-age child recognizes, on principle, that the needs of others must be recognized (Eisenberg & Fabes, 1998). As the child's ability to think in logically consistent ways develops, she comes to expect consistency between beliefs and actions, both her own and those of others (Kagan, 1984). A 9-year-old may resist a friend's suggestion that they shoplift some candy because she knows that action would not be in accord with her belief that stealing is wrong. This child refuses her friend's dare not just out of fear of punishment or internal anxiety and guilt but also because it is inconsistent with what she believes.

Because school-age children can think in logical terms, they more easily understand the rationales for correct behavior that adults provide. For example, a parent tells an 8-year-old, "You wouldn't want one of your friends to borrow your bike without asking, so you shouldn't do that to someone else." This statement makes sense to an 8-year-old, in part because he can now think in terms of logical propositions and in part because he can appreciate the feelings of others (Turiel, 1998). However, parental modeling continues to be the most powerful determinant of the morality children internalize. The child who has observed a parent borrow things without asking is likely to be more confused than impressed by the parent's moral directive. Given the importance of peers for school-age children, their moral values are also significantly influenced by the behavior modeled by friends they admire (Walker, Hennig, & Krettenauer, 2000).

During middle childhood, children begin to appreciate moral complexity and to develop more nuanced views of moral dilemmas. An 8- to 10-year-old frequently will consider both intentions and consequences in judging how wrong an act is. She distinguishes between acts that are morally wrong, "social-conventional" transgressions, and personal responses (Smetana, 1995). For example, an 8-year-old is likely to condemn another child's hitting or stealing as a moral violation, using words like "wrong," "bad," or "mean." By contrast, a child who violates social expectations by talking constantly and refusing to listen will not be judged as wrong but rather as "annoying" or "weird," or in violation of convention: "With him talking all the time, it's hard for the rest of us to do our work. The teacher's always telling him to be quiet." In a personal judgment about a child like this, a 9-year-old said, "I don't think he's bad for talking all the time, but I don't like being around him, so I usually try to sit far away from him."

Interesting research has examined school-age children's ideas about social exclusion. This issue makes a good basis for looking at the complexity of moral thinking in middle childhood because it bridges the moral, social, and personal domains. Groups of 6-, 9-, and 12-year-olds were asked about a range of possible justifications for excluding a child from a group. All children, regardless of age, judged as morally wrong the idea that a child could be excluded solely on the basis or race or gender. This judgment was made even when strong stereotypes were implied in the question. For example, children said it was wrong to exclude a boy from a dance class just because he was a boy. That would not be fair. Older children continued to emphasize fairness, but their ideas about who should be included in a group also expressed concerns how group functioning would be affected. For example, older boys might say that it would be better to choose the boy for the baseball cards collecting club because boys know more about baseball, and a girl might not be very interested and therefore would not be a good fit with the rest of the group (Killen & Stangor, 2001).

Compared with adolescents, school-age children tend to accept rules and authority. They assume that if a rule exists it must be there for a reason. This is a very different stance from that of a young adolescent, who analyzes adult rules and dictates for evidence of inconsistency. School-age children's general acceptance of authority makes them teachable and coachable. At the same time, since they tend to believe that authority is valid, they are often very uncomfortable with peers who openly defy authority.

School-age children are very aware of social norms. They are motivated to fit into their peer group and are very attuned to adult standards. They are particularly aware of rules and try to follow the rules of their teacher and school, at least in public. In general school-age children most often fit Kohlberg's (1984) level of moral development called the "Authority and Social Order Orientation." They tend to be conformist, going along with rules because their peers do. Although children may know the principle contained in a rule, they often follow rules unthinkingly because "that's what you're supposed to do." However, 9- and 10-year-olds *can* articulate reasons for rules as based on fairness, equality, and prevention of harm (Killen, Lee-Kim, McGlothlin, & Stangor, 2002).

Given this conformist moral orientation, school-age children do not like to be seen as "deviant." When a school-age child consistently ignores or violates school rules, his peers often stigmatize him and try to avoid him, because they do not want to be associated with wrongdoing. Children with untreated ADHD and behavioral disorders are often stigmatized by their peers. Peers worry that associating with the child with ADHD will cause them to get in trouble (Barkley, 2003).

SENSE OF SELF

The school-age child's sense of self is based on comparisons with others. Whereas the preschool child wishfully tries to imbue the self with power through fantasy expressed in play about adult roles or superheroes, the school-age child begins to evaluate herself in more realistic ways, particularly by comparing herself with her peers. By age 7 the child measures her abilities by ranking herself within her peer group. During middle childhood, "children become progressively more accurate in assessing their own competence in relation to their peers" (Harter, 1983b, p. 336). They know who is "the best" and "the worst," as well as gradations in between.

The school-age child is much more sensitive than the preschooler to the feedback she gets from peers. She thinks about her actions in the light of others' responses and mentally rehearses what she is going to do with an eye to how her peers are likely to respond. If her friends admire her ability at jump rope, she feels pride; if peers make fun of her mistakes, she is vulnerable to negative feelings—anxiety, embarrassment, self-doubt. Compared to the preschooler, then, her self-esteem depends more on her awareness of how she is perceived by others. However, the school-age child's self-esteem is only relatively dependent on her social status. The development of self-esteem in middle childhood is strongly related to a history of being accepted and supported by parents (Harter, 1999). Children with high self-esteem in earlier periods of development are likely to be more resilient in the face of teasing or rejection by peers than are children whose self-esteem has been damaged by insecure attachments or maltreatment.

Identification

School-age children, in contrast to preschoolers, take real people as heroes and role models. It is common for children to admire their parents, particularly the same-sex parent, with whom they identify. Since most elementary school teachers are women, girls frequently identify with teachers they admire. Children also attempt to imitate public figures such as sports stars. For example, a boy shooting baskets alone began to speak in a sportscaster's voice, describing himself as Michael Jordan: "Jordan takes the pass. He goes up, he's airborne! He scores!" This 10-year-old's identification with a great sports hero has much in common with the preschooler's identification with superhero characters. The difference is that the school-age child chooses real-life models and uses the identification to support the development of real-world skills.

The school-age child's increasing peer orientation also means that she takes older same-sex peers as role models and objects of identification. Often older siblings fill this role, as well. Younger school-age children admire the accomplishments and abilities of older peers. At the same time, an older child's skill in basketball seems more attainable to a younger child than becoming like Michael Jordan. Younger children watch older children to learn how to improve their skills and how to behave in new situations. Older children sometimes take pleasure in acting as mentors for younger ones. They enjoy being admired and like to demonstrate their skills. Often a younger child will risk doing something that makes him anxious if he knows an admired older peer has done it. Recently, the parent of a 10-year-old boy who was being referred to me said, "He didn't want to see you until we told him that Chris [a 14-year-old he looked up to] had seen you. He asked Chris, and Chris told him you were a cool guy. Then he had no problem coming."

Motivation to Achieve, Achievement, and Self-Esteem

The school-age child internalizes expectations for achievement based on identifications with parents and parents' explicit values about achievement. Research on how parents can positively influence the child's motivation to achieve identifies the following factors:

- Make expectations for achievement developmentally appropriate, so the child will feel competent in her efforts.
- Create a warm and supportive relationship with the child that encourages her to identify with parents as role models.
- Communicate expectations for achievement that are high but realistic, in terms of the child's potentials.
- Provide scaffolding and become directly involved in learning experiences for children at home. (Sénéchal & LeFevre, 2002; Eccles et al., 1998; Weinfield et al., 2002)

The school-age child evaluates himself by his degree of success in "getting good at" skills ranging from doing multiplication problems to mastering increasingly difficult levels of video games. His evaluation of his success makes particularly important contributions to self-esteem and overall valuation of self. The school-age child's motivation to put forth and realize goals is strongly influenced by previous successes and failures, by affective memories of how it felt to succeed or fail, and by internalized beliefs about his ability and efficacy (Bandura, 1994). How a child comes to feel about herself regarding her ability to succeed is an especially important aspect of school-age development, because future motivation to succeed depends a great deal on her accomplishments and internal evaluations of success during middle childhood (Eccles et al., 1998).

Compared to younger children, school-age children are more likely to respond to failure with negative judgments about the self. In part this derives from their more realistic understanding of failure and success, an understanding that is constantly reinforced by self-comparisons with other children (Eccles et al., 1998). However, normally developing school-age children generally do not view themselves as globally successful or unsuccessful. Rather, they assess their competence in separate domains. A child who knows she is an excellent student may assess herself as less adept in making friends. Even if a child does not feel competent in all areas, the ability to establish niches of competence contributes to self-esteem. By contrast, school-age children with histories of abuse or mental health problems such as depression, anxiety disorders, and ADHD may internalize views of self that emphasize lack of competence as well as beliefs that effort will not lead to success. Such negative views reduce the child's motivation to take on learning tasks and may lead to avoidance, which, in circular fashion, increases their sense of incompetence (Harter, 1998).

The Relationship between Self-Control and Self-Concept

School-age children put a strong emphasis on feeling and acting in control. By ages 8 or 9 the child tries to control his behavior in order to live up to his internal standards, not simply to please others. Feeling in control of one's emotions and behavior fosters self-esteem (Harter, 1998). A 9-year-old who breaks down and cries in response to losing a game later feels disturbed and embarrassed by his loss of control.

Similarly, a school-age child with learning disabilities becomes aware that she cannot control the way her brain works. She is aware of a required goal—to read a passage—and also realizes that she cannot do it. As she realizes what she cannot do and compares her own performance with peers who read with ease, her self-esteem declines. For learning-disabled children, as well as other children with less ability than their peers in pursuits important to school-age children, social comparison puts self-esteem at risk. Harter (1998) notes: "Thus, the very ability and penchant to compare the self with others makes one's self-concept vulnerable in those domains that are valued" (p. 572).

SELF-ESTEEM ISSUES OF A CHILD WITH LEARNING DISORDERS:
A BRIEF CASE EXAMPLE

Jill was an 8-year-old girl I saw in supportive psychotherapy to help her cope with serious learning disorders in reading, writing, and auditory processing. In sessions, Jill worked diligently on school-like tasks. She would laboriously write stories and bring in books to read to me. Her performance was slow, labored, and full of errors; yet, her choice of academic tasks demonstrated her strong motivation to succeed, her need to call attention to the problem, and her frustration over not being successful. Jill was aware of her learning problems and spoke about her frustration and desire to do better. Jill presented a vivid image of her struggle with learning disorders. As we talked about how she felt when she couldn't understand what the teacher was asking, I said that kids with a learning problem often blamed themselves and felt dumb. Jill said, "I don't blame myself. I blame my imaginary friend. What I do is when I don't know the answer I take a gun and shoot my imaginary friend." I said, "So you blame her for not knowing the answer?" "Yeah, if she can't tell the answer, I blast her." Jill was attempting to externalize the problem by blaming her imaginary companion. She knew very well that *she* didn't know the answer, but was using a typical school-age defense of displacing negative feelings about the self into fantasy.

Jill also tried to compensate for feelings of inadequacy caused by her learning disorders by identifying with boys. She made fun of the "wimpy" feminine girls in her class and claimed that she was the toughest girl. She said that boys were more fun to play with because they played "rough and tough." She was trying to disassociate herself from a gender stereotype of middle childhood—that girls are "good" in school—because she fell short of the academic skills girls are supposed to have; in compensation, she tried to fit herself into one of the male gender stereotypes—that boys are more physical and tough.

Capacity for Self-Observation

School-age children have much more capacity for self-observation than do younger children. They usually are at ease answering the question "What are you good at?" because they can take an outside perspective on themselves. They have an image of what they are like and are aware of their strengths and weaknesses (Harter, 1998). By contrast, a preschool child has trouble answering the same question, because she cannot take an outside perspective on herself. School-age children can also give concrete self-descriptions that demonstrate a more nuanced view of themselves: "I'm pretty friendly. I'm getting better at basketball. I'm bad at division. I used to write scratchy, but my handwriting is good now." School-age children can see themselves more realistically and accurately. As they move into the latter part of middle childhood, their self-evaluations tend to be increasingly consistent with the ways others see them (Harter, 1999). Self-knowledge increases across middle childhood (Flavell, Green, & Flavell, 2000). A recent interesting study documented this progress by focusing on children's understanding of where the knowledge resides—in one's parents or oneself? Children were asked such questions as "Who knows best what you are thinking?" and "Who knows best when you are hungry?" At age 6, over 70% of children said that an adult—most often a parent, sometimes a teacher—knew best what they were feeling. At age 10, ideas about the locus of self-knowledge had shifted dramatically, with 75% of 10-year-olds stating that *they* knew best what they were thinking or feeling (Burton & Mitchell, 2003).

In middle childhood, the self-image is based not simply on immediate ideas about the self but also on comparisons of present and past representations of the self. New cognitive abilities allow children to understand their earlier experiences in new ways. The ability to decenter in middle childhood allows the child to differentiate between past and present self-images, contributing to new views of the self (Gemelli, 1996). A child may say, "When I was 4, I used to think about robbers and monsters, and I'd be scared to go down to the basement. Now [at age 10], I still get that feeling when I go down there, but I know it's not real. I'm not a scaredy-cat like I was when I was 4." The ability to differentiate between past and present viewpoints has important implications for intervention with school-age children. In Chapter 4, I described an 8-year-old, Alex, whose continuing fears were rooted in experiences of abuse by his father when he was 3 and 4. The cognitive aspect of Alex's treatment involved helping him understand that he was responding to certain anxiety-producing situations from the perspective of a 3-year-old, and pointing out that now, as an 8-year-old, he knew much better how to appraise situations and get help.

Only near the very end of the school-age period can children begin to reflect on psychological reasons for their strengths or problems. For the most part, school-age children are oriented toward the external and concrete. Questions about motivations underlying their behavior are likely to be met with "I don't know." But school-age children can at least identify a problem or concern. This has implications for intervention. A school-age child can participate in setting goals. He can say, for example, "I wish I had more friends. Sometimes other kids tease me." This can open the way to conversations, either directly or in displacement, about the skills needed to get along with peers.

Gender and Sense of Self

At the beginning of middle childhood, at ages 6 or 7, the child increasingly adopts gender-specific behavior as defined by cultural prescriptions and avoids behavior associated with the opposite gender. This development coincides with the awareness of *gender constancy*, the understanding that gender cannot be changed. The child's implicit awareness that "I am a girl and I will always be a girl" leads to an insistence on behaving "like a girl, not like a boy," in terms of culturally defined characteristics. Gender identity now includes more specific information than the fact of being a girl or boy. In early childhood, families take a primary role in the socialization of gender (McHale et al., 2003). In middle childhood, particularly through observing older peers, the child continues to learn, for example, what girls are like, what girls like to do, what they do in certain situations. Identification with same-sex peers, relatives, and other adults, including media celebrities, furthers gender socialization.

As the school-age years proceed, children continue to elaborate gender roles. In general, girls value relationships and nurturance, whereas boys emphasize personal autonomy and competition. O'Brien (1992) describes a study of boys' and girls' interactional styles in middle childhood that illustrates these gender contrasts: "Girls' conversations are marked by expressions of acknowledgment and agreement and the regular exchange of speaking turns; boys interrupt each other, make demands and refuse to comply with others' demands, tell jokes or stories, and generally compete with each other for attention" (p. 339). These gender-based styles of social relating tend to reinforce gender segregation in school-age children, who report preferences for play with same-sex peers and find less pleasure in cross-sex play. Children who prefer playing with opposite-sex friends are likely to be stigmatized by their same-sex peers (Martin & Fabes, 2001).

While these broad constructions of male emphasis on autonomy and female emphasis of relatedness are useful metaphors for understanding gender differences, empirical studies show many more similarities than differences in the development of girls and boys (Hyde & Plant, 1995; Killen et al., 2002). O'Brien (1992) points out that older school-age children tend to recognize their similarities and the ways feminine and masculine behavior overlap, even while they maintain sex segregation in play. Rather than thinking of boys and girls as rigidly polarized in the development of the self, it is helpful to think of a "relational self" and an "autonomous self" as coexisting within each individual. Gender socialization influences how girls and boys balance these two competing self-orientations (Atwood & Safyer, 1993; Killen et al., 2002).

Precursors of Sexual Orientation in Middle Childhood?

Sexual orientation does not appear with clarity until sometime in early to late adolescence (Savin-Williams, 2001). This finding seems unsurprising, given that emerging sexuality has a physical basis in hormonal changes at puberty. Gay or lesbian orientation is ambiguous and fluid for many adolescents because powerful messages of homophobic prejudice create conflicts that may prevent them from exploring same-sex interests. Some research suggests that males become aware of same-sex attractions earlier in adolescence as compared with females. A significant number of lesbian and bisexual women report that same-sex attractions did not begin until adulthood (Diamond, 2000). However, in anecdotal accounts and retrospective studies some adults recall that their same-sex attractions began just before puberty, between the ages of 10 and 12. This is the same period when many children also become generally aware of heterosexual attractions.

It has been hypothesized that an ultimate gay, lesbian, or bisexual orientation is predicted in childhood by vague discomfort with one's gender, interest in opposite-gender activities, and the emergence of "sexual questioning" or same-sex attractions just before puberty (Bailey & Zucker, 1995). But, to date, no prospective longitudinal research has validated these ideas. A recent study suggested that older school-age children's doubts about their heterosexuality might be a link to a later sexual-minority orientation (Carver, Egan, & Perry, 2004). However, this study did not ask children *directly* about same-sex attractions. Instead, the researchers posed statements such as "Some girls think that they'll be a wife someday BUT Other girls don't think that they'll be a wife" (Carver et al., 2004, p. 45). Children who identified with the second half of this and similar statements were judged to be questioning heterosexuality. Whether such answers to these indirect questions predict a minority sexual orientation is impossible to determine. Without longitudinal studies that follow subjects from late school age to the end of adolescence, it remains unclear whether particular characteristics of school-age children, including presumed sexual questioning, are related to the development of sexual orientation. Savin-Williams (2001) argues that there are a number of different developmental trajectories to one's eventual sexual orientation. This makes it difficult to specify the middle childhood precursors of gay, lesbian, bisexual, or heterosexual identity.

Racial and Ethnic Awareness in Middle Childhood

Although children take in information about ethnicity during early childhood, they become more aware of their racial and ethnic identity during the elementary school years. At about the same time children attain gender constancy, they realize that ethnicity is also not changeable (Aboud, 1984). This is in part a function of general cognitive tendencies toward identifying and classifying differences. Implicit and explicit socialization experiences and exposure to different groups at school also increase ethnic awareness. Race, ethnicity, and gender strongly influence peer relationships. Just as boys and girls form separate groups, younger school-age children tend to choose as friends peers with whom they identify. This trend continues throughout the middle years. In spite of these patterns of choosing friends, there is evidence that prejudice based on stereotypes declines during middle childhood, as a result of improving cognitive ability to differentiate between learned stereotypes and personal experience. Unlike younger children, who egocentrically tend to identify with people like themselves, 8- and 9-year-olds take a more complex view of race and ethnic differences, seeing *human* attributes of people of different races and noting differences among people of the same race (Doyle & Aboud, 1995).

Antibias curricula in schools that build on the more complex thought of school-age children have had some success. For example, a program that encouraged open talk about race and ethnic differences and stereotypes, as well as the internal and personal qualities of people, led to reduced bias in 10-year-old children (Aboud & Fenwick, 1999). In schools with multicultural populations, children's awareness of their own ethnic identity is greater because they interact with peers who look different from themselves and speak different dialects or languages. In such settings, the tendency to form cliques based only on race or ethnic identification is somewhat disrupted by children who resist race-based group dynamics. School-age children in multicultural schools and camps are more likely to interact with one another across ethnic lines and to form friendships based on personal liking (Moore, 2002). By contrast, children living in homogeneous communities have less awareness and experience of ethnic differences and are more likely to believe racial stereotypes.

In general, minority children show greater awareness of race and ethnicity than do children who identify with the majority group (Verkuyten & Thijs, 2001). Minority children learn about their minority status and majority values through personal experiences, mass media, and exposure to institutions such as schools where majority norms dominate. Cross (1987) has shown that African American children with good self-esteem nevertheless may show strong interest in white cultural symbols and attitudes because they correctly perceive the status and power associated with them. This interest in the majority culture also indicates the tendency of many minority families to socialize their children to develop "bicultural competence" so that they can function in both the majority and minority cultures (McAdoo, 2001).

M. B. Spencer (1987) has argued that children in "castelike minorities," whose group faces discrimination and devaluation based on racist views in the majority society, may devalue their own ethnicity as they become aware of the majority culture's negative views. This awareness frequently occurs during the middle years, when new cognitive abilities and exposure to the wider world allow the child to realize that others can perceive her negatively because of categorical attributes that identify her has a member of a particular group. A recent large-scale study suggests how common this experience is for African American children: 67% indicated that they had been insulted or demeaned on the basis of race (Simons, Murry, McLoyd, Lin, Cutrona, & Conger, 2002). Many minority group members recall the first incidents of prejudice toward them as occurring in elementary school, as in the following case example:

A biracial child of a single white mother had lived in an ethnically mixed urban neighborhood during her early years. Although she identified with her mother's ethnicity at that time, she often saw her paternal grandparents, who were African American, and realized vaguely that she was a mix of black and white. When she was 9, her family moved to a small town where she was the only "nonwhite" child in her school. She was shocked when other children called her racial epithets and rejected her. To defend herself, she denied the black part of her identity and made up a new one, telling other children, "I'm Filipino!"

Although this example is about a biracial child, it reflects the realization that comes to most minority children—that they can be subject to social rejection on a categorical rather than a personal basis. As the result of progressive advances in perspective taking and general social knowledge during middle childhood, children become increasingly aware of stereotypes regarding race and ethnicity. This means that minority children increasingly are able to pick up on much more subtle messages of prejudice than overt derogation. Awareness of broadly held stereotypes and the ability to intuit prejudicial beliefs in individuals develops gradually between ages 6 and 10 (McKown & Weinstein, 2003). For example, a child in third grade, "may infer that her teacher expects less of children from her ethnic group; this observation may in turn affect how the child responds to the teacher's instructional strategies" (McKown & Weinstein, 2003, p. 498). When a child becomes aware that she is being viewed stereotypically by an adult in authority, she may not perform as well academically because she expects to be judged negatively. This scenario is most likely when the child is not buffered by countervailing forces, such as supportive parents and peers who encourage her to succeed (McKown & Weinstein, 2003).

During the school-age years, when self-esteem is strongly influenced by the child's sense of how well she is accepted by peers and by how adults in authority regard her, the minority child faces greater risks of either devaluing her minority identity, internalizing the stereotypical view that she is less competent, or giving up on academic pursuits because she believes she will not be evaluated fairly (Steele, 1997). In view of these risks, it is important for minority parents and other significant adults to stress the strengths and values of their ethnicity so that the child can react to racism and discrimination from the perspective of a positive ethnic identity, essentially realizing, "That's the way they feel about us. But that's their problem. I feel good about who I am" (Miller & MacIntosh, 1999). Mentoring programs that offer sustained relationships with older successful role models can also help offset risk (Barron-McKeagney, Woody, & D'Souza, 2001). Intervention can also incorporate positive perspectives on race and ethnicity. School-age minority children who present with low self-esteem should be assessed for conflicts about their racial identity and offered positive messages about their ethnicity by their parents and therapist or school social worker. Positive ethnic socialization is likely to be most powerful when the practitioner represents the same group as the child (Greene, 1992).

OVERVIEW OF DEVELOPMENTAL PROGRESS IN MIDDLE CHILDHOOD

Since the period of middle childhood covers a long time span (from 6 to 11 or 12), it may be useful to step back from the description of domains of development and to present a brief summary of the child's progress during this period. Near the end of this period, the child of 10 or 11 who has a history of successful mastery of developmental tasks and who has not yet entered puberty is likely to appear confident, competent, reasonable, and calm. He is capable of logical thought, can look at situations from multiple perspectives, and has many adaptive strategies of self-regulation. He has developed skills through concentration on learning and practice. Several years ago when I told a colleague who had grown children that my son was 10 years old, she exclaimed, "Ten-year-olds should be bronzed like baby shoes!" She went on to say that 10 is a "perfect age" because children are mature, self-controlled, relatively independent, and self-possessed. If they were "preserved" at 10, she said, they—and their parents—would not have to go through the struggles of adolescence.

Although middle childhood is generally seen as continuing up to age 11 or 12, during the last year or so of the period there are signs of the disequilibrium that characterizes early adolescence. The onset of puberty and the adolescent growth spurt begin for many children between 10 and 12, with girls, on average, being a year ahead of boys. While 11- and 12-year-olds retain the cognitive abilities they have developed over the course of middle childhood, the internal stresses of rapid physical growth, hormonal changes, sexual maturation, and sexual interest challenge the school-age child's capacity to maintain calm and self-control. Consequently, many 11-year-olds, compared with just a year earlier, are more active, defiant of authority, self-centered, and emotionally labile. The child's self-regulatory capacities, while still functioning well most of the time, cannot always withstand the new pressures of growth toward adolescence. The child of 11 or 12 has consolidated the developmental accomplishments of middle childhood but is moving into the transformations of self in adolescence.

APPENDIX 11.1. Summary of Middle Childhood Development, 6 to 11 or 12 Years of Age

Overall Tasks

• To develop and utilize a sense of calm, educability, and self-control
• To develop real-world skills and a sense of competence
• To establish oneself in the world of peers

Attachment

• Child uses autonomous coping rather than attachment seeking in situations of mild stress (6 years+)
• Rituals symbolizing attachment persist—bedtime routines, gestures of affection (6 years+)
• Proximity seeking may be activated in situations of severe stress or during transitions, such as entry into school (6 years+)
• Attachment needs are increasingly expressed in friendships with peers (6 years+)

Social Development

• Increasing orientation toward peers, development of friendships (6 years+)
• Social skills (sharing, negotiation, etc.) develop through peer interaction (6 years+)
• Development of peer group norms and status hierarchies (6 years+)
• Elaboration of gender roles and behavior (6 years+)
• Prosocial behavior, based on internalization of values and improved perspective taking (6 years+)
• Social perspective taking: increasingly clear understanding of others' viewpoints, social expectations, and social cues (6 years+)
• Awareness of the psychological intent of others (8–10 years)
• Holds two opposing viewpoints in mind at the same time (10–12 years)

Language and Communication

• Basic facility in syntax and grammar established (6–7 years)
• Gradually increasing understanding of nuances of meaning and more difficult grammatical features such as the passive voice (6–7 years+)
• Gradually increasing ability to put thoughts and feelings into words (6 years+)
• Narrative ability—child can tell an organized story (7 years+)
• Understanding of wordplay, jokes, figures of speech, metaphor (8–10 years)

Play and Fantasy

- Play is increasingly sublimated into a work orientation, emphasizing physical skills and intellectual competence (6–7 years+)
- Play continues to be an important source of pleasure and discharge, but now is increasingly ritualized into games (6 years+)
- Fantasy play is increasingly ritualized and rule-governed (6 years+)
- Uses of fantasy include displacement of feelings and wishes into imaginary scenarios and imagining the self in more competent or grown-up roles (6 years+)
- Interest in collections and hobbies (7–8 years+)
- Interest in games involving planning and strategy (10–12 years)

Cognitive Development

- Increasingly accurate perception of reality (reality testing) (6 years+)
- Reversibility—systematic ability to analyze perceptions by thinking back over them (6–7 years)
- Improving understanding of cause and effect; decline in magical thinking (6–7 years)
- Decentration: decline in egocentrism and increase in decentered thought allow child to distinguish between subjective and objective reality (6–7 years+)
- Concrete operations: processes of logic and reasoning can be applied to understand immediate reality (6–7 years+)
- Developmental spurt in cognitive functions at about age 7: spatial organization; visual organizational ability; time orientation; distinctions between parts and wholes; seriation; auditory processing (6–8 years)
- Memory: improved registration and categorization of memory contributes to mastery of academic tasks (6 years+)
- Executive processes: new skills in thinking about problem solving, sustaining attention to intellectual tasks (7–8 years+)

Self-Regulation

- Application of cognitive strategies to self-regulation: logical thinking; representational competence; conscious control of arousal and anxiety; using thinking to delay acting on impulses; conscious intent to stay focused on attainment of goals (6 years+)
- Internalization of values, expectations, rules, and social norms fosters self-control (6 years+)
- Psychological defense mechanisms become more effective in limiting anxiety (6 years+)

- Desire to receive approval of peers sets limits on impulsive behavior (6–7 years+)
- Capacity to see conflicting views and tolerate ambivalence improves self-control (10 years)

Moral Development

- Decentered thinking and perspective taking enable child to better understand and empathize with the needs of others (6 years+)
- Development of the conscience (superego) as an internal force controlling behavior (5–7 years)
- Cognitive understanding of rationales, rules, and norms of correct behavior (6–7 years+)
- Social conformity and acceptance of authority supports adherence to rules and expectations (6 years+)

Sense of Self

- Self-esteem based on awareness of competence, status in peer group (6–7 years+)
- Identification with parents, other adults, and peers as role models (6–7 years+)
- Capacity for self-control influences self-esteem and self-concept (6–7 years+)
- Increasing awareness of identity—personal characteristics, gender expectations, racial and ethnic identity (7 years+)
- Awareness of racism, negative stereotypes applied to the self (7–8 years+)
- Increasing capacity for self-observation (8 years+)
- Ability to make comparisons between past and present characteristics of the self (7–8 years+)
- Internalized values create need to gain self-esteem by pleasing oneself, not just others (8 years)

CHAPTER 12

Practice with School-Age Children

School-age children are usually referred because of problems that show up at school. Examples of typical presenting symptoms include the following:

- Behavioral and academic problems
- Attention/concentration problems
- Restlessness/hyperactivity
- Impulsive, aggressive, oppositional, or defiant behavior
- Poor peer relationships
- Social withdrawal/social immaturity/rejection by peers
- Generalized anxiety and separation anxiety

From a developmental perspective, these problems can be understood as difficulties in mastering the tasks of middle childhood. Often these symptoms represent problems in self-regulation, particularly overreliance on the defenses of early childhood rather than more mature and adaptive regulatory strategies. The child may be unable to consistently maintain the self-control, calmness, flexibility, and educability associated with middle childhood. Since the same symptoms can represent different problems, a careful assessment is necessary. Attention to the child's progress in different developmental domains helps specify areas of strength and areas requiring intervention.

ASSESSMENT

The assessment process for school-age children should recognize the increasing complexity of the interaction between the child's developmental progress and the increasingly complicated environments he enters.

Assessment should draw on multiple sources of information, including parents, other caregivers, and teachers as observers of the child, as well as on several observations. Only rarely can evaluation findings based on one session be considered reliable and complete. The child should be observed in multiple contexts, ideally both individually and in a family session, and also at home and at school. Scales of developmental level and symptomatology assess child behavior and specific problems. These include comprehensive instruments, such as the Child Behavior Checklist (Achenbach, 1991), and more specialized questionnaires on problems such as ADHD (attention-deficit/hyperactivity disorder), depression, and anxiety disorders. Self-report instruments that ask the child to assess himself should be viewed with caution. They often do not produce accurate information about the younger school-age child, because he tends to deny problems and frequently can figure out which answers will make him appear "normal" (Folman, 1995). After about age 9, children's self-reports tend to become more accurate (Kazdin & Weiz, 2003). While scales, symptom checklists, and structured interview protocols are helpful, they should not be considered as substitutes for observations and clinical interviews of the child. (For an excellent review of the range of assessment scales and structured interviews, see Netherton, Holmes, and Walker [1999].)

Evaluation of a school-age child should involve the following areas of assessment.

Developmental Level

Sarnoff (1976) defines psychopathology in the middle years as resulting from "the inability of the child to produce at appropriate times the pliability, calm and educability expected in a latency age child" (p. 186). If we observe this inability, then questions about the child's functioning in several developmental domains must be considered. Is she relying on omnipotent fantasies? Are her coping strategies and defenses more like those of a younger child? Does she remain more egocentric than expected? Does she withdraw from peers or show an inability to get along with them? Does she have difficulty regulating impulses? Are there cognitive or language deficits or academic difficulties that are suggestive of learning or language disorders?

History of Developmental Interferences

In taking the child's developmental and interactional history, possible developmental interferences—such as exposure to violence, chronic parental fighting, divorce, the loss of family members, abuse, and trauma—should be noted. Very often, the child's inability to proceed with normal development in middle childhood is tied to defenses and coping mechanisms established in response to anxiety-provoking experiences during early childhood. For example, a history of physical or sexual abuse may result in a child's using withdrawal into fantasy and dissociation as preferred defenses. Such children may appear quiet and shy but seem "normal" in that they do not have behavioral problems. However, when they begin school, their reliance on daydreaming and dissociation makes it hard for them to concentrate on learning. As with all emergency-based coping strategies, dissociation helped the child survive the abuse, but if it persists as a defense it will interfere with developmental tasks in middle childhood.

Reality Orientation

Assessment of orientation to reality helps determine the child's developmental level. Middle childhood is characterized by increasing appreciation of the demands of following rules, doing well in school, and being perceived as similar to one's peers. The school-age child is motivated to succeed and willing to practice to develop skills. It is useful to analyze whether she is giving priority to the demands of external reality (parents, school, peer relationships) or whether she is drawn toward magical thinking as a defense against feelings of inadequacy or vulnerability in the real world.

Problems That Interfere with Developmental Tasks in Middle Childhood: Language Disorders, Learning Disabilities, and Attention-Deficit/Hyperactivity Disorder

In many cultures, including the United States, adequate development during middle childhood is judged by the child's ability to master increasingly complex cognitive tasks. Success in these tasks is measured by the child's school performance. The evaluator of a school-age child needs to be alert for problems that may compromise the child's ability to learn. Three prominent contributors to academic difficulties are language disorders, learning disabilities, and ADHD.

Language Disorders

Language disorders are often diagnosed during the preschool years. Sometimes preschool children with language disorders are referred for evaluation because of behavioral problems, particularly with oppositional behavior, which may be at least partly the result of the child's ongoing frustration at not being able to understand or make herself understood. Language disorders include difficulty articulating words and problems with receptive or expressive language.

When we observe language problems, referral for a speech and language evaluation is necessary. Since hearing impairment is a common cause of language disorders, a hearing test may also be needed. If English is not the first language of the child, the referral request should ask for an assessment of the child's abilities in her first language, in order to distinguish between actual language disorders and problems associated with second-language acquisition (Canino & Spurlock, 2000).

Some children who have less overt language disorders may escape notice until they reach elementary school age. Rather than having an obvious articulation problem, these children may have trouble organizing what they want to say and appear to have trouble expressing themselves. Children who have a history of a language disorder during the preschool years often develop reading and writing disorders during school age. In particular, children with problems in receptive language are more likely to have learning disorders in the area of reading. Their difficulties differentiating speech sounds contribute to problems in "segmenting speech into phonemes" represented by the written alphabet and associating letter symbols with sounds (Lyon, Fletcher, & Barnes, 2003, p. 544). It has been hypothesized that reading/writing disorders are an extension of the neurobiological mechanisms underlying expressive and receptive language problems (Eden & Zeffiro, 1998).

Learning Disabilities

Learning disabilities (LD) tend to become evident when the child reaches school age and begins to have difficulty with specific academic tasks in the early grades. Neurobiological impairments involving problems with memory, logic, information processing, or visual–spatial organization usually underlie these academic problems (Lyon et al., 2003). A child may have difficulty taking in information, remembering it, mentally sorting it out or organizing it, or expressing it—or some combination of these. Learning disabilities represent specific rather than generalized developmental problems, in the sense that a child with LD may have normal intelligence and function well across most areas of development but have specific cognitive deficits that affect her ability to read, write, do math problems, remember information and instructions, or integrate information. It is beyond the purpose of this section to describe the whole range of learning disabilities, and instead I will illustrate their potential developmental impact and importance in evaluation by briefly discussing dyslexia.

Dyslexia, or "word recognition disability," is the most common learning disorder. The dyslexic child has difficulty decoding single words and organizing sequences of words. Her reading is slow and laborious. Because she must put so much energy into the cognitive task of decoding, her comprehension ability suffers. Without intervention, the dyslexic child faces an increasingly difficult struggle since school tasks assume proficiency in reading. In a general evaluation, a practitioner can ask parents about the child's reading ability and review report cards. One can ask a child to read a passage appropriate to her grade level aloud and observe for fluency, errors, and level of frustration. If this initial screening suggests a reading disability, the practitioner can refer the child for specialized testing by an educational psychologist. Some tests, such as the Decoding Skills Test, can identify dyslexia as early as grade 1, which allows for early intervention. (See Elbert [1999] for a discussion of tests for dyslexia and other learning disabilities.) Even when a practitioner is not a specialist in learning disabilities, her early identification of a reading problem can make an important difference in a young child's academic development. When dyslexia is diagnosed and effectively treated in the early elementary years, its long-term negative effects can be prevented (Foorman & Torgesen, 2001).

Assessing Learning Disabilities in the Context of Culture. In a multicultural society such as the United States, it is important to view the results of testing in the wider context of the child's culture, so that cultural differences are not mistaken for learning or language disorders. Students who speak English as a second language may not perform well on tests conducted in English. African American children who speak "black English" may be misdiagnosed because their language does not match the "standard English" of the test instruments. In assessing culturally diverse children it is necessary to look cautiously at the results of tests that have been normed on white middle-class children. If items on cognitive tests reflect real and assumptive worlds that are unfamiliar to the child, the child's actual cognitive abilities may not be elicited, and scores will be lower (Garcia Coll & Magnuson, 1999). Canino and Spurlock (2000) note: "Normal but underachieving culturally diverse students whose language at home differs from that used in school are often overrepresented in programs for the learning disabled" (p. 29). The best antidote to this problem is for the tester to be familiar with the culture of the child being tested so that she has a broader context for understanding a child's performance.

Secondary Effects of Learning Disabilities. Children with learning disabilities often become disruptive out of frustration with not being able to do academic tasks. But they may get labeled as kids with behavior problems and be referred for mental health evaluation. If testing shows clear learning or language disorders, specialized educational intervention—special periods with a teacher consultant, tutoring, language therapy, and so on—will be needed. Psychotherapy is obviously not the treatment of choice for academic skills disorders, but it is sometimes needed to help children deal with the emotional fallout of their learning problems.

Attention-Deficit/Hyperactivity Disorder

If a child's problems revolve around hyperactivity, difficulty concentrating, short attention span, tendency to get overstimulated easily, impulsivity, and distractibility, one needs to assess for ADHD. Because ADHD is 3–6 times more common in boys than girls (Barkley, 2003), I will use the male pronoun in the following discussion.

ADHD compromises the school-age tasks of learning to maintain calm, sustain attention, and think in organized sequences. A child with ADHD may start an activity or a learning task requiring these qualities with enthusiasm, but as his attention wanes, he cannot sustain the task through its various steps. Then off-task behavior, often perceived as disruptive, begins to emerge. Further, he has more difficulty than a normal child in inhibiting responses to stimuli extraneous to learning tasks, and thus is much more often distracted and off-task (Barkley, 2003). His learning often has a hit-or-miss quality, since he may not attend to directions or may rush through school work. Because kids with ADHD have more difficulty in inhibiting impulses, they often cannot wait for their turn, interrupt when others are talking, talk constantly about what they are thinking, and begin a task before they have finished listening to the directions. All these characteristics make it difficult for them to function well in school.

By the early elementary years, peers begin to avoid or reject the child with ADHD. The reasons for rejection include ADHD children's frequent interpersonal intrusiveness and violation of social boundaries, their unpredictable impulsiveness, their perceived failure to abide by "the rules"—which are so important to school-age children—and their perceived obliviousness to situational and social cues. Over time, the negative responses of others may contribute to a negative sense of self.

To make the ADHD diagnosis, symptoms must be present persistently *across* situations—at home and at school. If a parent reports symptoms of ADHD in a 7-year-old at home, but the teacher reports that the child is able to concentrate and complete work adequately and is not unusually active or fidgety, this criterion is not met, and the clinician should look for other explanations for the child's behavior at home. The following areas of evaluation will help clarify the ADHD diagnosis.

History. Parents will often recall a school-age child with ADHD as *always* having been hyperactive, impulsive, and inattentive. By contrast, the child whose ADHD-like symptoms are based on anxiety or on reactions to stress or trauma may be remembered as developing normally up to the time that ADHD symptoms began to show up. Obviously, it will not be easy to differentiate between these two types if the child and family have had chronic exposure to severe stressors, such as ongoing domestic and/or community violence, sustained poverty and homelessness, or living in a dangerous neighborhood. School-age children who were chronically traumatized during their earliest years may have such poor regulatory capacities that they appear to have ADHD. However, for these children, PTSD (posttraumatic stress disorder) is likely to be a more accurate and useful diagnosis (Glod & Teicher, 1996).

Another aspect of the history taking is to inquire about ADHD in the child's siblings, parents, and other relatives. There is evidence that the neurobiological deficits characterizing ADHD are genetically inherited, and it is not unusual to hear that one of the child's parents or other close relatives had symptoms of ADHD as a child (Barkley, 2003).

Observation. Very often, children with ADHD will appear more active, restless, fidgety, and will shift rapidly from one activity to another, even in a one-on-one situation in a practitioner's office. One's subjective impression will be that the child is "in overdrive" and doesn't seem able to slow down. Some children with milder ADHD, however, will not appear driven in the first office visit, possibly because the environment is novel and therefore more compelling of their attention, or because being in an office with one person is much less overstimulating for the child than being in a busy classroom. It is often very helpful, and eye-opening, for the practitioner to observe the child in the classroom.

Teachers' Reports. It is very useful to speak with the child's teacher to learn about the details of his classroom behavior. The descriptions of teachers often bring life to the general categories of impulsivity and hyperactivity: "In the space of 5 minutes, he tapped his pencil on the desk, dropped it on the floor three times, got out of his seat three times without—as far as I could tell—intending to go somewhere, and even when he was sitting still, he was kicking the seat of the student in front of him, not maliciously, just out of nervous energy."

Rating Scales. It is also useful to have parents, teachers, and other adults who interact regularly with the child fill out rating scales designed to assess for the symptoms of ADHD. The Revised Conners Parent and Teachers Rating Scale (Goyette, Conners, & Ulrich, 1978), the ADHD Rating Scale (DuPaul, 1991), and the ADD-H Comprehensive Teacher Rating Scale (ACTeRS) (Ullman, Sleator, & Sprague, 1984) are valuable tools for this aspect of assessment. Initial ratings can serve as baseline data, and parents and teachers can fill out the same scale to help assess the effectiveness of treatment.

Assess for Learning Disabilities. Either LD or ADHD can lead to similar symptoms. In the school setting, a learning disabled child may look like a child with ADHD as he reacts behaviorally to frustration or attempts to avoid academic tasks he is unable to do. But this child may not show the symptoms of ADHD in situations where his learning deficits are not exposed. However, there is a comorbidity rate of 20–30% between ADHD and learning disabilities (Barkley, 2003), which means that some children struggle with both conditions and that their development is doubly at risk. Therefore, if one condition is present, the clinician should consider evaluating for the other.

Treatment for ADHD. If information from these areas of inquiry converges on a diagnosis of ADHD, treatment combining parent training, cognitive-behavioral therapy, and medication is indicated. The stimulant medications commonly used to treat ADHD are quick-acting and, assuming the dosage is at a therapeutic level, can produce changes in the symptoms of many children within a few days. For many children medication can have a dramatic impact on the child's functioning, especially in terms of removing interferences to learning and changing the child's relationship with parents (Rapport, Denney, DuPaul, & Gardner, 1994). However, the best results come from interventions that combine behavior modification programs at home and at school, cognitive treatment to help the child self-monitor his behavior, and medication (Anastopoulos, 1999).

A Cautionary Note. The prevalence of ADHD in different cultures varies widely, from 3.8% in Holland to 19.8% in the Ukraine (Barkley, 2003). This suggests that cultural assumptions and values influence the perception of symptoms of the disorder. In the United States, where prevalence is estimated at 3–5% (American Psychiatric Association, 2000), ADHD has become a "popular" diagnosis in recent years. This popularity is related to increasing public awareness of the disorder as well as to trends in mental health care emphasizing brief treatment in managed care and pharmacological treatment. These trends may resonate with American cultural biases toward a quick and easy solution to problems. The practitioner must be aware that some parents will initiate an evaluation having already made the diagnosis themselves. Similarly, some teachers—especially those who must cope with many disruptive children in their classrooms—may press for an ADHD diagnosis and medication. While it is important to respect parents' and teachers' impressions, the clinician must do her own careful evaluation that covers the areas described above before making the diagnosis.

INTERVENTION

Some of the typical goals of therapy with school-age children are the following:

- To remove emotional barriers that prevent them from feeling competent in work and with peers
- To help them move from action-based modes of expression to modes involving language, thought, and fantasy
- To help them move away from the compensations of magical thinking and toward a more reality-oriented stance
- To help them develop coping strategies that permit them to maintain a capacity to learn

The developmental advances of middle childhood permit a broad array of intervention approaches and techniques, including the following.

Cognitive-Behavioral Interventions

School-age children's new cognitive skills—decentration, perspective taking, logical thinking, improved understanding of cause and effect—make possible interventions that help them make sense of stressful experiences. For example, in sexual abuse treatment a 9-year-old girl can cognitively grasp the accuracy of a statement that differentiates the abuser's motives and behavior from her own: "He is responsible for what he did to you. You did not cause it to happen, and it is not your fault." Further, the school-age child's capacity for decentered thinking can be drawn on to help her differentiate between herself in the abuse situation and her overall self. This opens the way to cognitive interventions that aim to strengthen the child's self-image and separate the abuse from her sense of self (Friedberg & McClure, 2002).

The older school-age child's ability to analyze cause-and-effect sequences and use reversible thought implies that he can sometimes understand the connections between thoughts and impulses and behavior, and can realize that a feeling may have caused him to act, as demonstrated in the following case example:

> Mark, a 10-year-old with many fears and inadequate defenses and coping skills, was provoking fights at school. His foster mother called me before his session and told me that he had been sent to the office for fighting the preceding day. I asked Mark what had happened, and he said, "Two guys jumped on me. They held me down and punched me." I began working backward, asking him how the fight got started. He said, "They told me 2 weeks ago that they were going to get me. So I saw them out in front waiting for the bus, and I knew they were waiting for me." I asked if they'd said anything to him, and he said, "No, maybe they didn't see me." When I said I was still not sure how the fight started, he said, "Well, I kicked one of them in the stomach." My approach was to go over this situation in detail, clarifying that his provocative aggression was based on his fear of being beaten up. This made him attack even though he hadn't

been attacked. Because he was afraid, he had put himself into the exact situation he feared. I expressed my concern that he'd put himself into a dangerous situation when he didn't need to. I said, "I don't like you to get hurt, and it makes me feel bad for you when you do something that makes other people want to hurt you." We also discussed alternative ways of responding. I asked, "What else could you do if you're worried about those guys?" We explored several possibilities: stay away from those kids; tell the teacher; stick with your friends so you feel safer; stay back until the bus comes and get on after they do, and don't sit by them. I also tried to help him appraise the severity of the threat in retrospect: "It's good to be careful and be ready to do something if they really do come after you, but if they threatened you 2 weeks ago and still hadn't done anything by yesterday, maybe they were just talking big." In subsequent sessions, I helped Mark identify situations with peers that tended to trigger his anxiety, and continued to examine more adaptive ways of responding. Using role plays, we practiced ways he could stand up for himself without attacking other children.

This cognitive approach models thinking through fears and gaining some control over them through the use of reasoning. It also asks the child to think before he acts, to consider alternative ways of responding, and to evaluate what happened (Kazdin, 2003). Although treatment focusing on the cognitive skills draws on the developing executive function in middle childhood, it does not require autonomous self-reflection or insight, abilities that are still beyond those of the school-age child. The therapist functions as a teacher or "auxiliary ego," helping the child utilize reasoning abilities and making suggestions of more adaptive ways to deal with anxiety (Chethik, 2000). The cognitive approach aims to facilitate development by calling attention to and exercising the school-age child's new ability to think things through. The therapist helps the child practice age-appropriate cognitive skills whose development has been impeded by maturational delays or by reliance on appraisal styles and coping mechanisms formed by early experiences of trauma or neglect (Holmbeck, Greenley, & Franks, 2003).

School-age children can also be engaged in behavioral treatment more easily than younger children. The school-age child's understanding of cause and effect enables him to conceptualize how rewards can be contingent on appropriate behavior. This understanding enables him to see the possible benefits of controlling defiant or aggressive behavior (Barkley, 1997). In behavior management programs involving token economies, the child's participation can be enlisted because he sees that he will be rewarded for changing his behavior. His firm knowledge of time supports his motivation because he can understand, for example, that if he does his homework without protest four out of five school nights he will earn a reward on the weekend. Such programs depend on the child's developing cognitive skills, including thinking logically, using cognitive strategies to control behavior, and self-monitoring. Further the child's active and externalizing orientation in middle childhood is likely to make him interested in a treatment program that emphasizes control over behavior rather than understanding of feelings.

Group Treatment

Group intervention is particularly appropriate for school-age children because of their compelling interest in peer relationships. School-age children think groups are "normal," in the sense that they spend a lot of time in groups at school. Groups can be helpful for children who have similar issues, such as difficulties in social skills, or similar experiences, such as parental divorce or incarceration of a parent. School-age groups have the potential to help children cope with internal difficulties and at the same time to increase their skills in relating to peers (Webb, 2003). Most children's groups focus around scripts and structured tasks, which from the child's perspective makes them seem similar to familiar classroom activities. Dealing with issues in a group has several advantages that derive from the developmental characteristics of middle childhood (Kalter, 1988; Kalter & Schreier, 1994):

- Children get support from one another. Especially when groups are composed of children at about the same level of development, they can identify with one another.
- The group provides "safety in numbers." Children do not feel singled out or stigmatized, as they often do initially in individual or family treatment.
- Being with peers who have similar situations or symptoms reduces conscience-driven anxiety about self-revelation.
- By becoming aware of other children's experiences, the individual child's experience is normalized.
- By observing how other group members have coped with or solved problems, children can expand their own range of coping devices.

Individual Play Therapy

Individual treatment that combines play, structured activities, and talk is an effective approach in middle childhood. However, practitioners beginning to work with school-age children often feel that the child is "resistant," or "lacks insight," or "doesn't seem to know he has problems." Such observations are largely accurate, and, from a developmental perspective, they are normative. School-age children usually do not talk about their problems in a sustained way. In the individual treatment situation, many children actively avoid talking about worries, painful experiences, and problems. This is consistent with the following characteristics of middle childhood:

- *External orientation.* School-age children are more oriented to the outer world than to their internal consciousness, and they tend more toward doing than toward feeling.
- *Defenses.* Their defense mechanisms are more adequate to prevent painful, forbidden, or anxious thoughts from coming into consciousness; they are also more adept at conscious suppression.
- *Conscience.* School-age children tend to resist talking about symptoms and problems—such as getting into fights, being disruptive in class, or defying a parent—because they are associated in the child's mind with being bad. Because the conscience is now internalized, badness is felt inside. Consequently, the child resists talking about problems in order to avoid feeling guilty.
- *Social awareness.* School-age children are very aware of what is appropriate socially and highly invested in being like everyone else—in being "normal." They often worry that their friends will find out they are in therapy. To have a problem is to feel abnormal, defective, or crazy.

> One day, I was waiting for an 8-year-old boy to come for his first appointment. I looked out of my office window and saw his mother pulling him bodily out of the car. He was crying and resisting. He had gotten himself together by the time they got into my office, I think because he didn't want to embarrass himself by crying. Partway through the hour, we were playing with puppets. He hid behind a chair and stuck his puppet up and said, "I'm not crazy." This gave me a chance to address his fear. I said, "Sometimes kids think I'll prove they're crazy, but that's a mistake— that's not why kids come to see me. They come because they have some worries, and I know how to help with worries."

Displacement

The school-age child tries to avoid difficult feelings and worries through conscious suppression, unconscious defenses, or displacement of personal experiences and inner concerns into play and fantasy. A child's "fictional" story about the content of a drawing or play scenario allows her to express worries or represent difficult experiences. Yet, displacement into play provides psychic protection for the child, allowing forbidden impulses, strong feelings, and conflicts to be looked at and experienced as if not connected to the self. Children can unconsciously use the displacement of symbolic play and action to describe their emotional dilemmas.

When we enter the child's fantasy world through the medium of play or other displacement activities such as drawing, storytelling, or therapeutic games, we can learn about the child's inner experience of his difficulties without requiring the child to talk directly about them. The practitioner must also learn to respond to the play and fantasy with displaced interpretations, so that the child's defenses are not challenged too strongly. An example of a displaced interpretation would be speak in universal terms about "how girls feel" instead of "how you feel"; or to talk about "another boy I knew who had some worries" and then tailor the story to fit the child's problems. In many cases the eventual goal will be to make connections between the play and the child's actual problems, including talking directly about the problems and helping the child understand how they began.

This chapter presents two examples to illustrate the use of displacement and other developmentally relevant approaches in work with school-age children. The first case presents a 7-year-old whose early history of chronic trauma threatened to interfere with the transition to middle childhood. The second demonstrates the ability of a child with previous adequate development to use the cognitive skills of middle childhood in coping with family stressors during two periods of treatment at 8 and 11 years of age.

WORKING TO MASTER THE TRAUMA OF REPEATED ABUSE: A CASE EXAMPLE

Michael was a 7-year-old boy in foster care who presented with manifest sadness, statements that he wished he was dead, and aggression and sexual behavior toward his younger biological sister, who lived in the same foster home. He was working at grade level in school and did not show behavior problems there. He was in an excellent foster care placement and had made a strong attachment to his foster mother.

Michael's early experience up to age 4 was chaotic. His father was physically and sexually abusive to him and his two sisters. He took nude pictures of them and prostituted his older sister, which Michael sometimes witnessed. The children also witnessed frequent violence between their mother and father. Both parents abused alcohol and cocaine. The children often were left alone while the parents were away at bars or procuring drugs. All three children were removed for neglect and abuse when Michael was 4. They were returned to their mother, but were removed again 4 months later when it was discovered that the father was living with the family and continuing to abuse the children. Michael's older sister was assessed as severely disturbed secondary to trauma and was placed in a residential setting. Michael and his younger sister returned to the same foster home and were eventually adopted by that family after parental rights were terminated.

A sexual abuse treatment agency referred Michael to the clinic where I was on staff because he was showing symptoms of depression and had threatened to hurt himself. Michael had been in sexual abuse treatment for 1 year. During this treatment, Michael had described a number of incidents of sexual abuse, primarily involving fondling of his genitals by his father. He revealed that his mother did nothing to protect him. Treatment had focused on direct educational interventions regarding sexual abuse. Michael was told that his father's behavior was wrong and that no adult had the right to sexually abuse a child. Additionally, the therapist worked with his foster parents to structure the home environment so that Michael and his sister would not be able to act sexually toward each other. The therapist and foster parents repeatedly defined appropriate boundaries and behavior for Michael and his sister.

This intervention had been very helpful to Michael. However, as he gained some control over impulses to act out sexually and aggressively, he became more anxious and depressed. The switch in emphasis from behavioral to emotional symptoms was an effect of intervention as well as development. He had been helped to remember and describe in words a number of traumatic experiences of sexual abuse, at a time when increasing cognitive capacities permitted better verbal encoding of memories. He had gained a perspective that emphasized the wrongness of the abuse and the responsibility of the perpetrators of abuse, at a time when internalization of moral values was proceeding. He had been helped to limit his sexualized behavior, at a time when the ability to exert self-control becomes an important component of the conscience and the sense of self.

Formulation of Presenting Symptoms

From a psychodynamic point of view, Michael had begun to rely less on "acting out" as a defense against anxiety. Acting out serves the defensive function of relieving unconscious tension through action. Acting out is very common response to trauma-based anxiety and environmental reminders of traumatic events. Michael's sexual abuse treatment had helped him gain some control over tendencies to act out. At the time of referral to me, his foster mother noted a significant decline in sexualized behavior. However, it appeared that chronic trauma in his experience had not been fully addressed. Consequently, even though Michael relied less on acting out as a means of discharging trauma-based anxiety, the anxiety remained internalized as depressive symptoms. Trauma is a risk factor in the development of depression (Pynoos et al., 1996). When the affective and cognitive symptoms of trauma persist, the child may become increasingly distressed and depressed because of his inability to control the symptoms (McFarlane, 1995). I hypothesized that for Michael the restriction of acting out as a means of discharge intensified the internalization of emotional symptoms, resulting in increased anxiety and depression.

Approaches to the Treatment of Trauma
in Middle Childhood

My approach to Michael's treatment was to see if he could use the emerging developmental abilities of middle childhood to reduce his depression, increase self-control, and master the traumas of his early years by creating a *trauma story* that would contain and reduce the affective power of the memories of trauma. Traumatized children—especially when the trauma is abuse by caregivers—often have not been helped by adults to process the experience verbally when it occurred (Fivush, 1998). In working with traumatized children we try to help them develop representational competence retrospectively. The experience of trauma overpowers coping capacities, supplanting thinking and words with raw and overwhelming affect. The sense of personal continuity and narrative memory are also severely disrupted, so that the child's representation of traumatic events is imagistic and distorted rather than an organized narrative. This is particularly likely, as was true for Michael, when trauma has been chronic (Terr, 1991). Even when children do have clear memories of traumatic events, the fearful arousal associated with the traumatic memory causes them to suppress or avoid the memory, often through acting-out behavior.

Helping the client put his story into words is a well-accepted principle in the treatment of traumatized adults. This principle holds for children too. We want to help traumatized children (1) develop an understanding of what happened; (2) create a narrative of the traumatic events that is coherent and as accurate as possible; (3) name the affects that accompanied the trauma; (4) label the traumatic events as *past* rather than current events, so that the trauma is thought of as an incident or series of incidents in the narrative of the child's past life, not a fearful lens for viewing the world; and (5) process the trauma from his current more advanced cognitive perspective, taking advantage of the fact that representational competence improves as cognitive development proceeds (this is particularly important for the child who was very young at the time of the trauma) (Salmon & Bryant, 2001).

However, technique with children needs to be adapted to the child's primary representational modes, including play, reenactment, and other types of symbolic expression. Very often, the play of traumatized children is disorganized and lacking in narrative, simply repeating over and over an image of the traumatic events. It becomes the therapist's job to help the child structure this seemingly chaotic play into a narrative that clarifies what happened, establishes sequences of cause and effect, and describes the child's affective reactions (Gil, 1991). Michael's case presents the process of helping a young school-age child move from play expression of concerns about trauma to describing traumatic events in words and creating a verbal narrative. I will not present the entire case narrative but rather will use sessions from the early months of treatment to illustrate the use of displacement techniques in the creation of a trauma story.

Posttraumatic Play in Michael's Early Sessions

In order to learn how Michael was remembering and constructing his traumatic experiences during the first 4 years of his life, I took a less directive approach than that taken by the therapist at the sexual abuse treatment agency. I encouraged Michael to play and hoped that by observing his play I would begin to learn how his traumatic experiences continued to influence his affects and view of the world. During the early sessions, Michael played while I watched. His play had many of the characteristics of posttraumatic play. It was driven, repetitive, and restricted in content. As he played with dinosaurs, the biting, roaring, and killing were unremitting in an amoral universe where everyone fought everyone else and there was no protection for anyone.

Michael's play symbolically demonstrated how adaptations to trauma can interfere with emerging developmental tasks. In early middle childhood, children learn that there is a social order that sets standards for behavior and a "social contract" that provides rewards for appropriate behavior. When a child has suffered gross violations of the social contract, as Michael had when his parents abused him, he experiences "a disruption of a belief in a socially modulated world" (Pynoos et al., 1996, p. 340). Michael's pessimism about this issue was reflected in his early play in treatment. There was no evident order in the play world he created, only repetitious violence. This play also reflected difficulties in creating a coherent narrative, an accomplishment that preschool children practice and school-age children achieve. As is typical of posttraumatic play, there was no developing story in Michael's play, but rather a single repetitive scenario involving a violent "bad guy" who never died.

Creating a Safe Therapeutic Environment

Unlike many children his age, Michael did not invite me to join the play. This was consistent with the self-reliant and mistrustful attitude he had developed in response to betrayal and abuse by his parents. A few times during the first few sessions I asked Michael to tell me about the dinosaurs—what made them so angry, why they were fighting each other. In response to these mild questions, Michael looked startled. This told me that he might be experiencing my questions as intrusive and perhaps that my simply noticing what he was doing made him anxious. Abused children frequently adopt a watchful, unobtrusive style, remaining quiet and self-contained in order to keep the abuser's attention away from them. It appeared that Michael was generalizing this style. Michael had adapted to the abusive situation by becoming hypervigilant and by overregulating affects. His need to feel in control, both of his environment and his feelings, had to be respected. In response, I tried to be friendly but undemanding. I realized that I would need to pace my interventions carefully and respond first to Michael's strengths before beginning to address his anxiety (Pearce & Pezzot-Pearce, 1997).

During these sessions Michael also spent time drawing. His drawings showed artistic talent. In contrast to his reactions to my questions about his play, he was at ease talking about the content of his drawings. Discussion of his artwork seemed a safe vehicle for building our relationship. His early drawings were about more neutral subjects than his play. He drew planet Earth with green land masses and blue oceans. Then he drew other planets. Over the first month of treatment, a routine developed in which Michael would begin the session by drawing several pictures, then play chaotically with dinosaurs or action figures. I suggested another element to this routine—a return to drawing at the end of the session. I did this because I wanted Michael to experience a sense of structure and control in our sessions. I did not want him to associate his therapy primarily with the posttraumatic play that heightened his anxiety, and I did not want him to leave sessions filled with anxiety. Traumatized children who are not helped to seal off traumatic material during a session are more likely to act out after the session. They may learn to view therapy as a time when they are flooded with affective arousal and resist coming to sessions.

Michael's Drawings: Identifying Developmental Strengths

In assessing any child, it is important to identify areas of strength and developmental adequacy. When Michael drew and talked about his drawings, he demonstrated many of the normal characteristics of a younger school-age child. He was calm and thoughtful. He would take a moment to look at what he had drawn, then comment on it. For example, after he had drawn the head of a bird, he pointed to the eye, which he had drawn as an outer circle of black, an inner area of yellow, and a black dot in the middle, and said, "That's the way a bird's eye looks." Then he said, "I couldn't get the beak right." Drawing seemed to symbolize the forces of progressive development in Michael, in contrast to his compulsive play, which symbolized an internal preoccupation with trauma. Drawing was a more neutral activity that was completely under his control. Consequently, he had more ability to defend against anxiety and posttraumatic reminders while drawing. His drawings covered many different subjects that interested him and reflected some of the cognitive abilities and interests of school-age children. He applied internal standards of accuracy to his work, as when he commented that he had not gotten the bird's beak right. He explained the content of his drawings in a coherent way and implicitly used them to create a sense of organization to his world. For example, he drew a careful picture of his room at home, showing the placement of his bed, chest of drawers, the location of the door and windows, and many other details. When we attempt to understand the meaning of children's drawings, it is essential to ask the child to explain the drawing, as opposed to assuming that we understand its meaning by looking at it. Often the child's verbal account clarifies concerns that are not obvious or only hinted at in the picture (Malchiodi, 1998). My asking about the picture of his bedroom led Michael to tell me that he didn't like to sleep in his room by himself and that he was glad his foster brother shared the room with him. I asked him what he was afraid of, and he was evasive. Nevertheless, drawing opened the way to his first words about the anxiety that was registered nonverbally in his play.

Drawing as a Displacement of Posttraumatic Anxiety

Another picture allowed us to expand the discussion of Michael's fears a bit. He drew an ocean scene. First, he drew a boy on a surfboard. Then, as he drew the line of the water across the page, a huge wave threatened to engulf the surfer. Near the wave, Michael drew a large shark's fin sticking above the water. Before completing the picture Michael made a revision. He changed the boy into a heavily armored dinosaur. This seemed a response to the dangers in the picture: he had given the boy on the surfboard some protection, perhaps making him invulnerable. In response to my questions, Michael explained that the dinosaur was not in danger from the wave because he could jump right over it. He explained that the sharks would not be able to hurt the dinosaur. It is helpful to watch the process of the drawing carefully—to note what a child draws first, emphasizes, does quickly and without care, what he erases, what he revises. When I asked Michael if he had changed the picture in the middle, he laughed and agreed. I asked why he had decided to change it. He pointed to the big wave and said, "At first this was going to be just plain water, and he was going to be a person. And then the fish was going to bite him." I said, "So, maybe it was looking like this person could get hurt out here by the sharks or the wave, but if you turn him into a dinosaur, he can keep himself safe because he's so strong and protected by his armor." In this drawing, he was able to peek at his feelings of vulnerability and then compensate for them. This picture suggested Michael's strong motivation to master his fears, which could more easily be expressed because of his complete control of what he drew.

Displaced Interpretations of Posttraumatic Play

After Michael began to feel comfortable talking about fearful themes in his pictures, it became possible for him to tolerate some commentary on his play. During the second month of treatment, he brought a collection of plastic action figures that included superheroes and villains from cartoon shows as well as the Teenage Mutant Ninja Turtles. I was pleased because I felt that his decision to bring these toys from home reflected his growing investment in our relationship. First we looked over the figures together. Then Michael launched into his usual play, with figures killing each other. After watching for several minutes, I noticed that one superhero figure was defeating all challengers. I asked who he was, and Michael said, "He's a bad guy." This figure was eaten by sharks and blown up by bombs, yet he continued to defeat the other figures. I said, "It seems like this bad guy can't be stopped or killed. He keeps coming back." The play continued with this theme. A few minutes later I told Michael I wanted to tell him a story that his play made me think of: "Sometimes if a kid has had bad things done to him by a grown-up and it keeps happening over and over again, the kid feels like the bad guy keeps coming back. Even when the kid is taken away from the person who was hurting him and begins to live with a family that takes care of him, sometimes a kid can still worry about getting hurt, even though he's safe now." Michael's response was to tell me a story about a kid he knew who had "a bad guy coming back." He said, "Now the bad guy doesn't know where he lives. I think his name was Michael."

Since his story mirrored mine, I decided to expand it. I told him that I had known a kid whose dad had hit him and touched his privates. His dad should not have done those things. But since the kid was living with his dad, he couldn't get away, so he always felt like his dad was like a bad guy who would always come back. Even when he was safe with a new family, he remembered the bad things his dad had done and felt scared. Although I was speaking in displacement about "another kid," I was tailoring my story to match the themes of Michael's play as his experience of chronic physical abuse. After this story, Michael's play changed. The bad guy figure was punished for his misdeeds. He was forced to swallow bombs, which blew up inside him. Then a Ninja Turtle figure killed him. Although the play was still violent, it had changed from hopeless posttraumatic play, in which the bad guy dominated, to the defeat of the bad guy. The triumph of a good guy—a Ninja Turtle who might be considered a self-representation—suggested that Michael could imagine a different outcome to the experience of being abused.

This theme continued in the next session, when for the first time he divided the dinosaurs into good guy and bad guy teams and then had the good guys repeatedly defeat the bad guys. There was more order in this play. The good and bad dinosaurs faced each other individually. After each fight, two more dinosaurs were brought forward. Compared with the chaotic play during the first few months of treatment, this play resembled a game with rituals and rules, and thus was more typical of a younger school-age boy's play. I asked Michael to take a break from play and told him a story about a kid who had played in a similar way. I said, "This kid always beat on the bad guys, and we figured out that he played that way because he was mad at someone who had hurt him. He wanted to punish that person, and his play was a way of imagining that." I told Michael that the therapist at the previous agency had told me that his father had hurt him. Michael agreed. I asked him to tell me about it, and he recounted some instances of his father's sexual abuse. He made clear that he had hated what had happened to him and that he thought his father had been wrong. Since Michael was able to talk about being sexually abused, I asked him to tell me other things that happened when he lived with his mom and dad. My aim was to expand the scope of our discussion in order to help develop a trauma story that would include more than sexual abuse.

Expanding the Trauma Story

Sometimes directive educational treatment for sexual abuse can be too narrow in scope. Sexually abused children often have been traumatized in other ways. It is important to observe for other traumatic events, even though the manifest problem is sexual abuse. Effective treatment gives the child a chance to fully represent his difficult experiences. Michael described many instances of his father's violent behavior. He had witnessed his father beat his mother and sisters many times. He said, "My dad chased my mom with a knife. One time he threw a glass at her and it broke on the wall." I asked how he had felt at these times. He said, "Sad. Scared too. I was afraid my mom would get killed. Sometimes he would bust down the door."

I asked if he still worried about getting hurt by his dad now, even though he was living with his foster family. He said that he wasn't worried because his dad didn't know where he lived. However, he indicated that he *was* afraid by immediately telling about a dream in which a man broke into his house, chased him and found him in every place he hid, and finally shot him. I said, "That was a very scary dream. It reminds me of how kids feel when grown-ups are doing bad things to them. The grown-ups are so strong that the kid can't really stop them, so all he can do is try to hide. But that's the reason you're not living with your dad anymore—because he did all those mean things." Michael agreed and then talked about times his father had slapped his face and spanked him with a belt. I empathized with his fear and said that his father was wrong to have hurt him, his sisters, and his mom.

At the end of this session, I said, "I'm really glad you could tell me about all this. Now I know what it was like for you. Now you're probably feeling a lot safer. I would like to keep talking about what you remember." My impression was that Michael gained some relief by talking about these memories of his father's violence and his fears. The emphasis of Michael's trauma story changed. Although his sexual abuse experiences had probably been traumatic, the more profound sources of his posttraumatic stress were his memories of being physically abused and witnessing his father's violence. He had been presenting his anxiety about violence and damage in his play since the very first session. As we continued to piece together his story over many sessions, I constantly tried to help him integrate his memories with the affects he had experienced. I made frequent comparisons between his past and present experiences, aiming to help him differentiate his fears from his present reality of living in a caring and protective family. In this work I was constantly aided by Michael's emerging developmental capacities to understand cause and effect, to take a decentered view of past events, and to think in more logical and organized ways about his experience.

USING DEVELOPMENTAL STRENGTHS: A CASE EXAMPLE

Stacey, age 8, was referred to me by her mother, Ms. Kline, within a few weeks after she decided to separate from Stacey's stepfather. Ms. Kline and her husband had been married for 2 years. Stacey's biological father had died in an auto accident when she was only 3 months old. Ms. Kline had raised Stacey and her older sister as a single parent until she married, when Stacey was 6 years old. Ms. Kline reported that Stacey had developed an affectionate relationship with her stepfather, Bill, and that she seemed depressed. Ms. Kline said Stacey and her sister had felt betrayed when they overheard their stepfather angrily say he was glad to be leaving the family. She was worried about the impact of Bill's angry statement, even though she had told the girls that the divorce was not their fault. Over the next month, Stacey frequently called him, but he often did not respond to her messages. Within 4 months he moved to another state and contacted her even less often.

Stacey demonstrated many of the qualities we expect in a school-age child who is developing adequately. She was thoughtful, calm, articulate, and self-possessed. She immediately showed a capacity to use displacement to represent her concerns, which seemed to center on anger about the divorce and feelings of abandonment. She drew two pictures: one was of an angry man whose head appeared to be exploding; the other was an idealized image of her family, including her stepfather, having a good time on the roller coaster at an amusement park. These pictures conveyed the reality of an angry divorce, followed by a denial in fantasy that expressed her wish that the family would be reunited and happy again. The choice of a roller coaster may also have expressed Stacey's anxious sense of the precariousness of her parents' relationship. Her work on these drawings was careful, demonstrating the motivation to do a good job that is typical of well-developing 8-year-olds. She was calm as she drew and as she explained the pictures, suggesting that she was expressing conflictual issues without consciously relating them directly to herself. This was a sign of adequate development in the area of self-regulation (Sarnoff, 1987). Although the picture of the angry man surely represented her stepfather and perhaps her own anger about the divorce, she simply explained, "This is a guy who's blowing his top." When I asked what had made him mad, she said, "Who knows?"

When I asked Stacey about the arguments her mother and stepfather were having, she looked very somber and explained calmly, "They're getting a divorce." When I suggested that many kids were upset about parents fighting and deciding to divorce, she denied being upset but admitted that her sister was. When I suggested that her second picture showed a time her family was happier and that now she and her sister might be sad, she ignored this comment and told me a story that she said she'd read in a book: "A prince wasn't getting along with his wife, so he ran away. A wizard turned him into a frog and put him in a pond, and his wife was in the pond and she was a frog too, so they got back together." I said that maybe she wished her mother and stepfather would get back together, and she responded in a rational tone, "My mom told me they're not," essentially stating the facts while avoiding acknowledgment of the reunion fantasy in her story.

Stacey showed the school-age child's ability to repress and compartmentalize painful affects. She was much more disturbed by the loss of her stepfather and her sense of an intact family than she let on. Her defenses and capacities for conscious suppression and self-distraction kept her sad and angry feelings at a distance. Her mother had explained the reasons for the divorce to her, and Stacey had a good cognitive understanding that her parents had been arguing frequently for over a year. At age 8, she did not seem to blame herself for the divorce, as egocentric preschool children tend to do. Her ability to observe the conflict from a relatively decentered perspective lessened fantasies of self-blame. Because of her strong identification with her mother, she did not, at least immediately after the separation, struggle with questions about which parent to be loyal to, which is a very common reaction of younger school-age children (Kelly, 2000). Stacey's primary reactions to the divorce focused first on an overall sense of deprivation and disruption and then increasingly on her anger and confusion regarding her sense of being betrayed by her stepfather. These became the main themes of a therapy lasting 6 months.

Displacement Activities in Intervention

During the first month of therapy, which coincided with exposure to several arguments between her mother and stepfather over the division of property, Stacey produced a "book" of drawings that she added to each week. The pictures symbolized Stacey's primary concerns about her parents' divorce. The first several pages showed sharks swimming in the ocean foraging for food. I commented that the sharks looked upset and possibly angry. Stacey said that they were very angry because there was not enough food. I offered a displaced interpretation, suggesting that when parents divorce and are fighting about who gets the house and furniture and money, kids sometimes worry that they won't have a place to live or money to buy food. In a subsequent session, a picture showed people living in houses near the ocean. Some of the people foolishly swam in the ocean and were attacked by the hungry sharks. In a later picture, the houses turned out to be sitting on earthquake faults and were destroyed. These images condensed Stacey's feelings of anger, deprivation, and fear. Even though she was consistently calm as she drew, the content of the pictures showed her internal sense that a disaster had befallen her and her family. In a parent session with Ms. Kline, I asked her to assure the children that she would be able to support them however the property settlement turned out. In a family session Ms. Kline empathized with their distress, saying that she was able to take care of them and that the conflicts she and her husband were having would diminish as the divorce was settled. I also attempted to discuss these issues with Stacey's stepfather, but he was unwilling to talk with me.

After her mother and I put her feelings of anger and disruption into words, Stacey stopped drawing, and we began to play Connect Four, a paper-and-pencil game that involves joining lines to form squares. We also played cards. In these games, she controlled everything. She shuffled the cards, dealt them, and acted as the authority on the rules. She was a good player who frequently beat me because of her skill; however, if she began to lose, she would look me in the eye with a defiant smile and openly cheat. I commented that she wanted to be in control, even to the point of cheating. She laughed and agreed. I asked if she would cheat if she were playing with a friend. She looked surprised and said, "No way." I had expected this answer, because it appeared that Stacey's game play in therapy had some special functions and that it was not subject to the same standards of fairness that would be used in play with a peer. This type of play continued over several sessions, with Stacey keeping running score sheets of her victories. I understood Stacey's pleasure in controlling the games as a reversal of her recent real experiences. I told her, "When I can't do anything to win, it reminds me of how kids feel when something happens that they can't stop from happening. Like if their parents decide to get a divorce. Maybe the kids don't want that to happen, but they can't stop the grown-ups from doing it. Or, like what's happened to you with your stepdad—I think you'd like to see him more, but he's so wrapped up in his own worries that he doesn't call you. I've known other kids this has happened to, and it made them really angry and sad." Stacey listened carefully and said, "I don't care that much." At this point she was unable to tolerate sad feelings. However, my comment about her stepfather's inconsistent behavior seemed to give permission for Stacey to express angry feelings more directly.

Displacement Play and Transference

School-age children often use competitive games in therapy to express strong emotions and transferences in activity that is displaced from the real situation of conflict. Just as the game is used as a safe vehicle for expressing negative feelings, the adult opponent in the game, the therapist, becomes a stand-in for significant adults. Since the context is "play," the child can displace toward the therapist feelings and impulses that she might be too anxious to express directly toward parents. Stacey was very angry at her stepfather. She felt frustrated by her inability to control when she could see him. These feelings were presented in our games through making fun of my inability to win and her insistence on controlling the game. At the same time, she was friendly toward me and looked forward to our sessions.

Therapy created for Stacey both a safe place to express anger and disappointment and a consistent relationship that symbolically took the place of her damaged relationship with her stepfather. These themes came through clearly in a note she wrote after a game:

> Stacey RULES at Connect Four against Douglas Davies! Cause he isn't too good! But don't tell him I said that. I think he would get mad, knowing his temper.
> Love, Stacey

Stacey's note simultaneously put me down and expressed affection for me. A few weeks later she expressed her love and anger toward her stepfather in transference to me even more directly when she made me a

Christmas card. She spent 10 minutes carefully col(
she had written, "Merry Christmas. Love, Stacey. (
the other side she had written, "You are so stupid!"
ously when I turned it over. I laughed with her an(
good trick. I said I was reminded of how kids do (
grown-ups and sometimes want to pay them ba(
have felt tricked by Bill. When he and your mom were toge...
nice to you and had fun doing things with you. Now he almost never sees
you. I think that's felt like a terrible trick."

Working Through Reactions to Parental Divorce

In the next session Stacey returned to her book of drawings. This time she drew a family living in a house that was in a safe place. The family—a mother and two daughters—seemed to represent her family in its new configuration, without a father. She said, "Before they were in a spot where an earthquake shook down their house, but this time they read about earthquakes in *National Geographic* and found a place where there weren't any quakes. Also they built a better house." I asked if they were still near the ocean with the sharks. She said, "Yeah, but they don't swim in the ocean now. Now they're smart. They learned not to swim there because the dad did and he was eaten by sharks." I said, "The dad?" In response she quickly undid the implied aggression toward her stepfather by saying, "Really, it was a very old man who had a heart attack in the water, and they ate him after he was dead." Compared to her first drawings, this depiction of a family showed some acceptance of the new composition of her family. Ms. Kline had told me that she and her husband had settled the divorce issues and were not arguing now. The image of the family as safe suggested Stacey was aware that the conflict had diminished. Her anger toward her stepfather was still strong, as represented in the father who was eaten by sharks; however, her anger was still not acceptable to her on a conscious level, so she denied it by modifying the story of who had been eaten by sharks. Nevertheless, her angry feelings were quite intense, as indicated by the next picture she drew, a river full of piranhas. Moving back into the displacement of transference, she threatened to draw me in the water with the piranhas. When I expressed mock alarm, she laughed and said, "All right, I won't put you in there. Let's play Connect Four."

During the first 3 months of treatment, Stacey used displacement through drawing and games to symbolically approach her feelings about the loss of her stepfather. Through a combination of displaced and direct interpretation I helped her acknowledge her feelings in their real context. Gradually, during the next 3 months she was able to talk about her disappointment and anger directly. She began to complain about her stepfa-

failure to see her regularly. She was critical of him for making promises and failing to keep them. When he told her he would be moving away to attend a distant university, she continued to describe her mixed feelings in sessions. She said she wished he would stay but accepted his explanation that he needed to complete his education. She continued to be angry at him, and I felt that her anger was in part a defense against sad feelings. However, Stacey denied this when I suggested it. In fact, talking directly about her feelings about the divorce and her stepfather's move over several sessions seemed to accomplish some working through of the disruption of her life. This was evident in her mother's reports that she was happier. Her affect in sessions was more buoyant, and the controlling play declined. During the termination process, I asked Stacey what advice she might give other kids whose parents were divorcing. Her answer implicitly expressed the school-age child's tendency to use cognitive strategies to regulate affect: "Tell them to think that it happened for a good reason."

Work with an Older School-Age Child: Stacey's Second Treatment

Two-and-a-half years later, Ms. Kline called to ask me to see Stacey, who was now 11. Ms. Kline told me that she was planning to marry again within a few months and that Stacey seemed angry and anxious. She was often rude and sarcastic toward her mother and sometimes toward her mother's fiancé. She was arguing constantly with her older sister. It appeared that Stacey was worried about her mother's upcoming marriage, and that her previous experience of divorce and loss formed the context of her anxiety. When her mother made plans to marry again, Stacey felt threatened by the possible repetition of making an attachment to a father and then losing him.

Because of their advanced cognitive abilities, older school-age children are capable of analyzing problems within their families and realistically worrying or being angry about them. Since these concerns are conscious, though kept private, it is often possible to move fairly quickly from displacement to direct discussion of the problems, especially when, as was true for Stacey, the child has had a previous relationship with the therapist. Even though many school-age children are unwilling to initiate a discussion of problems, they are often responsive when a therapist puts the problem into words accurately.

In the second round of therapy, occurring 2 years after the first, Stacey's way of presenting and working on her concerns showed similarities and differences from the first treatment. She still utilized the displacement of a transference relationship, alternating between seeking my interest and approval and playfully acting rude and rejecting me. This transference revealed both sides of her ambivalence about her mother's remarriage—she wanted a father but resisted that wish because of her anxiety about loss. She still chose to play Connect Four and card games with me. This seemed to be Stacey's way of reestablishing our relationship and affirming its continuity.

Despite these similarities in presentation, there were also important differences that reflected her gains in development during the intervening 2 years. Stacey was more consciously aware of what was bothering her than she had been 2 years previously. With some help, she could discuss her worries, as opposed to expressing them in displacement. When we played games, she always played fairly. She might playfully make fun of me when I lost, but she did not cheat or change the rules. Because she was able to think about what was bothering her and to tolerate ambivalent feelings more easily, she had less need to hide her concerns from herself via displacement. This did not mean that she could talk with ease about her worries. But she responded more readily when I commented on transference behavior or directly brought up concerns about her mother's remarriage.

Although older school-age children often resist talking directly about problems, they frequently agree with direct interpretations that are phrased in concrete terms and presented with empathy for the child's feelings. Once the therapist has established a solid relationship with an older school-age child, direct interpretation can be used to help the child organize and understand emotionally painful experiences and memories. For example, early in the second period of treatment, I tried to help Stacey connect her anxiety about her mother's new relationship with her memories of the divorce. I said, "Other kids I've known have been mad and worried when their mom decides to get married again. That's because they start thinking about the divorce and they don't want to go through that again. I think it was sad and upsetting for you when Bill and your mom divorced. You never knew your real dad, and Bill was the closest to a dad you ever had. But he didn't see you much after he moved out and then he moved away. That really hurt your feelings." Stacey listened thoughtfully and said, "You're right." When I said directly that I thought she and her sister were worried the new marriage would also end in divorce and they would have to go through the same painful feelings all over again, Stacey said, "I bet he'll be gone in 3 months." This comment confirmed my impression that Stacey was consciously thinking about the possibility of another loss.

Stacey brought up other related concerns. She described her mother's fiancé, Andy, as "nice" but said she didn't really know him very well. She described the pressure she felt from her mother to become close to him. I said, "It takes a long time to get to know someone well. Just because your mom is excited about marrying Andy doesn't mean you have to feel the same way right away. It seems like you like him, but you want to get to know him better." Stacey looked thoughtful and agreed. I also suggested that since she was worried that the relationship might not endure, it was normal for her to be cautious about getting close to Andy. Stacey was also alert to changes in her mother. For example, she complained that her mother wanted Stacey and her sister to be on their best behavior when Andy was around. I commented that since her mom's relationship with Andy was still new, maybe she was extrasensitive to anything that might cause a problem. I also said, however, that if they were going to be a family she and her sister should feel free to be themselves with Andy.

Developmental Guidance

In a parent guidance session, Ms. Kline expressed concern that Stacey and her sister were speaking rudely and sarcastically to both herself and Andy. I suggested that Stacey was showing her anxiety about the remarriage. I also pointed out that her anxiety intersected with developmentally normal behavior common in 11-year-olds: as school-age children begin the transition to adolescence, they frequently become more contentious and critical of their parents. This reflects the child's unconscious awareness that her coming developmental tasks involve differentiating the self from parents and learning to function more autonomously (Blos, 1979). In describing this process to Ms. Kline, I pointed out that a normal aspect of development in preadolescents was being intensified by the stress of Stacey's fears that her mother's new marriage would fail.

Utilizing the Older Child's Cognitive Abilities

When I told Stacey that her mother had said she was saying rude things particularly to Andy, Stacey immediately agreed and said, "Yeah, my sister and I are trying to drive him away." I asked how she thought they could do that. She said, "Maybe he'll be disgusted by us bad kids and give up." This gave me a chance to revisit issues from the first treatment. I told her that perhaps she and her sister had *felt* they had driven Bill, their first stepfather, away, even though that was not the reason for the divorce. If a kid feels that, I said, she might think it's better to show how bad she can be *before* the marriage. Stacey said that she liked Andy but that she really did not want to go through another divorce.

This second treatment particularly made use of Stacey's cognitive abilities. At age 11, she could assess similar and different aspects of a situation that seemed the same. She became anxious when her mother decided to remarry because she was afraid of a repetition of divorce. But she also was able to compare the differing personalities of her previous stepfather and her new stepfather. Her new stepfather, she gradually realized, was more emotionally attuned to her and more interested in her school and sports activities. As Stacey differentiated Andy from Bill, she became less anxious about their relationship. After her mother and Andy were married, I continued to see Stacey periodically, each time reviewing her reactions to her mother's new marriage.

In the second short-term treatment when Stacey was 11, it was easier to move from displacement activities to direct discussion of problems than had been true during the first treatment. In part this was because there were differences in the presenting problems. Stacey's anxiety over her mother's remarriage was not as acute and painful as her distress over the divorce. However, Stacey's ability to approach problems cognitively, control the intensity of her feelings, and tolerate ambivalence had increased as a result of ongoing development between ages 8 and 11. Consequently, she had less need to disguise her thoughts and feelings through displacement.

A Developmental Perspective on Intervention

Stacey's case is a good illustration of "intermittent therapy," a model in which the therapist provides intervention when difficulties occur, terminates when the problems are resolved, and remains available for future therapy. The intermittent treatment model is appropriate for children because they are developing rapidly and may need help at different points in development. After a child and parents have been helped to master a particular developmental hurdle, then therapy can cease, with the understanding that it may resume when a new hurdle presents itself.

I saw Stacey in the first intervention for about 6 months, until she had begun to cope with the divorce and loss of her stepfather. When her anxiety about loss resurfaced 2 years later in reaction to her mother's plans to remarry, I saw her again for about 6 months. In this model, the therapist works to establish a positive attachment relationship with the parent and child in order to support their relationship and the child's development. The therapeutic relationship then becomes used in the same way a child uses the attachment relationship: at times of stress, confusion, or anxiety, the parent and child can draw on the attachment relationship with the therapist for "refueling," guidance or clarification. Intermittent treatment is especially likely to be needed when a child has experienced trauma or loss, because at each new level the child may need to reprocess the trauma or loss from the perspective of her new level of development. The practitioner who thinks developmentally can create treatment plans and interventions that respond to the child's emerging developmental tasks and skills.

Observation Exercises

1. Spend 2–3 hours observing a group of elementary-school children. Preferably observe in three contexts: the regular classroom, the playground at recess, and a special class such as gym or music.

   a. Choose one child and observe his behavior in class and interaction with peers at recess. In class, look for attentional capacities and interest in work. On the playground, look for social abilities, place in status hierarchies, and general level of involvement with peers.

   b. Observe for gender-based behavior. Do girls and boys play in segregated groups, as the developmental literature of middle childhood suggests? Do you see instances of sustained interactions between boys and girls? Do you observe differences in the themes of boys' versus girls' play and interactions?

   c. Observe for behavior that reflects the social and moral values of school-age children. For example, do you see evidence of social rejection or stigmatization? Instances of prosocial behavior? Reactions to children who show difficulties controlling impulses? Controversies over rules or "correct" behavior? Negotiation of controversies?

2. Observe for developmental progress across middle childhood by spending 1 hour observing first graders (ages 6–7) and 1 hour observing fourth graders (ages 9–10). What differences do you see in the areas of social skills, peer orientation, physical abilities, and self-regulation?

CHAPTER 13

Conclusion:
Developmental Knowledge
and Practice

For a concluding review of the implications of developmentally based practice, I will return to the case of Jared, the toddler who struggled with ongoing fearful reactions to witnessing his father's abuse of his mother (see Chapters 7 and 8). Like many traumatized young children who experience frequent hyperarousal, Jared had begun to adopt the defense of aggression as a means of warding off danger when he felt anxious. He was aggressive both at home and at child care. His development was at risk because he was beginning to rely on aggression as a means of coping with anxiety, and also because others were already reacting negatively to his aggression. From a transactional perspective, the angry and distressed responses of child care providers and peers to his aggression fueled his anxiety and insecurity, reinforcing his sense that he needed to be aggressive to feel safe. The influence of anxiety on his perceptions and the negative feedback he was receiving created a risk that he would adopt an impulsive and aggressive style that would severely limit his possibilities for adaptive development.

Although Jared's mother was very invested in him, unwittingly she was also reinforcing his aggressive behavior. When he would hit her at home, she would become sad but would not stop him. She felt unable to set limits on him. Her sense of helplessness, based on her own traumatic abuse, prevented her from giving Jared the protection (in this case from his own impulses) he needed in order to feel secure. Their individual experiences of trauma were being carried into their relationship. The pattern of domestic violence was being repeated, this time with Jared in the abusive role. I was concerned that if she did not set limits on his aggression, he would continue to use it to cope with anxious or angry feelings and even would be at risk to become an abuser himself.

APPLYING PRACTICE KNOWLEDGE AND SKILLS

What resources and strengths can we find in the child and parent or parents to help a child like Jared cope with trauma? How does developmental knowledge that integrates maturational, transactional, and ecological perspectives inform intervention planning? What skills do practitioners need to translate this knowledge into intervention strategies? My work with Jared was informed by a knowledge of the developmental capabilities of older toddlers, by an analysis of how Jared's posttraumatic defenses and symptoms were interfering with the development of self-regulation, by an understanding of the crucial importance of attachment in supporting developmental progress, by an awareness that Jared's interactions in the world outside his family—in this case, the child care center—would also influence his development, and by my training in play therapy and toddler–parent intervention.

Assessment of Strengths

For work on Jared's behalf, two sources of strength were present. The first was his mother's investment in him, including her capacity for empathy, and the presence of some attachment strategies that they could use to relieve his distress. Mrs. Taylor was capable of carrying out one of the new functions of attachment that emerge during the toddler period—helping the child construct an understanding of the world through explanation, clarification, and reassurance. The second resource was Jared's developmental capabilities in the areas of symbolic play and language. In the first two sessions, Mrs. Taylor told the story of her husband's breaking the door, sending shattered glass cascading over herself and Jared. Jared's play in response to this story (having a dinosaur break down a door and bite a baby) demonstrated that he had age-appropriate resources for understanding and communicating about his experience. His receptive language ability permitted him to take in his mother's words, and his capacity for symbolic play allowed him to represent what the experience had meant to him.

Developmental Knowledge and Intervention Planning

Developmental understanding informed the intervention approach and goals in the following ways:

- *Attachment perspective.* Understanding of the continuing salience of attachment for toddlers led to a choice of the parent–child treatment. Especially when a young child has been traumatized, the security provided by the attachment relationship is the most critical resource. With these issues in mind, I established strengthening the child–parent attachment as a primary goal of intervention.
- *Maturational perspective.* Jared's capacity to represent his fears and memories in play made it possible for his mother and me to learn specifically how he had constructed the experiences of witnessing his father's violence. His emerging language ability made it possible for him to process his traumatic experiences through verbal understanding. A second goal of intervention was to use these developmental capacities to help him gain some mastery of trauma by interpreting his play as representing frightening memories, by putting them into words, by locating them in the past rather than in the present, and by offering verbal reassurance. This goal implicitly aimed to take advantage of areas of strength—play and language—in order to undo the maladaptive rigidity of a developmental function—regulation of affect and impulse—that had been compromised by trauma. I hoped that if Jared could be helped to think about his experiences and fears at a higher cognitive level in language and if his sense of security in the attachment could increase, then he would be able to move beyond a reliance on his aggressive defenses, which had great potential to interfere with his later development.
- *Ecological perspective.* It is necessary to be aware of all of the child's environments—home, child care, school—and to be ready to intervene when a setting outside the home has the potential to interfere with a child's development. There was a real risk that Jared's aggression would cause him to be identified as a mean or uncontrollable child by his child care providers. A third intervention goal was to consult with his caregivers to help them understand his aggressive behavior in the context of his traumatic exposure to violence and to ask them to give the treatment some time to work before dismissing him from the program. This intervention was helpful to his teachers because it enabled them to see his previously unexplained behavior in a new context. I also suggested some ways that Jared could be helped to feel more secure in the day care setting.

EVER-PRESENT COMPLICATIONS IN PRACTICE

While it is useful to articulate practice guidelines in the abstract, it is also important to realize that each child and each family must be approached with a respect for the unique ways they express their distress, the unique barriers that prevent them from resolving problems, and the unique resources they can use to move to a more adaptive pathway of development. I have tried to convey this idea throughout the book by presenting many case examples that demonstrate individualized applications of developmental practice principles.

Often these barriers and resources become evident when intervention reaches a plateau or sticking point. Then the practitioner must look for new ways to intervene. In the case of Jared, Mrs. Taylor had been very successful at verbalizing the meaning of Jared's play and reassuring him. But an impasse developed as it became evident that Mrs. Taylor was unable to set limits on his aggression toward her. She had trouble understanding that her inability to stop Jared from hitting her was contradicting her verbal assurances that violence would not occur in their family again. I believed that Jared would not feel confident in the attachment relationship until his mother could show him that she could keep herself safe.

Fortunately, Jared's play in sessions became a vehicle for helping Mrs. Taylor understand his need for limits. Jared pretended to have a party and served his mother and me coffee and cake. But when his mother asked for another cup, he pretended to pour "burning hot" coffee onto her leg. When she pretended to cry, Jared moved out of pretend and began hitting her hard on the leg with a Lincoln Log. He was hurting her, but she did not stop him. I intervened by taking the Lincoln log from Jared, telling him that I did not allow hurting. I would not let him hurt his mother, and I would not let him be hurt. Jared struggled with me for a moment and looked frightened. His mother took him on her lap and comforted him.

This incident allowed Mrs. Taylor to examine her own responses to Jared's aggression. She realized that she was making things worse by taking his aggression and pretending to cry. I pointed out that when I restrained him he had shown us that beneath the aggressive tough guy was a frightened 2-year-old who needed to feel safe and protected on his mother's lap. Her reflections on her sense of helplessness in the face of Jared's aggression ushered in a period of work lasting several months on her own traumatization. Gradually, as part of this work, she recognized that she had projected aspects of her relationship with her husband onto her relationship with Jared. As Mrs. Taylor consciously separated the two relationships, she saw more clearly that Jared's aggression needed to be handled with firm limits. Her new firmness, combined with her ongoing empathic responsiveness, allowed Jared to relax his hyperalert, aggressive defense. Her firmness signaled to him that he did not have to constantly test her ability to be protective. His aggressive behavior gradually diminished.

INTERVENTION AND DEVELOPMENTAL OUTCOME

Intervention that is timely and effective can have an important positive impact on a child's subsequent development. Although the child's relationships with his or her parents, the balance of risk and protective factors, and experiences in school and with peers will have much more cumulative influence on a child's development than will intervention, timely intervention can be an important turning point. It can help a child move away from a maladaptive pathway and onto a more adaptive one that has long-term implications for development.

I worked with Jared and his mother early in my social work career. I ran into Mrs. Taylor a few times over the years and was able to learn how Jared's development had proceeded. It had not been without problems. He struggled to learn to read in the early grades and began to develop low self-esteem about his school performance. Both his academic abilities and self-esteem improved after he was diagnosed with a learning disorder and appropriate special education was provided. However, in the areas of most concern during the treatment—regulation of affect and impulse and adaptive use of relationships—Jared had done well. A few years ago, Mrs. Taylor sent me a note, and it was a shock to learn that Jared had just turned 21. She described him as a caring, calm, and humorous person who has a good relationship with his girlfriend. She wrote that his driven aggression had stopped during our treatment when he was 3 and had never resurfaced.

References

Aber, J. L., & Allen, J. P. (1987). Effects of maltreatment on young children's socioemotional development: An attachment theory perspective. *Developmental Psychology, 23,* 406–414.

Aboud, F. E. (1984). Social and cognitive bases of ethnic identity constancy. *Journal of Genetic Psychology, 145,* 227–229.

Aboud, F. E., & Fenwick, V. (1999). Exploring and evaluating school-based Interventions to reduce prejudice. *Journal of Social Issues, 55,* 767–786.

Achenbach, T. M. (1991). *Manual for the child behavior checklist/4–18 and 1991 profile.* Burlington, VT: University of Vermont, Department of Psychiatry.

Ackerman, B. P., Izard, C. E., Schoff, K., Youngstrom, E. A., & Kogos, J. (1999). Contextual risk, caregiver emotionality, and the problem behaviors of six- and seven-year-old children from economically disadvantaged families. *Child Development, 70,* 1415–1427.

Adams, J. W., & Snowling, M. J. (2001). Executive function and reading impairments in children reported by their teachers as "hyperactive." *British Journal of Developmental Psychology, 19,* 293–306.

Adolph, K. E. (1997). Learning in the development of infant locomotion. *Monographs of the Society for Research in Child Development, 62,* 1–140.

Adolph, K. E., Vereijken, B., & Shrout, P. E. (2003). What changes in walking and why. *Child Development, 74,* 475–497.

Ainsworth, M. D. S. (1967). *Infancy in Uganda: Infant care and the growth of love.* Baltimore: Johns Hopkins University Press.

Ainsworth, M. D. S. (1982). Attachment: Retrospect and prospect. In C. M. Parkes & J. Stevenson-Hinde (Eds.), *The place of attachment in human behavior* (pp. 3–30). New York: Basic Books.

Ainsworth, M. D. S., Blehar, M. C., Waters, E., & Wall, S. (1978). *Patterns of attachment: A psychological study of the Strange Situation.* Hillsdale, NJ: Erlbaum.

Aisenberg, E., & Mennen, F. E. (2000). Children exposed to community violence: Issues for assessment and treatment. *Child and Adolescent Social Work Journal, 17,* 341–360.

Akhtar, N., Jipson, J., & Callanan, N. A. (2001). Learning words through overhearing. *Child Development, 72,* 416–430.

Al-Mateen, C. S. (2002). Effects of witnessing violence on children and adolescents. In D. H. Schetky & E. P. Benedek (Eds.), *Principles and practice of child and adolescent forensic psychiatry* (pp. 213–224). Washington, DC: American Psychiatric Publishing.

Albano, A. M., Chorpita, B. F., & Barlow, D. H. (2003). Childhood anxiety disorders. In E. J. Mash & R. J. Barkley (Eds.), *Child psychopathology* (2nd ed., pp. 279–329). New York: Guilford Press.

Albright, K. J. (2002). Scaffolding parental functioning in the context of serious mental illness: Roles and strategies for the infant mental health specialist. In J. J. Shirilla & D. J. Weatherson (Eds.), *Case studies in infant mental health: Risk, resiliency, and relationships* (pp. 153–176). Washington DC: Zero to Three.

Altermatt, E. R., Pomerantz, E. M., Ruble, D. N., Frey, K. S., & Greulich, F. K. (2002). Predicting changes in children's self-perceptions of academic competence: A naturalistic examination of evaluative discourse among classmates. *Developmental Psychology, 38*, 903–917.

Amato, P. R. (2001). Children of divorce in the 1990s: An update of the Amato and Keith (1991) meta-analysis. *Journal of Family Psychology, 15*, 355–370.

American Academy of Pediatrics, Committee on Communications. (1995). Media violence. *Pediatrics, 95*, 949–951.

American Psychiatric Association (2000). *Diagnostic and statistical manual of mental disorders* (4th ed., text rev.). Washington, DC: Author.

Anastopoulos, A. D. (1999). Attention deficit/hyperactivity disorder. In S. D. Netherton, D. Holmes, & C. E. Walker (Eds.), *Child and adolescent psychological disorders: A comprehensive textbook* (pp. 98–117). New York: Oxford University Press.

Anda, R. F., Whitfield, C. L., Felitti, V. J., Chapman, D., Edwards, V. J., Dube, S. R., Williamson, D. F. (2002). Adverse childhood experiences, alcoholic parents, and later risk of alcoholism and depression. *Psychiatric Services, 53*, 1001–1009.

Anglin, J. M. (1993). Vocabulary development: A morphological analysis. *Monographs of the Society for Research in Child Development, 58* (10, Serial No. 238).

Anthony, E. J. (1986). Terrorizing attacks on children by psychotic parents. *Journal of the American Academy of Child Psychiatry. 25*, 326–335.

Armstrong, F. D., Blumberg, M. J., & Toledano, S. R. (1999). Neurobehavioral issues in childhood cancer. *School Psychology Review, 28*, 194–203.

Arndorfer, R. E., & Miltenberger, R. G. (1993). Functional assessment and treatment of challenging behavior: A review with implications for early childhood. *Topics in Early Childhood Special Education, 13*, 82–105.

Ashman, S. B., Dawson, G., Panagiotides, H., Yamada, E., & Wilkinson, C. W. (2002). Stress hormone levels of children of depressed mothers. *Development and Psychopathology, 14*, 333–349.

Aspendorpf, J. B. (1993). Beyond temperament: A two-factorial coping model of the development of inhibition during childhood. In K. H. Rubin & J. B. Aspendorpf (Eds.), *Social withdrawal, inhibition, and shyness in childhood* (pp. 265–289). Hillsdale NJ: Erlbaum.

Atwood, R., & Safyer, A. W. (1993). The autonomous self vs. the relational self: Implications of clinical assessment and treatment in child psychotherapy. *Journal of Analytic Social Work, 1*, 39–54.

Bailey, J. M., & Zucker, K. J. (1995). Childhood sex-typed behavior and sexual orientation: A conceptual analysis and quantitative review. *Developmental Psychology, 31*, 43–55.

Baldwin, A. L., Baldwin, C. P., Kasser, R., Zax, M., Sameroff, A., & Seifer, R. (1993). Contextual risk and resiliency during late adolescence. *Development and Psychopathology, 5,* 741–761.

Baldwin, D. (1995). Understanding the link between joint attention and language. In C. Moore & P. J. Dunham (Eds.), *Joint attention: Its origins and role in development* (pp. 131–158). Hillsdale, NJ: Erlbaum.

Bandura, A. (1994). *Self-efficacy: The exercise of control.* New York: Freeman.

Barakat, L. P., Kazak, A. E., Gallager, P. R., Meeske, K., & Stuber, M. (2000). Posttraumatic stress symptoms and stressful life events predict the long-term adjustment of survivors of childhood cancer and their mothers. *Journal of Clinical Psychology in Medical Settings, 7,* 189–196.

Barkley, R. A. (1997). *Defiant children: A clinician's manual for parent training* (2nd ed.). New York: Guilford Press.

Barkley, R. A. (2003). Attention deficit/hyperactivity disorder. In E. J. Mash & R. A. Barkley (Eds.), *Child psychopathology* (2nd ed., pp. 75–143). New York: Guilford Press.

Barnett, D., Ganiban, J., & Cicchetti, D. (1999). Maltreatment, negative expressivity, and the development of Type D attachments from 12 to 24 months of age. In J. I. Vondra & D. Barnett (Eds.), Atypical attachment in infancy and early childhood among children at developmental risk. *Monographs of the Society for Research in Child Development, 64* (Serial No. 258), 97–118.

Baron-Cohen, S. (2001). Theory of mind and autism: A review. *International Review of Research in Mental Retardation, 23,* 169–184.

Barron-McKeagney, T., Woody, J. D., D'Souza, H. J. (2001). Mentoring at-risk Latino children and their parents: Impact on social skills and problem behaviors. *Child and Adolescent Social Work Journal, 18,* 119–136.

Bartholomew, K., & Horowitz, L. M. (1991). Attachment styles among young adults: A test of a four category model. *Journal of Personality and Social Psychology, 61,* 226–244.

Barton, M. L., & Robins, D. (2000). Regulatory disorders. In C. H. Zeanah, Jr. (Ed.), *Handbook of infant mental health* (2nd ed., pp. 311–325). New York: Guilford Press.

Bartsch, K., & Wellman, H. M. (1995). *Children talk about the mind.* New York: Oxford University Press.

Bates, E., Camaioni, L., & Volterra, V. (1975). The acquisition of performatives prior to speech. *Merrill–Palmer Quarterly, 21,* 205–226.

Bates, E., Reilly, J., Wulfeck, B., Dronkers, N., Opie, M., Fenson, J., Kriz, S., Jeffries, R., Miller, L., & Herbst, K. (2001). Differential effects of unilateral lesions on language production in children and adults. *Brain and Language, 79,* 223–265.

Bates, J., & Bayles, K. (1988). Attachment and the development of behavior problems. In J. Belsky & T. Nezworski (Eds.), *Clinical applications of attachment* (pp. 253–299). Hillsdale, NJ: Erlbaum.

Bates, J. E., Wachs, T. D., & Emde, R. N. (1994). Toward practical uses for biological concepts of temperament. In J. E. Bates & T. D. Wachs (Eds.), *Temperament: Individual differences at the interface of biology and behavior* (pp. 275– 306). Washington, DC: American Psychological Association.

Bauer, P. (1996). Recalling past events: From infancy to early childhood, *Annals of Child Development, 11,* 25–71.

Bandmaster, R. F., & Senders, P. S. (1988). Identity development and the role structure of children's games. *Journal of Genetic Psychology, 52,* 163–176.

Baumrind, D. (1993). The average expectable environment is not good enough: A response to Scarr. *Child Development, 64,* 1299–1317.

Bauserman, R. (2002). Child adjustment in joint-custody versus sole-custody arrangement: A meta-analytic review. *Journal of Family Psychology, 16,* 91–102.

Bayley, N. (1993). *Bayley scales of infant development* (2nd ed.). San Antonio, TX: Psychological Corporation.

Bell, C. C., & Jenkins, E. J. (1993). Community violence and children on Chicago's southside. *Psychiatry, 56,* 46–54.

Bell, S. M., & Ainsworth, M. D. S. (1972). Infant crying and maternal responsiveness. *Child Development, 43,* 1171–1190.

Bennett, D. S., Bendersky, M., & Lewis, M. (2002). Children's intellectual and emotional-behavioral adjustment at 4 years as a function of cocaine exposure, maternal characteristics, and environmental risk. *Developmental Psychology, 38,* 648–658.

Bennett, J. W., Jr., & Davies, D. (1981). Intervention and adaptation in the third year: The mother–child dialogue. *Journal of Child Psychotherapy, 7,* 19–32.

Benoit, D., & Parker, K. (1994). Stability and transmission of attachment across three generations. *Child Development, 65,* 1444–1456.

Berg-Nielsen, T. S., Vikan, A., & Dahl, A. A. (2002). Parenting related to child and parental psychopathology: A descriptive review of the literature. *Clinical Child Psychology and Psychiatry, 7,* 529–552.

Bergmann, T., & Freud, A. (1965). *Children in the hospital.* New York: International Universities Press.

Berk, L. E. (1992). Children's private speech: An overview of theory and the status of research. In R. M. Diaz & L. E. Berk (Eds.), *Private Speech: From social interaction to self-regulation* (pp. 17–53). Hillsdale, NJ: Erlbaum.

Berkowitz, L. (1993). *Aggression: Its causes, consequences, and control.* New York: McGraw-Hill.

Berman, S. (1979). The psychodynamic aspects of behavior. In J. Noshpitz (Ed.), *Handbook of child psychiatry: Vol. 2. Disturbances in development* (pp. 3–28). New York: Basic Books.

Bernstein, V. J., Hans, S. L., & Percansky, C. (1991). Advocating for the young child in need through strengthening the parent–child relationship. *Journal of Clinical Child Psychology, 20,* 28–41.

Bertenthal, B. I., & Clifton, R. K. (1998). Perception and action. In W. Damon, D. Kuhn, & R. S. Siegler (Eds.), *Handbook of child psychology* (5th ed.): *Vol. 2. Cognition, perception, and language* (pp. 51–102). New York: Wiley.

Bertenthal, B. I., & Von Hofsten, C. (1998). Eye, head, and trunk control: The foundation for manual development. *Neuroscience and Biobehavioral Reviews, 22,* 515–520.

Bialystok, E. (2001). *Bilingualism in development: Language, literacy, and cognition.* New York: Cambridge University Press.

Bisanz, J., & LeFevre, J. (1990). Strategic and nonstrategic processing in the development of mathematical cognition. In D. F. Bjorklund (Ed.), *Children's strategies: Contemporary views of cognitive development* (pp. 213–244). Hillsdale, NJ: Erlbaum.

Black, M., Nair, P., Schuler, M., Keane, V., Snow, L., & Rigney, B. (1997). Risk factors for disruption in primary caregiving among infants of substance abusing women. *Child Abuse and Neglect, 21,* 1039–1051.

Bloom, L. (1991). *Language development from two to three*. New York: Cambridge University Press.

Bloom, L. (1998). Language acquisition in its developmental context. In W. Damon, D. Kuhn, & R. S. Siegler (Eds.), *Handbook of child psychology* (5th ed.): *Vol. 2. Cognition, perception, and language* (pp. 309–370). New York: Wiley.

Bloom, L., Margulis, C., Tinker, E., & Fujita, N. (1996). Early conversations and word learning: Contributions from child and adult. *Child Development, 67,* 3154–3175.

Blos, P. (1979). *The adolescent passage*. New York: International Universities Press.

Blos, P., Jr., & Davies, D. (1993). Extending the intervention process: Report of a distressed family with a damaged newborn and a vulnerable preschooler. In E. Fenichel & S. Provence (Eds.), *Development in jeopardy: Clinical responses to infants and families* (pp. 51–92). Madison, CT: International Universities Press.

Blount, R. L., Davis, N., Powers, S.W., & Roberts, M. C. (1991). The influence of environmental factors and coping style on children's coping and distress. *Clinical Psychology Review, 2,* 193–116.

Bolger, K. E., & Patterson, C. J. (2001). Developmental pathways from child maltreatment to peer rejection . *Child Development, 72,* 549–568.

Bolger, K. E., Patterson, C. J., Thompson, W. W., & Kupersmidt, J. B. (1995). Psychosocial adjustment among children experiencing persistent and intermittent family economic hardship. *Child Development, 66,* 1107–1129.

Bond, M. H. (1993). Emotions and their expression in Chinese culture. *Journal of Nonverbal Behavior, 17,* 245–262.

Borkowski, J. G., & Muthukrishna, N. (1995). Self-regulation of learning and performance: Issues and educational applications. In F. Weinert & W. Schneider (Eds.), *Memory performance and competencies: Issues in growth and development* (pp. 283–300). Hillsdale, NJ: Erlbaum.

Bowlby, J. (1969). *Attachment and loss: Vol 1. Attachment*. New York: Basic Books.

Bowlby, J. (1973). *Attachment and loss: Vol 2. Separation*. New York: Basic Books.

Bowlby, J. (1978). Attachment theory and its therapeutic implications. *Adolescent Psychiatry, 6,* 5–33.

Bowlby, J. (1980). *Attachment and loss: Vol 3. Loss*. New York: Basic Books.

Bowlby, J. (1988). *A secure base: Parent–child attachment and healthy human development*. New York: Basic Books.

Bradley, R. H., & Corwyn, R. F. (2002). Socioeconomic status and child development. *Annual Review of Psychology, 53,* 371–399.

Bradley, S. J. (2000). *Affect regulation and the development of psychopathology*. New York: Guilford Press.

Brazelton, T. B. (1990). Saving the bathwater. *Child Development, 61,* 1661–1671.

Brazelton, T. B. (1992). *Touchpoints: Your child's emotional and behavioral development*. Reading, MA: Addison-Wesley.

Brazelton, T. B. (1996). A window on the newborn's world: More than two decades of experience with the Neonatal Behavioral Assessment Scale. In S. J. Meisels & E. Fenichel (Eds.), *New visions for the developmental assessment of infants and young children* (pp. 127–146). Washington, DC: Zero to Three.

Brazelton, T. B., Nugent, J. K., & Lester, B. M. (1987). Neonatal behavioral assessment scale. In J. D. Osofsky (Ed.), *Handbook of infant development* (2nd ed., pp. 780–817). New York: Wiley.

Brazelton, T. B., & Yogman, M. Y. (1986). Introduction: Reciprocity, attachment and effectance: Anlage in early infancy. In T. B. Brazelton & M. Y. Yogman (Eds.), *Affective development in infancy* (pp. 1–9). Norwood, NJ: Ablex.

Bretherton, I. (1987). New perspectives on attachment relations: Security, communication and internal working models. In J. D. Osofsky (Ed.), *Handbook of infant development* (2nd ed., pp. 1061–1100). New York: Wiley.

Bretherton, I., & Munholland, K. A. (1999). Internal working models in attachment relationships: A construct revisited. In J. Cassidy & P. R. Shaver (Eds.), *Handbook of attachment: Theory, research, and clinical applications* (pp. 89–114). New York: Guilford Press.

Bricker, D., Squires, J., Mounts, L., Potter, L., Nickel, R., & Farrell, J. (1995). *Ages and stages questionnaires: A parent-completed, child-monitoring system.* Baltimore: Brookes.

Briere, J. (1992). *Child abuse trauma: Theory and treatment of the lasting effects.* Newbury Park, CA: Sage.

Brody, G. H., Dorsey, S., Forehand, R., & Armistead, L. (2002). Unique and protective contributions of parenting and classroom processes to the adjustment of African American children living in single-parent families. *Child Development, 73,* 274–286.

Broidy, L. M., Nagin, D. S., Tremblay, R. E., Bates, J. E., Brame, B., Dodge, K. A., Fergusson, D., Horwood, J. L., Loeber, R., Laird, L., Lynam, D. R., Moffitt, T. E., Pettit, G. S., & Vitaro, F. (2003). Developmental trajectories of childhood disruptive behaviors and adolescent delinquency. *Developmental Psychology, 39,* 222–245.

Bronfenbrenner, U. (1979). *The ecology of human development: Experiments by nature and design.* Cambridge, MA: Harvard University Press.

Brooks-Gunn, J., Han, W.-J., & Waldfogel, J. (2002). Maternal employment and child cognitive outcomes in the first three years of life: The NICHD study of early child care. *Child Development, 73,* 1052–1072.

Brownell, C., & Carringer, M. (1990). Changes in cooperation and self-other differentiation during the second year. *Child Development, 61,* 838–848.

Bruner, J. S. (1985). Vygotsky: A historical and conceptual perspective. In J. V. Wertsch (Ed.), *Culture, cognition and communication: Vygotskian perspectives* (pp. 21–34). New York: Cambridge University Press.

Bruner, J. S., & Lucariello, J. (1989). Monologue as narrative recreation of the world. In K. Nelson (Ed.), *Narratives from the crib* (pp. 73–97). Cambridge, MA: Harvard University Press.

Budwig, N., & Wiley, A. (1995). What language reveals about children's categories of personhood. In L. L. Sperry & P. A. Smiley (Eds.), *Exploring young children's concepts of self and other through conversation* (pp. 21–32). *New Directions in Child Development,* No. 69. San Francisco: Jossey-Bass.

Buka, S. L., Stichick, T. L., Birdthistle, I., & Earls, F. (2001). Youth exposure to violence: Prevalence, consequences. *American Journal of Orthopsychiatry, 71,* 298–310. Burton, S., & Mitchell, P. (2003). Judging who knows best about yourself: Developmental change in citing the self across middle childhood. *Child Development, 74,* 426–443.

Bushman, B. J., & Heusmann, L. R. (2001). Effects of televised violence on aggression. In D. Singer & J. Singer (Eds.), *Handbook of children and the media* (pp. 223– 254). Thousand Oaks, CA: Sage.

Buss, K. A., & Goldsmith, H. H. (1998). Fear and anger regulation in infancy:

Effects on the temporal dynamics of affective expression. *Child Development, 69,* 359–374.

Byng-Hall, J. (1995). Creating a more secure family base: Some implications of attachment theory for family therapy. *Family Process, 34,* 45–58.

Byng-Hall, J. (1999). Family and couple therapy: Toward greater security. In J. Cassidy & P. R. Shaver (Eds.), *Handbook of attachment: Theory, research, and clinical applications* (pp. 625–645). New York: Guilford Press.

Campbell, S. B. (1990). *Behavioral problems in preschool children.* New York: Guilford Press.

Campbell, S. B. (2002). *Behavioral Problems in Preschool Children* (2nd ed.). New York: Guilford Press.

Campo, A. T., & Rohner, R. P. (1992). Relationships between perceived parental acceptance–rejection, psychological adjustment, and substance abuse among young adults. *Child Abuse and Neglect, 16,* 429–440.

Campos, J. J., Anderson, D. I., Barbu-Roth, M. A., Hubbard, E. M., Hertenstein, M. J., & Witherington, D. (2000). Travel broadens the mind. *Infancy, 1,* 149–219.

Campos, J. J., Kermoian, R., Witherington, D., & Chen, H. (1997). Activity, attention, and developmental transitions in infancy. In P. J. Lang (Ed.), *Attention and orienting: Sensory and motivational processes* (pp. 393–415). Mahwah, NJ: Erlbaum.

Canino, I. A., & Spurlock, J. (2000). *Culturally diverse children and adolescents: Assessment, diagnosis and treatment* (2nd ed.). New York: Guilford Press.

Carver, P. R., Egan, S. K., & Perry, D. G. (2004). Children who question their heterosexuality. *Developmental Psychology, 40,* 43–53.

Case, R. (1985). *Intellectual development: From birth to adulthood.* Orlando, FL: Academic Press.

Case, R. (1998). The development of conceptual structures. In W. Damon, D. Kuhn, & R. S. Siegler (Eds.), *Handbook of child psychology* (5th ed.): Vol. 2. Cognition, perception, and language (pp. 745–800). New York: Wiley.

Cassidy, J. (1994). Emotion regulation: Influences of attachment relationships. In N. A. Fox (Ed.), The development of emotion regulation: Biological and behavioral considerations. *Monographs of the Society for Research in Child Development, 59* (Serial No. 240), 228–249.

Cassidy, J., & Berlin, L. (1994). The insecure/ambivalent pattern of attachment: Theory and research. *Child Development, 65,* 971–991.

Castle, J., Groothues, C., Bredenkamp, D., Beckett, C., O'Connor, T., Rutter, M., & the E.R.A. Study Team (1999). Effects of qualities of early institutional care on cognitive attainments. *American Journal of Orthopsychiatry, 69,* 424–437.

Caughy, M. O., O'Campo, P. J., Randolph, S. M., & Nickerson, K. (2002). The influence of racial socialization practices on the cognitive and behavioral competence of African American preschoolers. *Child Development, 73,* 1611–1625.

Ceballo, R., & McLoyd, V. C. (2002). Social support and parenting in poor, dangerous neighborhoods. *Child Development, 73,* 1310–1321.

Center for the Child Care Workforce. (2001). *Current data on child care salaries and benefits in the United States.* Washington, DC: Author.

Cerel, J., Fristad, M. A., Weller, E. B., & Weller, R. A. (1999). Suicide-bereaved children and adolescents: A controlled longitudinal examination. *Journal of the American Academy of Child and Adolescent Psychiatry,38,* 672–679.

Cerel, J., Fristad, M. A., Weller, E. B., & Weller, R. A. (2000). Suicide bereaved children and adolescents II: Parental and family functioning. *Journal of the American Academy of Child and Adolescent Psychiatry, 39*, 437–444.

Chang, P. (1990). Psychosocial needs of long-term cancer survivors: A review of the literature. *Pediatrician, 18*, 20–24.

Charman, T., Baron-Cohen, S., Swettenham, J., Baird, G., Cox, A., & Drew, A. (2001). Testing joint attention, imitation, and play as infancy precursors to language and theory of mind. *Cognitive Development, 15*, 481–498.

Chen, E., Zeltzer, L. K., Craske, M. G., & Katz, E. R. (2000). Children's memories for painful cancer treatment procedures: Implications for distress. *Child Development, 71*, 933–947.

Cheour, M., Ceponiene, R., Lehtokoski, A., Luuk, A., Allik, J., Alho, K., & Naatanen, R. (1998). Development of language-specific phoneme representations in the infant brain. *Nature Neuroscience, 1*, 351–353.

Chess, S., & Thomas, A. (1986). *Temperament in clinical practice.* New York: Guilford Press.

Chethik, M. (2000). *Techniques of child therapy: Psychodynamic approaches* (2nd ed.). New York: Guilford Press.

Children's Defense Fund. (1998). *The state of America's children yearbook 1998.* Washington, DC: Author.

Children's Defense Fund. (2002). *The state of children in America's union: A 2002 action guide to leave no child behind.* Washington, DC: Author.

Children's Defense Fund. (2003). *State budget cuts create a growing child care crisis for low-income working families.* Washington, DC: Author.

Child Welfare League of America. (1998). *Alcohol and other drugs survey of state child welfare agencies.* Washington, DC: Author.

Chisholm, K., Carter, M. C., Ames, E. W., & Morison, S. J. (1995). Attachment security and indiscriminately friendly behavior in children adopted from Romanian orphanages. *Development and Psychopathology, 7*, 283–284.

Cicchetti, D., & Beeghly, M. (1987). Symbolic development in maltreated toddlers. *New Directions for Child Development, 36*, 5–29.

Cicchetti, D., & Toth, S. (1995). A developmental psychopathology perspective on child abuse and neglect. *Journal of the American Academy of Child and Adolescent Psychiatry, 34*, 541–565.

Clarke-Stewart, K. A., & Hayward, C. (1996). Advantages of father custody and contact for the psychological well-being of school age children. *Journal of Applied Developmental Psychology, 17*, 239–270.

Cobb, C. L. H. (1996). Adolescent–parent attachments and family problem-solving. *Family Process, 35*, 57–82.

Coie, J. D., & Dodge, K. A. (1998). Aggression and antisocial behavior. In W. Damon & N. Eisenberg (Eds.), *Handbook of child psychology* (5th ed.). *Vol. 3: Social, emotional and personality development* (pp. 779–862). New York: Wiley.

Cole, M., & Cole, S. R. (1989). *The Development of Children.* New York: Scientific American Books.

Coley, R. L., & Chase-Lansdale, P. L. (1998). Adolescent pregnancy and parenthood: Recent evidence and future directions. *American Psychologist, 53*, 152–166.

Collins, R., Mascia, J., Kendall, R., Golden, O., Schock, L., & Parlakian, R. (2003). Promoting mental health in child care settings: Caring for the whole child. *Zero to Three, 23*, 39–45.

Collins, W. A., Maccoby, E. E., Steinberg, L. Hetherington, E. M., & Bornstein, M. H. (2000). Contemporary research on parenting: The case for nature *and* nurture. *American Psychologist, 55,* 218.

Conger, R. D., McLoyd, V. C., Wallace, L. E., Sun, Y., Simons, R. L., & Brody, G. H. (2002). Economic pressure in African-American families: A replication and extension of the family stress model. *Developmental Psychology, 38,* 179–195.

Crain, R. M. (1996). The influences of age, race, and gender on child and adolescent multidimensional self-concept. In B. A. Bracken (Ed.), *Handbook of self-concept* (pp. 395–420). New York: Wiley.

Crawford-Brown, C . J., & Rattray, J. M. (2001). Parent–child relationships in Caribbean families. In N. B. Webb (Ed.), *Culturally diverse parent–child and family relationships: A guide for social workers and other practitioners* (pp. 89–106). New York: Columbia University Press.

Crick, N. R., Casas, J. F., & Nelson, D. A. (2002). Toward a more comprehensive understanding of peer maltreatment: Studies of relational victimization. *Current Directions in Psychological Science, 11,* 98–101.

Crittenden, P. M. (1992a). Children's strategies for coping with adverse environments: An interpretation using attachment theory. *Child Abuse and Neglect, 16,* 329–343.

Crittenden, P. M. (1992b). Quality of attachment in the preschool years. *Development and Psychopathology, 4,* 209–241.

Crockenberg, S. (1988). Social support and parenting. In H. Fitzgerald, B. Lester & M. Yogman (Eds.), *Theory and research in behavioral pediatrics* (pp. 141– 174). New York: Plenum Press.

Crockenberg, S., & Leerkes, E. (2000). Infant social and emotional development in family context. In C. H. Zeanah, Jr. (Ed.), *Handbook of infant mental health* (2nd ed., pp. 60–90). New York: Guilford Press.

Cross, W. E., Jr. (1985). Black identity: Rediscovering the distinction between personal identity and reference group orientation. In M. B. Spencer, G. K. Brookins, & W. R. Allen (Eds.), *Beginnings: The social and affective development of black children* (pp. 152–172). Hillsdale, NJ: Erlbaum.

Cross, W. E., Jr. (1987). A two-factor theory of black identity: Implications for the study of identity development in minority children. In J. S. Phinney & M. J. Rotherham (Eds.), *Children's ethnic socialization: Pluralism and Development* (pp. 117–133). Newbury Park, CA: Sage.

Cummings, E. M., & Davies, P. (1996). Emotional security as a regulatory process in normal development and the development of psychopathology. *Development and Psychopathology, 8,* 123–139.

Cummings, E. M., & Davies, P. (1994). *Children and marital conflict.* New York: Guilford Press.

Cummings, E. M., & Davies, P. T. (1999). Depressed parents and family functioning: Interpersonal effects and children's functioning and development. In T. Joiner & J. C. Coyne (Eds.), *The interactional nature of depression* (pp. 299– 327). Washington, DC: American Psychological Association.

Darwish, D., Esquivel, G. B., Houtz, J. C., & Alfonso, V. C. (2001). Play and social skills in maltreated and non-maltreated children in peer interactions. *Child Abuse and Neglect, 25,* 13–31.

Davies, D. (1991). Intervention with male toddlers who have witnessed parental violence. *Families in Society, 72,* 515–524.

Davies, D. (1992). Psychotherapy of a preschool cancer survivor: Promoting mastery and understanding. *Child and Adolescent Social Work, 9,* 289–305.

Davies, P. T., Harold, G. T., Goeke-Morey, M. C., & Cummings, E. M. (2002). Child emotional security and interparental conflict. *Monographs of the Society for Research in Child Development, 67* (3, Serial No. 270).

DeBellis, M. D., Baum, A. S., Birmaher, B., Keshavan, M. S., Eccard, C. H., Boring, A. M., Jenkins, F. J., & Ryan, N. D. (1999a). A. E. Bennett Research Award. Developmental traumatology. Part I: Biological stress systems. *Biological Psychiatry, 45,* 1259–1270.

DeBellis, M. D., Keshavan, M. S., Clark, D. B., Casey, B. J., Giedd, J. N., Boring, A. M., Frustaci, K., & Ryan, N. D. (1999b). A. E. Bennett Research Award. Developmental traumatology. Part II: Brain development. *Biological Psychiatry, 45,* 1271–1284.

DeCasper, A. J., & Fifer, W. P. (1980). Of human bonding: Newborns prefer their mother's voices. *Science, 208,* 1172–1176.

DeGangi, G. (2000). *Pediatric disorders of regulation in affect and behavior: A therapist's guide to assessment and treatment.* San Diego: Academic Press.

DeLoache, J. S., Miller, K. F., & Pierroutsakos, S. L. (1998). Reasoning and problem solving. Damon, D. Kuhn, & R. S. Siegler (Eds.), *Handbook of child psychology* (5th ed.): *Vol. 2. Cognition, perception, and language* (pp. 801–850). New York: Wiley.

DeMulder, E. K., & Radke-Yarrow, M. (1991). Attachment with affectively ill and well mothers: Concurrent behavioral correlates. *Development and Psychopathology, 3,* 227–242.

Demos, V. (1986). Crying in early infancy: An illustration of the motivational function of affect. In T. B. Brazelton & M. Y. Yogman (Eds.), *Affective development in infancy* (pp. 39–73). Norwood, NJ: Ablex.

Denby, R., Rindfleisch, N., & Bean, G. (1999). Predictors of foster parents' satisfaction and intent to continue to foster. *Child Abuse and Neglect, 23,* 287–303.

Denham, S. A., Blair, K. A., DeMulder, E., Levitas, J., Sawyer, K., Auerbach-Major, S., & Queenan, P. (2003). Preschool emotional competence: Pathway to social competence? *Child Development, 74,* 238–256.

Dennis, S. (1992). Stage and structure in the development of children's spatial representations. In R. Case (Ed.), *The mind's staircase: Exploring the conceptual underpinnings of children's thought and knowledge* (pp. 229–245). Hillsdale, NJ: Erlbaum.

Dews, S., Winner, E., Kaplan, J., Rosenblatt, E., Hunt, M., Lim, K., McGovern, A., Qualter, A., & Smarsh, B. (1996). Children's understanding of the meaning and function of verbal irony. *Child Development, 67,* 3071–3085.

Diamond, L. M. (2000). Sexual identity, attractions, and behavior among sexual minority women over a 2–year period. *Developmental Psychology, 36,* 241–250.

Dionnne, G., Tremblay, R., Boivin, M., Laplante, D., & Perusse, D. (2003). Physical aggression and expressive vocabulary in 19–month-old twins. *Developmental Psychology, 39,* 261–273.

Dishion, T. J., Andrews, D. W., & Crosby, L. (1995). Antisocial boys and their friends in early adolescence: Relationship characteristics, quality, and interactional process. *Child Development, 66,* 139–151.

Dishion, T. J., Patterson, G. R., & Griesler, P. C. (1994). Peer adaptations in the development of antisocial behavior: A confluence model. In L. R. Huesmann (Ed.), *Current perspectives on aggressive behavior* (pp. 61–95). New York: Plenum Press.

Dishion, T. J., Patterson, G. R., & Kavanagh, K. A. (1992). An experimental test of the coercion model: Linking theory, measurement and intervention. In J. McCord & R. E. Tremblay (Eds.), *Preventing antisoical behavior: Interventions from birth through adolescence* (pp. 253–282). New York: Guilford Press.

Dodge, K. A., Lansford, J. E., Burks, V. S., Bates, J. E., Pettit, G. S., Fontaine, R., & Price, J. M. (2003). Peer rejection and social information-processing factors in the development of aggressive behavior problems in children. *Child Development, 74,* 374–393.

Dodge, K. A., Pettit, G. S., & Bates, J. E. (1994). Effects of physical maltreatment on the development of peer relations. *Development and Psychopathology, 6,* 43–55.

Donahue, P. J., Falk, B., & Provet, A. G. (2000). *Mental health consultation in early childhood.* Baltimore: Brookes.

Dowdney, L. (2000). Annotation: Childhood bereavement following parental death. *Journal of Child Psychology and Psychiatry, 41,* 819–830.

Doyle, A. B., & Aboud, F. E. (1995). A longitudinal study of white children's prejudice as a social-cognitive development. *Merrill–Palmer Quarterly, 41,* 209–228.

Dozier, M., Albus, K., Fisher, P. A., & Sepulveda, S. (2002). Interventions for foster parents: Implications for developmental theory. *Development and Psychopathology, 14,* 843–860.

Duncan, G., Brooks-Gunn, J., & Klebanov, P. (1994). Economic deprivation and early development. *Child Development, 65,* 296–318.

Dunn, B. (1993). Growing up with a psychotic mother: A retrospective study. *American Journal of Orthopsychiatry, 63*(2), 177–189.

Dunn, J. (1987). The beginnings of moral understanding: Development in the second year. In J. Kagan & S. Lamb (Eds.), *The emergence of morality in young children* (pp. 91–111). Chicago: University of Chicago Press.

Dunn, J., Brown, J., & Beardsall, L. (1991). Family talk about feeling states and children's later understanding of others' emotions. *Developmental Psychology, 27,* 448–455.

Dunn, J., & Cutting, A. L. (1999). Understanding others, and individual differences in friendship interactions in young children. *Social Development, 8,* 201–219.

Dunn, J., Cutting, A. L., & Fisher, N. (2002). Old friends, new friends: Predictors of children's perspective on their friends at school. *Child Development, 73,* 621–635.

Dunn, J., Davies, L. C., O'Connor, T. G., & Sturgess, W. (2001). Family lives and friendships: The perspectives of children in step-, single-parent, and nonstep families. *Journal of Family Psychology, 15,* 272–287.

Dunn, J., & Hughes, C. (2001). "I got some swords and you're dead": Violent fantasy, antisocial behavior, friendship, and moral sensibility in young children. *Child Development, 72,* 491–505.

DuPaul, G. J. (1991). Parent and teacher ratings of ADHD symptoms: Psychometric properties in a community-based sample. *Journal of Clinical Child Psychology, 20,* 245–253.

Easterbrooks, M. A., & Goldberg, W. A. (1990). Security of toddler-parent attachment: Relation to children's sociopersonality functioning during kindergarten. In M. T. Greenberg, D. Cicchetti, & E. M. Cummings (Eds.), *Attachment in the preschool years: Theory, research and intervention* (pp. 221–224). Chicago: University of Chicago Press.

Eccles, J. S., Wigfield, A., & Schiefele, U. (1998). Motivation to succeed. In W. Damon & N. Eisenberg (Eds.), *Handbook of child psychology: Vol. 3. Social, emotional and personality development* (pp. 1017–1095). New York: Wiley.

Eckenrode, J., Laird, M., & Doris, J. (1993). School performance and disciplinary problems among abused and neglected children.*Developmental Psychology, 29*, 53–62.

Edelman, P. (1997). The worst thing Bill Clinton has done. *The Atlantic Monthly, 253*, 43–58.

Eden, G. F., & Zeffiro, T. A. (1998). Neural systems affected in developmental dyslexia revealed by functional neuroimaging. *Neuron, 21*, 279–282.

Edleson, J. L. (1999a). Children's witnessing of adult domestic violence. *Journal of Interpersonal Violence, 14*, 839–870.

Edleson, J. L. (1999b). The overlap between child maltreatment and woman battering. *Violence Against Women, 5*, 134–154.

Egeland, B., Carlson, E., & Sroufe, L. A. (1993). Resilience as process. *Development and Psychopathology. 5*, 517–528. Eisenberg, N. (2000). Emotion, regulation, and moral development. *Annual Review of Psychology, 51*, 665–697.

Eisenberg, N., & Fabes, R. A. (1998). Prosocial development. In W. Damon & N. Eisenberg (Eds.), *Handbook of child psychology* (5th ed.). Vol. 3. *Social, emotional and personality development* (pp. 701–778). New York: Wiley.

Eisenberg, N., Fabes, R. A., Guthrie, I. K., Murphy, B. C., Maszk, P., Holmgren, R., & Suh, K. (1996). The relations of regulation and emotionality to problem behavior in elementary school children. *Development and Psychopathology, 8*, 141–162.

Eisenberg, N., Fabes, R. A., Shepard, S. A., Guthrie, I. K., Murphy, B. C., Reiser, M. (1999). Parental reactions to children's negative emotions: Longitudinal relations to quality of children's social functioning. *Child Development, 70*, 513–534.

Eisler, R., & Levine, D. S. (2002). Nurture, nature, and caring: We are not prisoners of our genes. *Brain and Mind, 3*, 9–52.

Elbert, J. C. (1999). Learning and motor skills disorders. In S. D. Netherton, D. Holmes, & C. E. Walker (Eds.), *Child and adolescent psychological disorders: A comprehensive textbook* (pp. 24–50). New York: Oxford University Press.

Elicker, J., Egeland, M., & Sroufe, L. A. (1992). Predicting peer competence and peer relationships in childhood from early parent–child relationships. In R. D. Parke & G. W. Ladd (Eds.), *Family–peer relationships: Modes of linkage* (pp. 77– 106). Hillsdale, NJ: Erlbaum.

Elkind, D. (1994). *A sympathetic understanding of the child* (3rd ed.). Boston: Allyn & Bacon.

Elkind, D., & Weiner, I. B. (1978). *Development of the child.* New York: John Wiley & Sons.

Elkind, D., & Weiss, J. (1967). Studies in perceptual development III: Perceptual exploration. *Child Development, 38*, 1153–1161.

Emde, R. N. (1989). The infant's relationship experience: Developmental and affective aspects. In A. J. Sameroff & R. N. Emde (Eds.), *Relationship disturbances in early childhood: A developmental approach* (pp. 33–51). New York: Basic Books.

Emde, R. N. (1992). Social referencing research: Uncertainty, self and the search for meaning. In S. Feinman (Ed.), *Social referencing and the social construction of reality* (pp. 79–94). New York: Plenum Press.

Emde, R. N., Biringen, A., Clyman, R. B., & Oppenheim, D. (1991). The moral self in infancy: Affective core and procedural knowledge. *Developmental Review, 11*, 251–270.

Emde, R. N., & Buchsbaum, H. K. (1990). "Didn't you hear my mommy?": Autonomy *with* connectedness in moral self emergence. In D. Cicchetti & M. Beeghly (Eds.), *The self in transition: Infancy to childhood* (pp. 35–60). Chicago: University of Chicago Press.

Emery, R. E. (1999). *Marriage, divorce, and children's adjustment* (2nd ed.). Thousand Oaks, CA: Sage.

Engel, S. (1995). *The stories children tell: Making sense of the narratives of childhood.* New York: Freeman.

Engel, S. (1996). The guy who went up the steep nicken: The emergence of story-telling during the first three years. *Zero to Three, 17,* 1–9.

Erickson, J. (1996). The Infant–Toddler Developmental Assessment (IDA): A family-centered transdisciplinary assessment process. In S. J. Meisels & E. Fenichel (Eds.), *New visions for the developmental assessment of infants and young children* (pp. 27–52). Washington, DC: Zero to Three.

Erickson, M. T. (1993). Rethinking Oedipus: An evolutionary perspective of incest avoidance. *American Journal of Psychiatry, 150,* 411–415.

Erickson, S. J., & Steiner, H. (2000). Trauma spectrum adaptation: Somatic symptoms in long-term pediatric cancer survivors. *Psychosomatics, 41,* 339–346.

Erickson, S. J., & Steiner, H. (2001). Trauma and personality correlates in long term pediatric cancer survivors. *Child Psychiatry & Human Development, 31,* 195–213.

Erikson, E. H. (1963). *Childhood and society* (2nd ed.). New York: Norton.

Estes, D., Wellman, H. M., & Wooley, J. D. (1989). Children's understanding of mental phenomena. In H. Reese (Ed.), *Advances in child development and behavior* (pp. 41–86). New York: Academic Press.

Evans, G. W., & English, K. (2002). The environment of poverty: Multiple stressor exposure, psychophysiological stress, and socioemotional adjustment. *Child Development, 73,* 1238–1248.

Ewen, D., Blank, H., Hart, K., & Schulman, K. (2002). *State developments in child care, early education, and school-age care 2001.* Washington, DC: Children's Defense Fund.

Fanshel, D., Finch, S. J., & Grundy, J. F. (1990). *Foster children in life course perspective.* New York: Columbia University Press.

Federman, J. (Ed.). (1997). Executive summary. *National television violence study, Vol. 2.* Santa Barbara, CA: The Center for Communication and Social Policy, University of California, Santa Barbara.

Fein, D. J., & Lee, W. S. (2003). The impacts of welfare reform on maltreatment in Delaware. *Children and Youth Services Review, 25,* 85–113.

Fein, E. (1991). Issues in foster family care: Where do we stand? *American Journal of Orthopsychiatry, 61*(4), 578–583.

Feinstein, C., & Berger, K. (1987). The chronically ill or disabled child. In J. Noshpitz (Ed.), *Basic Handbook of Child Psychiatry* (Vol. 5, pp. 122–131). New York: Basic Books.

Feldman, R., Weller, A., Sirota, L., & Eidelman, A. I. (2002). Skin-to-skin contact (Kangaroo Care) promotes self-regulation in premature infants: Sleep–wake cyclicity, arousal modulation, and sustained exploration. *Developmental Psychology, 38,* 194–207.

Fick, A. C., Osofsky, J. D., & Lewis, M. L. (1997). Perceptions of violence: Children, parents, and police officers. In J. D. Osofsky (Ed.), *Children in a violent society.* New York: Guilford Press.

Field, T. (1992). Infants of depressed mothers. *Development and Psychopathology, 4,* 49–66.

Field, T. (1998). Maternal depression effects on infants and early interventions. *Preventive Medicine, 27,* 200–203.

Field, T. (2000). Infant massage therapy. In C. H. Zeanah, Jr. (Ed.), *Handbook of infant mental health* (2nd ed., pp. 494–500). New York: Guilford Press.

Findlater, J. E., & Kelly, S. (1999). Child protective services and domestic violence. *The Future of Children, 9,* 84–96.

Finkelhor, D. (1995). The victimization of children: A developmental perspective. *American Journal of Orthopsychiatry, 65,* 177–193.

Fisher, A. G., Murray, E. A., & Bundy, A. C. (1991). *Sensory integration theory and practice.* Philadelphia: Davis.

Fivush, R. (1997). Event memory in childhood. In N. Cowan (Ed.), *The development of memory in childhood* (pp. 139–162). Sussex: Psychology Press.

Fivush, R. (1998). Children's recollections of traumatic and nontraumatic events. *Development and Psychopathology, 10,* 699–716.

Flavell, J. H. (2000). Development of children's knowledge about the mental world. *International Journal of Behavioral Development, 24,* 15–23.

Flavell, J. H., Green, F. L., & Flavell, E. R. (1995). The development of children's knowledge about attentional focus. *Developmental Psychology, 31,* 706–712.

Flavell, J. H., Green, F. L., & Flavell, E. R. (2000). Development of children's awareness of their own thoughts. *Journal of Cognition and Development, 1,* 97–112.

Flavell, J. H., & Miller, P. H. (1998). Social cognition. In W. Damon, D. Kuhn, & R. S. Siegler (Eds.), *Handbook of child psychology:* (5th ed.). Vol. 2: Cognition, perception, and language (pp. 851–898). New York: Wiley.

Fleck-Henderson, A. (2000). Domestic violence in the child protection system: Seeing double. *Children and Youth Services Review, 22,* 333–354.

Foley, M. A., Harris, J. F., & Hermann, S. (1994). Developmental comparisons of the ability to discriminate between memories for symbolic play enactments. *Developmental Psychology, 30,* 206–217.

Folman, R. D. (1995). *Resiliency and vulnerability among abused and neglected children in foster care.* Unpublished dissertation, University of Michigan, Ann Arbor, Michigan.

Folman, R. D. (1998). "I was tooken": How children experience removal from their parents preliminary to placement into foster care. *Adoption Quarterly, 2,* 7–35.

Fonagy, P., Redfern, S., & Charman, T. (1997). The relationship betweeen belief-desire reasoning and a projective measure of attachment security (SAT). *British Journal of Developmental Psychology, 15,* 51–61.

Fong, R. (2003). *Culturally competent practice with immigrant and refugee children and families.* New York: Guilford Press.

Foorman, B. R., & Torgesen, J. (2001). Critical elements of classroom and small-group instruction promote reading success in all children. *Learning Disabilities Research and Practice, 16,* 203–212.

Ford, J., & Kidd, P. (1998). Early childhood trauma and disorders of extreme stress as predictors of treatment outcome with chronic posttraumatic stress disorder. *Journal of Traumatic Stress, 11,* 743–761.

Foster, E. M. (2002). Trends in multiple and overlapping disadvantages among Head Start enrollees. *Children and Youth Services Review, 24,* 933–954.

Fraiberg, S. (1974). The clinical dimension of baby games. *Journal of the American Academy of Child Psychiatry, 13,* 202–220.

Fraiberg, S. (1980). Clinical assessment of the infant and his family. In S. Fraiberg (Ed.), *Clinical studies in infant mental health: The first year of life* (pp. 23–48). New York: Basic Books.

Fraiberg, S., Adelson, E., & Shapiro, V. (1975). Ghosts in the nursery: A psychoanalytic approach to the problems of impaired mother–infant relationships. *Journal of the American Academy of Child Psychiatry. 14,* 387–421.

Fraser, M. W., Richman, J. M., & Galinsky, M. J. (1999). Risk, protection, and resilience: Toward a conceptual framework for social work practice. *Social Work Research, 23,* 131–143.

Freud, A. (1963). The concept of developmental lines. *Psychoanalytic Study of the Child, 18,* 245–266.

Freud, A. (1965). *Normality and pathology in childhood: Assessments of development.* New York: International Universities Press.

Freud, A. (1966). *The ego and the mechanisms of defense* (rev. ed.). New York: International Universities Press.

Freyd, J. J. (1996). *Betrayal trauma: The logic of forgetting childhood abuse.* Cambridge, MA: Harvard University Press.

Friedberg, R. D., & McClure, J. M. (2002). *Clinical practice of cognitive therapy with children and adolescents: The nuts and bolts.* New York: Guilford Press.

Friedman, J. M., & Polifka, J. E. (1996). *The effects of drugs on the fetus and nursing infant.* Baltimore: Johns Hopkins University Press.

Frijda, N., & Mesquita, B. (1994). The social roles and functions of emotion. In S. Kitayama & H. Marcus (Eds.), *Emotion and culture* (pp. 51–87). Washington, DC: American Psychological Association.

Fuligni, A. J., Yip, T., & Tseng, V. (2002). The impact of family obligation on the daily activities and psychological well-being of Chinese American adolescents. *Child Development, 73,* 302–314.

Fuller, T. L., & Wells, S. J. (2003). Predicting maltreatment recurrence among CPS cases with alcohol and other drug involvement. *Children and Youth Services Review, 25,* 553–569.

Furstenberg, F. F., Jr., Cook, T., Eccles, J., Elder, G. H., & Sameroff, A. J. (1999). *Managing to make it: Urban families and adolescent success.* Chicago: University of Chicago Press.

Galdston, R. (1979). Disorders of early parenthood: Neglect, deprivation, exploitation and abuse of little children. In J. D. Noshpitz (Ed.), *Basic handbook of child psychiatry* (Vol. 2, pp. 581–593). New York: Basic Books.

Garbarino, J. (1995). The American war zone: What children can tell us about living with violence. *Journal of Developmental and Behavioral Pediatrics, 16,* 431–435.

Garbarino, J., Dubrow, N., Kostelny, K., & Pardo, C. (1992). *Children in danger: Coping with the consequences of community violence.* San Francisco: Jossey-Bass.

Garcia, E. C. (2001). Parenting in Mexican American families. In N. B. Webb (Ed.), *Culturally diverse parent–child and family relationships: A guide for social workers and other practitioners* (pp. 157–180). New York: Columbia University Press.

Garcia Coll, C., & Magnuson, K. (1999). Cultural influences on child development: Are we ready for a paradigm shift? In A. S. Masten (Ed.), *Cultural processes in child development: The Minnesota Symposia on Child Psychology* (Vol. 29, pp. 1–24). Mahwah, NJ: Erlbaum.

Garfinkel, I., McLanahan, S. S., Tienda, M., & Brooks-Gunn, J. (2001). Fragile families and welfare reform: An introduction. *Children and Youth Services Review, 23,* 277–301.

Gemelli, R. (1996). *Normal child and adolescent development*. Washington, D.C.: American Psychiatric Press. Gershoff, E. T. (2002). Corporal punishment by parents and associated child behaviors and experiences: A meta-analytic review. *Psychological Bulletin, 128*, 539–579.

Gil, E. (1991). *The healing power of play*. New York: Guilford Press.

Gilkerson, L., & Stott, F. (2000). Parent–child relationships in early intervention with infants and toddlers with disabilities and their families. In C. H. Zeanah, Jr. (Ed.), *Handbook of infant mental health (2nd ed., pp. 457–471). New York: Guilford Press.

Gilliam, W. S., & Mayes, L. C. (2000). Developmental assessment of infants and toddlers. In C. H. Zeanah, Jr. (Ed.), *Handbook of infant mental health* (2nd ed., pp. 236–248). New York: Guilford Press.

Glaser, D. (2002). Emotional abuse and neglect (psychological maltreatment): A conceptual framework. *Child Abuse and Neglect, 26*, 697–714.

Gleason, W. J. (1995). Children of battered women: Developmental delays and behavioral dysfunction. *Violence and Victims, 10*, 153–159.

Glod, C. A., & Teicher, M. H. (1996). Relationship between early abuse, posttraumatic stress disorder, and activity levels in prepubertal children. *Journal of the American Academy of Child and Adolescent Psychiatry, 35*, 1384–1393.

Goodlin-Jones, B. L., Burnham, M. M., Gaylor, E. E., & Anders, T. F. (2001). Night waking, sleep–wake organization, and self-soothing in the first year of life. *Journal of Developmental and Behavioral Pediatrics, 22*, 226–233.

Goodman, S. H., & Gotlib, I. H. (1999). Risk for psychopathology in the children of depressed mothers: A developmental model for understanding mechanisms of transmission. *Psychological Review, 106*, 458–490.

Goyette, C. H., Conners, C. K., & Ulrich, R. F. (1978). Normative data on Revised Conners Parent and Teacher Rating Scales. *Journal of Abnormal Child Psychology, 6*, 221–236.

Greig, A., & Howe, D. (2001). Social understanding, attachment security of preschool children and maternal mental health. *British Journal of Developmental Psychology, 19*, 381–393.

Greenberg, M., & Speltz, M. (1988). Attachment and the ontogeny of conduct problems. In J. Belsky & T. Nezworski (Eds.), *Clinical applications of attachment* (pp. 177–218). Hillsdale, NJ: Erlbaum.

Greene, B. A. (1992). Racial socialization as a tool in psychotherapy with African-American children. In L. A. Vargas & J. D. Koss-Chioino (Eds.), *Working with culture* (pp. 63–84). San Francisco: Jossey-Bass.

Greenspan, S. I., & Greenspan, N. T. (1985). *First Feelings: Milestones in the development of your baby and child*. New York: Viking.

Greenspan, S. I., & Meisels, S. J. (1996). Toward a new vision for the developmental assessment of infants and young children. In S. J. Meisels & E. Fenichel (Eds.), *New visions for the developmental assessment of infants and young children* (pp. 11–26). Washington, DC: Zero to Three.

Grossman, K. E., Grossman, K., & Zimmerman, P. (1999). A wider view of attachment and exploration: Stability and change during the years of immaturity. In J. Cassidy & P. R. Shaver (Eds.), *Handbook of attachment: Theory, research, and clinical applications* (pp. 760–786). New York: Guilford Press.

Grusec, J. E., Goodnow, J. J., & Kuczynski (2000). New directions in analyses of parenting contributions to children's acquisition of values. *Child Development, 71*, 205–211.

Gunnar, M. R., Bruce, J., & Grotevant, H. D. (2000). International adoption of institutionally reared children: Research and policy. *Development and Psychopathology, 12,* 677–693.

Gunnar, M. R., Morison, S. J., Chisholm, K., & Schuder, M. (2001). Salivary cortisol levels in children adopted from Romanian orphanages. *Development and Psychopathology, 13,* 611–628.

Haden, C. A., Haine, R. A., & Fivush, R. (1997). Developing narrative structure in parent–child reminiscing across the preschool years. *Developmental Psychology, 33,* 295–307.

Haight, W. L. (1999). The pragmatics of caregiver–child pretending at home: Understanding culturally specific socialization practices. In A. Goncu (Ed.), *Children's engagement in the world: Sociocultural perspectives* (pp. 128–147). New York: Cambridge University Press.

Haith, M. M., & Benson, J. B. (1998). Infant cognition. In W. Damon, D. Kuhn, & R. S. Siegler (Eds.), *Handbook of child psychology* (5th ed.): *Vol. 2. Cognition, perception, and language* (pp. 199–254). New York: Wiley.

Halpern, R. (1993). Poverty and infant development. In C. H. Zeanah, Jr. (Ed.), *Handbook of infant mental health* (pp. 73–86). New York: Guilford Press.

Hamilton, C. E. (2000). Continuity and discontinuity of attachment from infancy through adolescence. *Child Development, 71,* 690–694. Hanish, L. D., & Guerra, N. G. (2002). A longitudinal analysis of patterns of adjustment following peer victimization. *Development and Psychopathology, 14,* 69–89.

Hart, S., Binggeli, N., & Brassard, M. (1998). Evidence of the effects of psychological maltreatment. *Journal of Emotional Abuse, 1,* 27–58.

Harter, S. (1983). Developmental perspectives on the self-system. In E. M. Hetherington (Ed.), *Handbook of child psychology* (4th ed.). Vol. 4: Socialization, personality and social development (pp. 275–385). New York: Wiley.

Harter, S. (1998). The development of self-representations. In W. Damon & N. Eisenberg (Eds.), *Handbook of child psychology: Vol. 3. Social, emotional and personality development* (pp. 553–618). New York: Wiley.

Harter, S. (1999). *The construction of the self: A developmental perspective.* New York: Guilford Press.

Hartup, W. W. (1992). Peer relations in early and middle childhood. In V. B. Van Hasselt & M. Hersen (Eds.), *Handbook of social development: A lifespan perspective* (pp. 257–281). New York: Plenum Press.

Hartup, W. W. (1996). The company they keep: Friendships and their developmental significance. *Child Development, 67,* 1–13.

Hawley, T. L., Halle, T. G., Drasin, R. E., & Thomas, N. G. (1995). Children of addicted mothers: Effects of the 'crack epidemic' on the caregiving environment and the development of preschoolers. *American Journal of Orthopsychiatry, 65,* 364–379.

Hay, D. F. (1994). Prosocial development. *Journal of Child Psychology and Psychiatry, 35,* 29–71.

Hay, D. F., Castle, J., & Davies, L. (2000). Toddlers' use of force against familiar peers: A precursor of serious aggression? *Child Development, 71,* 457–467.

Hay, D. F., Castle, J., Davies, L., Demetriou, H,, & Stimson, C. A. (1999). Prosocial action in very early childhood. *Journal of Child Psychology and Psychiatry and Allied Disciplines, 40,* 905–916.

Hellige, J. B. (1994). *Hemispheric asymmetry: What's right and what's left.* Cambridge, MA: Harvard University Press.

Henning, K., Leitenberg, H., Coffey, P., Turner, T., & Bennett, R. (1996). Long-term psychological and social impact of witnessing violent physical conflict between parents. *Journal of Interpersonal Violence, 11*, 35–51.

Hesse, E. (1999). The adult attachment interview: Historical and current perspectives. In J. Cassidy & P. R. Shaver (Eds.), *Handbook of attachment: Theory, research, and clinical applications* (pp. 395–433). New York: Guilford Press.

Hesse, E., & Main, M. (1999). Second-generation effects of unresolved trauma in nonmaltreating parents: Dissociated, frightened, and threatening parental behavior. *Psychoanalytic Inquiry, 19*, 481–540.

Hetherington, E. M., & Kelly, J. (2002). *For better or for worse: Divorce reconsidered.* New York: Norton.

Hewitt, S. K. (1999). *Assessing allegations of sexual abuse in pre-school children: Understanding small voices.* Newbury Park, CA: Sage.

Hildyard, K. L., & Wolfe, D. A. (2002). Child neglect: Developmental issues and outcomes. *Child Abuse and Neglect, 26*, 679–695.

Hirshberg, L. M. (1998). Infant mental health consultation to early intervention programs. *Zero to Three, 18*, 19–23.

Hirschfeld, L. A. (1996). Seeing race. *Michigan Today, 28*, 2–3.

Hofer, M. A. (1995). Hidden regulators: Implication for a new understanding of attachment, separation, and loss. In S. Golberg, R. Muir, & J. Kerr (Eds.), *Attachment theory: Social, developmental, and clinical perspectives* (pp. 203–230). Hillsdale, NJ: Analytic Press.

Holmbeck, G. N., Greenley, R. N., & Franks, E. A. (2003). Developmental issues and considerations in research and practice. In A. E. Kazdin & J. R. Weisz (Eds.), *Evidence-based psychotherapies for children and adolescents* (pp. 21–41). New York: Guilford Press.

Hooper, S. R., Swartz, C., Wakely, M., deKruif, R., & Montgomery, J. (2002). Executive functions in elementary school children with and without problems in written expression. *Journal of Learning Disabilities, 35*, 59–68.

Horowitz, M. J. (1986). *Stress response syndromes* (2nd ed.). Northvale, NJ: Jason Aronson.

Howes, C. (1992). Sequences in the development of competent play with peers: Social and social pretend play. *Developmental Psychology, 28*, 961–974.

Howes, C. (1999). Attachment relationships in the context of multiple caregivers. In J. Cassidy & P. R. Shaver (Eds.), *Handbook of attachment: Theory, research, and clinical applications* (pp. 671–687). New York: Guilford Press.

Howes, C., & Ritchie, S. (1998). Changes in child–teacher relationships in a therapeutic preschool program. *Early Education and Development, 10*, 411–422.

Howse, R. B., Calkins, S. D., Anastopoulos, A. D., Keane, S. P., & Shelton, T. (2003). Regulatory contributors to children's kindergarten achievement. *Early Education and Development, 14*, 101–119.

Hudson, J. A. (1993). Understanding events: The development of script knowledge. In M. Bennett (Ed.), *The child as psychologist: An introduction to the development of social cognition* (pp. 142–167). New York: Harvester Wheatsheaf.

Huesmann, L. R., Moise-Titus, J., Podolski, C.-L., & Eron, L. D. (2003). Longitudinal relations between children's exposure to TV violence and their aggressive and violent behavior in young adulthood. *Developmental Psychology, 39*, 201–221.

Hughes, C. (2002). Executive functions and development: Why the interest? *Infant and Child Development, 11*, 69–71.

Hughes, C., & Graham, A. (2002). Measuring executive functions in childhood: Problems and solutions. *Child and Adolescent Mental Health, 7,* 131–142.

Hughes, C., White, A., Sharpen, J., & Dunn, J. (2000). "Hard to manage" preschoolers' peer problems, and possible social and cognitive influences. *Journal of Child Psychology and Psychiatry, 41,* 169–179.

Hughes, D. (2003). Correlates of african american and latino parents' messages to children about ethnicity and race: A comparative study of racial socialization. *American Journal of Community Psychology, 31,* 15–33.

Huppi, P. S., Schuknecht, B., Boesch, C., Bossi, E., Felbinger, J., Fusch, C., & Herschkowitz, N. (1996). Structural and neurobehavioral delay in postnatal brain development of preterm infants. *Pediatric Research, 39,* 895–901.

Huttenlocher, J. (1999). Language input and language growth. In N. Fox, L. Leavitt, & J. Warhol (Eds.), *The role of early experience in development* (pp. 69–82). Skillman, NJ: Johnson & Johnson.

Huttenlocher, J., Haight, W., Bryk, A., Seltzer, M., & Lyons, T. (1991). Early vocabulary growth: Relation to language input and gender. *Developmental Psychology, 27,* 236–248.

Huttenlocher, P. R., & Dabholkar, A. S. (1997). Regional differences in synaptogenesis in the human cerebral cortex. *Journal of Comparative Neurology, 387,* 167–178.

Hyde, J. S., & Plant, E. A. (1995). Magnitude of psychological gender differences: Another side to the story. *American Psychologist, 50,* 159–161.

Institute of Medicine. (1996). *Fetal alcohol syndrome.* Washington, DC: National Academy Press.

Isabella, R. A., & Belsky, J. (1991). Interactional synchrony and the origins of mother–infant attachment: A replication study. *Child Development, 62,* 373–384.

Jackson, J. F. (1993). Multiple caregiving among African Americans and infant attachment: The need for an emic approach. *Human Development, 35,* 87–102.

Janowsky, J. S., & Carper, R. (1996). Is there a neural basis for cognitive transitions in school age children? In A. J. Sameroff & M. M. Haith (Eds.), *The five to seven year shift: The age of reason and responsibility* (pp. 33–62). Chicago: University of Chicago Press.

Jenkins, J. M., & Astington, J. W. (2000). Theory of mind and social behavior: Causal models tested in a longitudinal study. *Merrill–Palmer Quarterly, 46,* 203–220.

Johnson, J. G., Smailes, M., Cohen, M., Brown, J., & Bernstein, D. P. (2000). Associations between four types of childhood neglect and personality disorder symptoms during adolescence and early adulthood: Findings of a community-based longitudinal study. *Journal of Personality Disorders, 14,* 171–187.

Johnson, M. H. (1998). The neural basis of cognitive development. In W. Damon, D. Kuhn, & R. S. Siegler (Eds.), *Handbook of child psychology* (5th ed.): *Vol. 2. Cognition, perception, and language* (pp. 1–50). New York: Wiley.

Johnson, M. H. (1997). *Developmental cognitive neuroscience.* Cambridge, MA: Blackwell.

Johnson, R. M., Kotch, J. B., Catellier, D. J., Winsor, J. R., Dufort, V., Hunter, W., & Amaya-Jackson, L. (2002). Adverse behavioral and emotional outcomes from child abuse and witnessed violence. *Child Maltreatment, 7,* 179–186.

Johnston, J. R. (1995). Research update: Children's adjustment in sole custody

families compared to joint custody families and principles for custody decision making. *Family Conciliation Courts Review, 33,* 415–425.

Kagan, J. (1981). *The second year: The emergence of self-awareness.* Cambridge, MA:
Harvard University Press.

Kagan, J. (1984). *The nature of the child.* New York: Basic Books.

Kagan, J. (1989). Temperamental contributions to social behavior. *American Psychologist, 44,* 668–674.

Kagan, J., Kearsley, R. B., & Solano, P. R. (1978). *Infancy: Its place in human development.* Cambridge, MA: Harvard University Press.

Kagan, J., Resnick, J. S., Clark, C., Snidman, N., & Garcia Coll, C. (1984). Behavioral inhibition to the unfamiliar. *Child Development, 55,* 2212–2225.

Kail, R. V., & Salthouse, T. A. (1994). Processing speed as a mental capacity. *Acta
Psychologica, 86,* 199–225.

Kaiser, B., & Rasminsky, J. S. (1999). *Meeting the Challenge: Effective Strategies for
Challenging Behaviours in Early Childhood Environments.* Ottawa: Canadian
Child Care Federation.

Kalter, N. (1988). *Time-limited developmental facilitation groups for children of divorce:
Early elementary school manual.* Ann Arbor, MI: Author.

Kalter, N., & Schreier, S. (1994). Developmental facilitation groups for children of
divorce: The elementary school model. In C. W. LeCroy (Ed.), *Handbook of
child and adolescent treatment manuals* (pp. 307–342). New York: Lexington
Books.

Kamerman, S. B. (2000). Parental leave policies: An essential ingredient in early
childhood education and care policies. *Social Policy Report, 14,* 3–15.

Kates, W. G., Johnson, R. L., Rader, M. W., & Strieder, F. H. (1991). Whose child is
this? Assessment and treatment of children in foster care. *American Journal of
Orthopsychiatry, 61,* 584–591.

Katz, L. F., & Woodin, E. M. (2002). Hostility, hostile detachment, and conflict
engagement in marriages: Effects on child and family functioning. *Child
Development, 73,* 636–652.

Kaufman, J., & Charney, D. (2001). Effects of early stress on brain structure and
function: Implications for understanding the relationship between child maltreatment and depression. *Development and Psychopathology, 13,* 451–471.

Kaufman, J., & Zigler, E. (1996). Child abuse and social policy. In E. Zigler, S.
Kagan, & N. Hall (Eds.), *Children, families, and government: Preparing for the
twenty-first century* (pp. 233–255). Cambridge, UK: Cambridge University
Press.

Kaufman Kantor, G., & Little, L. (2003). Defining the boundaries of child neglect:
When does domestic violence equate with parental failure to protect? *Journal
of Interpersonal Violence, 18,* 338–355.

Kaye, K. (1982). *The mental and social life of babies: How parents create persons.* Chicago: University of Chicago Press.

Kaye, K., & Fogel, A. (1980). The temporal structure of face-to-face communication between mothers and infants. *Developmental Psychology, 16,* 454–464.

Kazdin, A. E. (2003). Problem solving skills and parent management training for
conduct disorder. In A. E. Kazdin & J. R. Weisz (Eds.), *Evidence-based psychotherapies for children and adolescents* (pp. 241–262). New York: Guilford
Press.

Kazdin, A. E., & Weisz, J. R. (2003). Introduction: Context and background of evidence-based psychotherapies for children and adolescents. In A. E. Kazdin &

J. R. Weisz (Eds.), *Evidence-based psychotherapies for children and adolescents* (pp. 241–262). New York: Guilford Press.

Keller, H., Lohaus, A., Volker, S., Cappenberg, M., & Chasiotis, A. (1999). Temporal contingency as an independent component of parenting behavior. *Child Development, 70,* 474–485.

Kellman, P. J., & Banks, M. S. (1998). Infant visual perception. In W. Damon, D. Kuhn, & R. S. Siegler (Eds.), *Handbook of child psychology* (5th ed.): *Vol. 2. Cognition, perception, and language* (pp. 103–146). New York: Wiley.

Kelly, J. B. (2000). Children's adjustment in conflicted marriage and divorce: A decade review of research. *Journal of the American Academy of Child and Adolescent Psychiatry, 39,* 963–973.

Kelly, J. B., & Lamb, M. E. (2000). Using child development research to make appropriate custody and access decisions for young children. *Family and Conciliation Courts Review, 38,* 297–312.

Kelly, J. B., & Lamb, M. E. (2003). Developmental issues in relocation cases involving young children: When, whether, and how? *Journal of Family Psychology, 17,* 193–205.

Killen, M., Lee-Kim, J., McGlothlin, H., & Stangor, C. (2002). How children and adolescents evaluate gender and racial exclusion. *Monographs of the Society for Research in Child Development, 67*(Serial No. 271), 1–119.

Killen, M., Pisacane, K., Lee-Kim, J., & Ardila-Rey, A. (2001). Fairness or stereotypes? Young children's priorities when evaluating group exclusion and inclusion. *Developmental Psychology, 37,* 587–596.

Killen, M., & Stangor, C. (2001). Children's social reasoning about inclusion and exclusion in gender and race peer group contexts. *Child Development, 72,* 174–186.

Kinnard, E. M. (2001). Perceived and actual academic competence in maltreated children. *Child Abuse and Neglect, 25,* 33–45.

Klinger, L. G., Dawson, G., & Renner, P. (2003). Autistic disorder. In E. J. Mash & R. A. Barkley (Eds.), *Child psychopathology* (2nd ed., pp. 409–454). New York: Guilford Press.

Kochanska, G. (1994). Beyond cognition: Expanding the search for the early roots of internalization and conscience. *Developmental Psychology, 30,* 20–22.

Kochanska, G. (2001). Emotional development in children with different attachment histories: The first three years. *Child Development, 72,* 474–490.

Kochanska, G. (2002). Committed compliance, moral self, and internalization: A mediational model. *Developmental Psychology, 38,* 339–351.

Kochanska, G., Aksan, N., & Koenig, A. (1995). A longitudinal study of the roots of preschoolers' conscience: Committed compliance and emerging internalization. *Child Development, 66,* 1752–1769.

Kochanska, G., Casey, R., & Fukumoto, A. (1995). Toddler's sensitivity to standard violations. *Child Development, 66,* 643–656.

Kochanska, G., Coy, K. C., & Murray, K. T. (2001). The development of self-regulation in the first 4 years of life. *Child Development, 72,* 1091–1111.

Kochanska, G., & Murray, K. T. (2000). Mother–child mutually responsive orientation and conscience development: From toddler to early school age. *Child Development, 71,* 417–431.

Kochanska, G., Murray, K. T., & Harlan, E. T. (2000). Effortful control in early childhood: Continuity and change, antecedents, and implications for social development. *Developmental Psychology, 36,* 220–232.

Kohlberg, L. (1984). *Essays on moral development: Vol. 2. The psychology of moral development.* New York: Harper & Row.

Kopp, C. B. (1982). Antecedents of self-regulation: A developmental perspective. *Developmental Psychology, 18,* 199–214.

Kopp, C. B., & Kaler, S. R. (1989). Risk in infancy: Origins and implications. *American Psychologist, 44*(2), 224–230.

Korenman, S., Miller, J., & Sjaastad, J. (1995). Long-term poverty and child development in the United States: Results from the NLSY. *Children and Youth Services Review, 17,* 127–155.

Koverola, C., & Heger, A. (2003). Responding to children exposed to domestic violence: Research informing practice and policy. *Journal of Interpersonal Violence, 18,* 331–337.

Kozol, J. (1991). *Savage inequalities: Children in America's schools.* New York: Crown.

Kreppner, J. M., O'Connor, T. G., Rutter, M., & the English and Romanian Adoptees Study Team. (2001). Can inattention/overactivity be an institutional deprivation syndrome? *Journal of Abnormal Child Psychology, 29,* 513–528.

Kuhl, P. K. (1999). The role of experience in early language development: Linguistic experience alters the perception and production of speech. In N. Fox, L. Leavitt, & J. Warhol (Eds.), *The role of early experience in development* (pp. 101–126). Skillman, NJ: Johnson & Johnson.

Kurtz, P. D., Gaudin, J. M., Wodarski, J. S., & Howing, P. T. (1993). Maltreatment and the school aged child: School performance consequences. *Child Abuse and Neglect, 17,* 581–589.

Ladd, G. W. (1990). Having friends, keeping friends, making friends, and being liked by peers in the classroom: Predictors of children's early school adjustment? *Child Development, 61,* 1081–1100.

Ladd, G. W. (1999). Peer relationships and social competence during early and middle childhood. *Annual Review of Psychology, 50,* 333–359.

Ladd, G. W., Kochenderfer, B. J., & Coleman, C. C. (1996). Friendship quality as a predictor of young children's early school adjustment. *Child Development, 67,* 1103–1118.

Larsson, I., & Svedin, C. G. (2002). Teachers' and parents' reports on 3- to 6-year-old children's sexual behavior—a comparison. *Child Abuse and Neglect, 25,* 247–266.

Laursen, B., Hartup, W. W., & Koplas, A. L. (1996). Towards understanding peer conflict. *Merrill–Palmer Quarterly, 42,* 76–102.

Leach, P. (1978). *Your baby and child.* New York: Knopf.

Leathers, S. J. (2002). Foster children's behavioral disturbance and detachment from caregivers and community institutions. *Children and Youth Services Review, 24,* 239–268.

Lee, M.-Y. (2001). Marital violence: Impact on children's emotional experiences, emotional regulation and behaviors in a post-divorce separation situation. *Child and Adolescent Social Work Journal, 18,* 137–163.

Lehmann, P. (2000). Posttraumatic stress disorder (PTSD) and child witnesses to mother-assault: A summary and review. *Children and Youth Services Review, 22,* 275–306.

Leonard, K. E., Eiden, R. D., Wong, M. M., Zucker, R. A., Puttler, L. I., Fitzgerald, H. E., Hussong, A., Chassin, L., & Mudar, P. (2000). Developmental perspectives on risk and vulnerability in alcoholic families. *Alcoholism: Clinical and Experimental Research, 24,* 238–240.

Leslie, L. K., Landsverk, J., Ezzet-Lofstrom, R., Tschann, J. M., Slymen, D. J., & Garland, A. F. (2000). Children in foster care: Factors influencing outpatient mental health service use. *Child Abuse and Neglect, 24,* 465–476.

Lester, B. M., Boukydis, C. F. Z., & Twomey, J. E. (2000). Maternal substance abuse and child outcome. In C. H. Zeanah, Jr. (Ed.), *Handbook of infant mental health* (2nd ed., pp. 161–175). New York: Guilford Press.

Lester, B. M., LaGasse, L., & Brunner, S. (1997). Data base of studies on prenatal cocaine exposure and child outcome. *Journal of Drug Issues, 27,* 487–499.

Lester, B. M., LaGasse, L., & Seifer, R. (1998). Cocaine exposure and children: The meaning of subtle effects. *Science, 282,* 633–634.

Levendosky, A. A., & Graham-Bermann, S. A. (2000). Behavioral observations of parenting in battered women. *Journal of Family Psychology, 14,* 80–94.

Levine, D. S. (2002). Introduction to the special issue on brain development and caring behavior. *Brain and Mind, 3,* 1–7.

LeVine, R. A., & Miller, P. M. (1990). Commentary. *Human Development, 33,* 73–80.

Lewis, M. L. (2000). The cultural context of infant mental health: The developmental niche of infant–caregiver relationships. In C. H. Zeanah, Jr. (Ed.), *Handbook of infant mental health* (2nd ed., pp. 91–108). New York: Guilford Press.

Lewis, M. L., & Brooks-Gunn, J. (1979). *Social cognition and the acquisition of self.* New York: Plenum.

Lewis, R. (1966). *Miracles: Poems by children of the English-speaking world.* New York: Simon & Schuster. Liben, L. S., & Bigler, R. S. (2002). The developmental course of gender differentiation: Conceptualizing, measuring, and evaluating constructs and pathways. *Monographs of the Society for Research in Child Development, 67*(Serial No. 269), 1–146.

Lieberman, A. F. (1992). Infant–parent psychotherapy with toddlers. *Development and Psychopathology, 4,* 559–574.

Lieberman, A. F. (1993). *The emotional life of the toddler.* New York: Free Press.

Lieberman, A. F., & Pawl, J. H. (1990). Disorders of attachment and secure base behavior in the second year of life: Conceptual issues and clinical interventions. In M. T. Greenberg, D. Cicchetti, & E. M. Cummings (Eds.), *Attachment in the preschool years: Theory, research and intervention* (pp. 375–397). Chicago: University of Chicago Press.

Lieberman, A. F., & Pawl, J. H. (1993). Infant–parent psychotherapy. In C. H. Zeanah, Jr. (Ed.), *Handbook of infant mental health* (pp. 427–442). New York: Guilford Press.

Lieberman, A. F., Silverman, R., & Pawl, J. H. (2000). Infant–parent psychotherapy: Core concepts and current approaches. In C. H. Zeanah, Jr. (Ed.), *Handbook of infant mental health* (2nd ed., pp. 472–484). New York: Guilford Press.

Lieberman, A. F., & Zeanah, C. H. (1999). Contributions of attachment theory to infant–parent psychotherapy and other interventions with infants and young children. In J. Cassidy & P. R. Shaver (Eds.), *Handbook of attachment: Theory, research, and clinical applications* (pp. 555–574). New York: Guilford Press.

Lillo-Martin, D. (1996). Modality effects and modularity in language acquisition: The acquisition of American sign language. In T. Bhatia & W. Ritchie (Eds.), *Handbook of language acquisition.* New York: Academic Press.

Lindsey, D., & Martin, S. K. (2003). Deepening child poverty: The not so good news about welfare reform. *Children and Youth Services Review, 25,* 165–173.

Locke, J. L. (1993). *The child's path to spoken language.* Cambridge, MA: Harvard University Press.

Lozoff, B., Jimenez, E., Hagen, J., Mollen, E., & Wolf, A. W. (2000). Poorer behavioral and developmental outcome more than 10 years after treatment for iron deficiency in infancy. *Pediatrics, 105,* E51.

Luciana, M., & Nelson, C. A. (1998). The functional emergence of prefrontally-guided working memory systems in four- to eight-year-old children. *Neuropsychologia, 36,* 273–293.

Lupien, S. J., King, S., Meaney, M. J., & McEwen, B. S. (2001). Can poverty get under your skin? Basal cortisol levels and cognitive function in children from low and high socioeconomic status. *Development and Psychopathology, 13,* 653–676.

Luthar, S. S., Cicchetti, D., & Becker, B. (2000). The construct of resilience: A critical evaluation and guidelines for future work. *Child Development, 71,* 543–562.

Luthar, S. S., & Zigler, E. (1991). Vulnerability and competence: A review of research on resilience in childhood. *American Journal of Orthopsychiatry, 61,* 6–22.

Lynch, M., & Cicchetti, D. (1998). An ecological–transactional analysis of children and contexts: The longitudinal interplay among child maltreatment, community violence, and children's symptomatology. *Development and Psychopathology, 10,* 235–257.

Lyon, G. R., Fletcher, J. M., Barnes, M. C. (2003). Learning disabilities. In E. J. Mash & R. A. Barkley (Eds.), *Child psychopathology* (2nd ed., pp. 520–588). New York: Guilford Press.

Lyons-Ruth, K. (1996). Attachment relationships among children with aggressive behavior problems: The role of disorganized early attachment patterns. *Journal of Clinical and Consulting Psychology, 64,* 64–73.

Lyons-Ruth, K., & Jacobvitz, D. (1999). Attachment disorganization: Unresolved loss, relational violence, and lapses in behavioral and attentional strategies. In J. Cassidy & P. R. Shaver (Eds.), *Handbook of attachment: Theory, research, and clinical applications* (pp. 520–554). New York: Guilford Press.

Lyons-Ruth, K., & Zeanah, Jr., C. H. (1993). The family context of infant mental health: I. Affective development in the primary caregiving relationship. In C. H. Zeanah, Jr. (Ed.), *Handbook of infant mental health* (pp. 14–37). New York: Guilford Press.

Lyons-Ruth, K., Zeanah, C. H., & Benoit, D. (2003). Disorder and risk for disorder during infancy and toddlerhood. In E. J. Mash & R. A. Barkley (Eds.), *Child psychopathology* (2nd ed., pp. 589–631). New York: Guilford Press.

MacFarlane, J. (1975). Olfaction in the development of social preferences in the human neonate. In M. Hoffer (Ed.), *Parent–infant interaction.* Amsterdam: Elsevier.

Macfie, J., Cicchetti, D., & Toth, S. L. (2001). The development of dissociation in preschool-aged children. *Development and Psychopathology, 13,* 233–254.

Magai, C. (1999). Affect, imagery, and attachment: Working models of interpersonal affect and socialization of emotion. In J. Cassidy & P. R. Shaver (Eds.), *Handbook of attachment: Theory, research, and clinical applications* (pp. 787–802). New York: Guilford Press.

Mahler, M. S., Pine, F., & Bergman, A. (1975). *The psychological birth of the human infant.* New York: Basic Books.

Main, M., & Cassidy, J. (1988). Categories of response to reunion with the parent at age six: Predictable from infant attachment classifications and stable over a one-month period. *Developmental Psychology, 24,* 415–426.

Main, M., & Hesse, E. (1990). Parents' unresolved traumatic experiences are related to infant disorganized attachment status: Is frightened and or/frightening parental behavior the linking mechanism? In M. T. Greenberg, D. Cicchetti & E. M. Cummings (Eds.), *Attachment in the preschool years: Theory, research and intervention* (pp. 161–184). Chicago: University of Chicago Press.

Main, M., Kaplan, N., & Cassidy, J. (1985). Security in infancy, childhood and adulthood: A move to the level of representation. In I. Bretherton and E. Waters (Eds.), Growing points of attachment theory and research. *Monographs of the Society for Research in Child Development. 50*(1–2, Serial No. 209), 66–106.

Main, M., & Morgan, H. (1996). Disorganization and disorientation in infant strange situation behavior: Phenotypic resemblance to dissociative states? In L. K. Michelson & W. J. Ray (Eds.), *Handbook of Dissociation: Theoretical, empirical, and clinical perspectives* (pp. 107–138). New York: Plenum Press.

Main, M., & Solomon, J. (1990). Procedures for identifying infants as disorganized/disoriented during the Ainsworth Strange Situation. In M. T. Greenberg, D. Cicchetti, & E. M. Cummings (Eds.), *Attachment in the preschool years: Theory, research and intervention* (pp. 121–160). Chicago: University of Chicago Press.

Malchiodi, C. A. (1998). *Understanding children's drawings.* New York: Guilford Press.

Maldonado-Duran, M., & Sauceda-Garcia, J. (1996). Excessive crying in infants with regulatory disorders. *Bulletin of the Menninger Clinic, 60,* 62–78.

Maluccio, A. N., & Ainsworth, F. (2003). Drug use by parents: A challenge for family reunification practice. *Children and Youth Services Review, 25,* 511–533.

Marshak, L. E., Seligman, M., & Prezant, F. (1999). *Disability and the family life cycle.* New York: Basic Books.

Martin, C. L., & Fabes. R. A. (2001). The stability and consequences of young children's same-sex peer interactions. *Developmental Psychology, 37,* 431–446.

Marvin, R. S., & Britner, P. A. (1999). Normative development: The ontogeny of attachment. In J. Cassidy & P. R. Shaver (Eds.), *Handbook of attachment: Theory, research, and clinical applications* (pp. 44–67). New York: Guilford Press.

Marx, M. H., & Henderson, B. B. (1996). A fuzzy trace analysis of categorical inferences and instantial associations as a function of retention interval. *Cognitive Development, 11,* 551–569.

Maslin-Cole, C., & Spieker, S. J. (1990). Attachment as a basis for independent motivation: A view from risk and nonrisk samples. In M. T. Greenberg, D. Cicchetti, & E. M. Cummings (Eds.), *Attachment in the preschool years: Theory, research and intervention* (pp. 245–272). Chicago: University of Chicago Press.

Masten, A. S., Best, K. M., & Garmezy, N. (1990). Resilience and development: Contributions from the study of children who overcome adversity. *Development and Psychopathology, 2,* 425–444.

Masten, A. S., & Coatsworth, J. D. (1998). The development of competence in favorable and unfavorable environments: Lessons from research on successful children. *American Psychologist, 53,* 205–220.

McAdoo, H. P. (2001). Parent and child relationships in African American families. In N. B. Webb (Ed.), *Culturally diverse parent–child and family relationships: A guide for social workers and other practitioners* (pp. 89–106). New York: Columbia University Press.

McClosky, L., Figueredo, A., & Koss, M. (1995). The effects of systemic family violence on children's mental health. *Child Development, 66,* 1239–1261.

McCubbin, M., Balling, K., Possin, P., Frierdich, S., & Byrne, B. (2002). Family resiliency in childhood cancer. *Family Relations, 51,* 103–111.

McDonough, S. C. (2000). Interaction guidance: An approach for difficult-to-engage families. In C. H. Zeanah, Jr. (Ed.), *Handbook of infant mental health* (2nd ed., pp. 485–493). New York: Guilford Press.

McFadyen, A. (1994). *Special care babies and their developing relationships.* New York: Routledge.

McGreevy, A. (1990). Treasures of children: Collections then and now: or treasures of children revisited. *Early Child Development & Care, 63,* 33–36.

McHale, S. M., Crouter, A. C., & Tucker, C. J. (2001). Free-time activities in middle childhood: Links with adjustment in early adolescence. *Child Development, 72,* 1764–1778.

McHale, S. M., Crouter, A. C., & Whiteman, S. D. (2003). The family contexts of gender development in childhood and adolescence. *Social Development, 12,* 125–148.

McKown, C., & Weinstein, R. S. (2003). The development and consequences of stereotype consciousness in middle childhood. *Child Development, 74,* 498–515.

McLoyd, V. C. (1998). Socioeconomic disadvantage and child development. *American Psychologist, 53,* 185–204.

Meins, E. (1997). *Security of attachment and social development of cognition.* Hove, UK: Psychology Press.

Meins, E., Fernyhough, C., Russell, J., & Clark-Carter, D. (1998). Security of attachment as a predictor of symbolic and mentalising abilities: A longitudinal study. *Social Development, 7,* 1–24.

Meisels, S. J. (1996). Charting the continuum of assessment and intervention. In S. J. Meisels & E. Fenichel (Eds.), *New visions for the developmental assessment of infants and young children* (pp. 27–52). Washington, DC: Zero to Three.

Meltzoff, A. (1995). Understanding the intentions of others: Re-enactment of intended acts by 18–month-old children. *Developmental Psychology, 31,* 838–850.

Meltzoff, A. N. (1988). Infant imitation after a 1–week delay: Long term memory for novel acts and multiple stimuli. *Developmental Psychology, 24,* 470–476.

Meltzoff, A. N., & Borton, R. W. (1979). Intermodal matching by human neonates. *Nature, 282,* 403–404.

Messer, S. C., & Beidel, D. C. (1994). Psychosocial correlates of childhood anxiety disorders. *Journal of the American Academy of Child and Adolescent Psychiatry, 33,* 975–983.

Mezey, J. (2003). Threatened progress: U.S. in danger of losing ground on child care for low-income working families. *CLASP Policy Brief. Child Care and Early Education Series* (Brief No. 2, 1-7). Washington, DC: Center for Law and Social Policy.

Mezey, J. (2004). Five reasons why the Senate should adopt the Snowe–Dodd Amendment to increase child care funding. *CLASP Policy Brief. Child Care and Early Education Series* (Brief No. 4-22). Washington, DC: Center for Law and Social Policy.

Mezey, J., Schumacher, R., Greenberg, M. H., Lombardi, J., & Hutchins, J. (2002). *Unfinished agenda: Child care for low-income families since 1996. Implications for federal and state policy.* Washington, DC: Center for Law and Social Policy.

Miller, D. B., & MacIntosh, R. (1999). Promoting resilience in urban African American adolescents: Racial socialization and identity as protective factors. *Social Work Research, 23,* 159–169.

Miller, J., Gold, M. S., & Silverstein, J. (2003). Pediatric overeating and obesity: An epidemic. *Psychiatric Annals, 33,* 94–99.

Miller, L. S., Wasserman, G. A., Neugebauer, R., Gorman-Smith, D., & Kamboukos, D. (1999). Witnessed community violence and antisocial behavior in high-risk urban boys. *Journal of Clinical Child Psychology, 28,* 2–11.

Minde, K. (2000). Prematurity and serious medical conditions in infancy: Implications for development, behavior, and intervention. In C. H. Zeanah, Jr. (Ed.), *Handbook of infant mental health* (2nd ed., pp. 176–194). New York: Guilford Press.

Minuchin, S. (1974). *Families and family therapy.* Cambridge, MA: Harvard University Press. Moore, V. A. (2002). The collaborative emergence of race in children's play: A case study of two summer camps. *Social Problems, 49,* 58–78.

Moffitt, T. E., & Caspi, A. (1998). Annotation: Implications of violence between Intimate partners for child psychologists and psychiatrists. *Journal of Child Psychology and Psychiatry and Allied Disciplines, 39,* 137–144.

Morelli, G. A., & Tronick, E. Z. (1991). Efé multiple caretaking and attachment. In J. L. Gewirtz & W. M. Kurtines (Eds.), *Intersections with attachment* (pp. 41–52). Hillsdale, NJ: Erlbaum.

Morgan, C. M., Tanofsky-Kraff, M., Wilfley, D. E., & Yanovski, J. A. (2002). Childhood obesity. *Psychiatric Clinics of North America, 11,* 257–278.

Morison, S. J., Ames, E. W., & Chisholm, K. (1995). The development of children adopted from Romanian orphanages. *Merrill–Palmer Quarterly, 41,* 411–430.

Morison, S. J., & Ellwood, A.-L. (2000). Resiliency in the aftermath of deprivation: A second look at the development of Romanian orphanage children. *Merrill–Palmer Quarterly, 46,* 717–737.

Moses, A. (1999). Exposure to violence, depression, and hostility in a sample of inner city high school youth. *Journal of Adolescence, 22,* 21–32.

Moss, E., Rousseau, D., Parent, S., St. Laurent, D., & Saintong, J. (1998). Correlates of attachment at school age: Maternal reported stress, mother–child interaction, and behavior problems. *Child Development, 69,* 1390–1405.

Mulhern, R. K., Wasserman, A. L., Friedman, A. G., & Fairclough, D. (1989). Social competence and behavioral adjustment of children who are long-term survivors of cancer. *Pediatrics, 83,* 18–25.

Mullen, E. M. (1995). *Mullen scales of early learning: AGS edition.* Circle Pines, MN: American Guidance Service.

Nadel, J., Carchon, I., Kervalla, C., Marcelli, D., & Reserbat-Planty, D. (1999). Expectancies for social contingency in 2–month-olds. *Developmental Science, 2,* 164–173.

Nathanson, A. I. (1999). Identifying and explaining the relationship between parental mediation and children's aggression. *Communication Research, 26,* 124–143.

National Association for Bilingual Education. (2002, February). NABE's legislative priorities for the 108th Congress. Retrieved from *http://www.nabe.org/policy.asp*.

National Center for Addiction and Substance Abuse. (1998). *No safe haven: Children of substance-abusing parents*. New York: Columbia University.

National Research Council. (1993). *Understanding child abuse and neglect*. Washington, DC: National Academy Press.

Naylor, P., Cowie, H., & del Rey, R. (2001). Coping strategies of secondary school children in response to being bullied. *Child Psychology & Psychiatry Review, 6*, 114–120.

Neitzel, C., & Stright, A. D. (2003). Mothers' scaffolding of children's problem solving: Establishing a foundation of academic self-regulatory competence. *Journal of Family Psychology, 17*, 147–159.

Nelson, C. A. (1999). Neural plasticity and human development. *Current Directions in Psychological Science, 8*, 42–45.

Nelson, C. A. (2000a). Neural plasticity and human development: The role of early experience in sculpting memory systems. *Developmental Science, 3*, 115–136.

Nelson, C. A. (2000b). The neurobiological bases of early intervention. In J. P. Shonkoff & S. J. Meisels (Eds.), *Handbook of early childhood intervention* (2nd ed., pp. 204–227). Cambridge, UK: Cambridge University Press.

Nelson, C. A., & Carver, L. J. (1998). The effects of stress and trauma on brain and memory: A view from developmental cognitive neuroscience. *Development and Psychopathology, 10*, 793–809.

Nelson, K. (1989). Monologue as representation of real-life experience. In K. Nelson (Ed.), *Narratives from the crib* (pp. 27–72). Cambridge, MA: Harvard University Press.

Netherton, S. D., Holmes, D., & Walker, C. E. (Eds.). (1999). *Child and adolescent psychological disorders: A comprehensive textbook* New York: Oxford University Press.

Newton, R. R., Litrownik, A. J., Landsverk, J. A. (2000). Children in foster care: Disentangling the relationship between problem behaviors and number of placements. *Child Abuse and Neglect, 24*, 1363–1374.

NICHD Early Childhood Research Network. (1997). Child care in the first year of life. *Merrill–Palmer Quarterly, 43*, 340–360.

NICHD Early Childhood Research Network. (2003). Does quality of child care affect child outcomes at age 4½? *Developmental Psychology, 39*, 451–469.

Nickman, S. L., Silverman, P. J., & Normand, C. (1998). Children's construction of a deceased parent: The surviving parent's contribution. *American Journal of Orthopsychiatry, 68*, 126–134.

Ninio, A. (1995). Expression of communicative intents in the single-word period and the vocabulary spurt. In K. Nelson & Z. Reger (Eds.), *Children's language* (Vol. 8, pp. 103–124). Hillsdale, NJ: Erlbaum.

Nix, R. L., Pinderhughes, E. E., Dodge, K. A., Bates, J. E., Pettit, G. S., & McFadyen-Ketchum, S. A. (1999). The relation between mothers' hostile attribution tendencies and children's externalizing behavior problems: The mediating role of mothers' harsh discipline practices. *Child Development, 70*, 896–909.

Nowakowski, R. S., & Hayes, N. L. (1999). CNS development: An overview. *Development and Psychopathology, 11*, 395–417.

O'Brien, M. (1992). Gender identity and sex roles. In V. B. Van Hasselt & M.

Hersen. (Eds.), *Handbook of social development: A lifespan perspective* (pp. 325–345). New York: Plenum Press.

O'Connor, T. G., & Rutter, M. (2000). Attachment disorder behavior following early severe deprivation: Extension and longitudinal follow-up. *Journal of the American Academy of Child and Adolescent Psychiatry, 39,* 703–712.

O'Connor, T. G., Rutter, M., Beckett, C., Keaveney, L., Kreppner, J. M., & the English and Romanian Adoptees Study Team. (2000). The effects of global severe privation on cognitive competence: Extension and longitudinal follow-up. *Child Development, 71,* 376–390.

O'Donnell, D. A., Schwab-Stone, M. E., & Muyeed, A. Z. (2002). Multidimensional resilience in urban children exposed to community violence. *Child Development, 73,* 1265–1282.

Olweus, D. (1993). *Bullying in schools: What we know and what we can do.* Oxford, UK: Basil Blackwell.

O'Neill, R. E., Horner, R. H., Albin, R. W., Storey, K., & Sprague, J. R. (1996). *Functional assessment and program development for problem behavior: A practical handbook.* Belmont, CA: Wadsworth.

Oppenheim, D., Nir, A., Warren, S., & Emde, R. N. (1997). Emotion regulation in mother–child narrative co-construction: Associations with children's narratives and adaptation. *Developmental Psychology, 33,* 284–294.

Osofsky, J. D. (1996). Introduction. In J. D. Osofsky & E. Fenichel (Eds.), *Islands of safety: Assessing and treating young victims of violence* (pp. 5–8). Washington, DC: Zero to Three.

Osofsky, J. D., & Thompson, M. D. (2000). Adaptive and maladaptive parenting: Perspectives on risk and protective factors. In J. P. Shonkoff & S. J. Meisels (Eds.), *Handbook of early intervention* (2nd ed., pp. 54–75). New York: Cambridge University Press.

Ou, Y. S., & McAdoo, H. P. (1993). Socialization of Chinese American children. In H. P. McAdoo (Ed.), *Ethnicity: Strength in diversity* (pp. 245–270). Newbury Park, CA: Sage.

Ozonoff, S., & Jensen, J. (1999). Specific executive function profiles in three neurodevelopmental disorders. *Journal of Autism and Developmental Disorders, 29,* 171–177.

Paarlberg, K. M., Vingerhoets, A. J. J. M., Passchier, J., Dekker, G. A., & van Giegn, H. P. (1995). Psychosocial factors and pregnancy outcome: A review with emphasis on methodological issues. *Journal of Psychosomatic Research, 39,* 563–595.

Paik, H., & Comstock, G. A. (1994). The effects of television violence on antisocial behavior: A meta-analysis. *Communication Research, 21,* 516–546.

Paley, V. G. (1981). *Wally's stories: Conversations in the kindergarten.* Cambridge, MA: Harvard University Press.

Paley, V. G. (1986). *Mollie is three: Growing up in school.* Chicago: University of Chicago Press.

Paley, V. G. (1988). *Bad guys don't have birthdays: Fantasy play at four.* Chicago: University of Chicago Press.

Parker, S. J., & Zuckerman, B. S. (1990). Therapeutic aspects of the assessment process. In S. J. Meisels & J. P. Shonkoff (Eds.), *Handbook of early intervention* (pp. 370–369). New York: Cambridge University Press.

Parrott, S., & Mezey, J. (2003). *Bush administration projects that the number of children receiving child care subsidies will fall by 200,000 during the next five years: Actual loss in subsidies likely would be far greater.* Washington, DC: Center for Law and Social Policy/Center on Budget and Policy Priorities.

Patterson, G. R. (1982a). *A social learning approach: 3. Coercive family process.* Eugene, OR: Castalia.

Patterson, G. R. (1982b). Self-control and self-regulation in childhood. In T. Field & A. Huston-Stein (Eds.). *Review of human development* (pp. 222–241). New York: Wiley.

Patterson, G. R., DeBaryshe, B. D., & Ramsey, E. (1989). A developental perspective on antisocial behavior. *American Psychologist, 44*, 329–335.

Pauli-Pott, U., Becker, K., Mertesacker, T., & Beckmann, D. (2000). Infants with "colic"—Mothers' perspectives on the crying problem. *Journal of Psychosomatic Research, 48*, 125–132.

Paulsell, D., Nogales, R., & Cohen, J. (2003). Quality child care for infants and toddlers from families with low incomes: Lessons learned from three communities. *Zero to Three, 23*, 4–10.

Pearce, J. W., & Pezzot-Pearce, T. D. (1997). *Psychotherapy of abused and neglected children.* New York: Guilford Press.

Peisner-Feinberg, E. S., Burchinal, M. R., Clifford, R. M., Culkin, M. L., Howes, C., Kagan, S. L., & Yazejian, N. (2001). The relation of preschool child-care quality to children's cognitive and social developmental trajectories through second grade. *Child Development, 72*, 1534–1553.

Pelligrini, A. D., & Jones, I. (1993). Play, toys and language. In J. H. Goldstein (Ed.), *Toys, play and child development* (pp. 27–44). Cambridge, UK: Cambridge University Press.

Pelligrini, A. D., & Smith, P. K. (1998). Physical activity play: The nature and function of a neglected aspect of play. *Child Development, 69*, 577–598.

Penzerro, R. M., & Lein, L. (1995). Burning their bridges: Disordered attachment and foster care discharge. *Child Welfare, 74*, 351–366.

Perner, J., Kain, W., & Barchfield, P. (2002). Executive control and higher-order theory of mind in children at risk of ADHD. *Infant and Child Development, 11*, 141–158.

Perry, B. D. (1994). Neurobiological sequelae of childhood trauma: Post-traumatic stress disorders in children. In M. Murberg (Ed.), *Catecholamine function in post-traumatic stress disorder: Emerging concepts* (pp. 233–255). Washington, DC: American Psychiatric Press.

Perry, B. D. (1997). Incubated in terror: Neurodevelopmental factors in the "cycle of violence." In J. D. Osofsky (Ed.), *Children in a violent society* (pp. 124–149). New York: Guilford Press.

Perry, B. D. (2002a). Childhood experience and the expression of genetic potential: What childhood neglect tells us about nature and nurture. *Brain and Mind, 3*, 79–100.

Perry, B. D. (2002b). Neurodevelopmental impact of violence in childhood. In D. H. Schetky & E. P. Benedek (Eds.), *Principles and practice of child and adolescent forensic psychiatry* (pp. 191–203). Washington, DC: American Psychiatric Publishing.

Peterson, L., Reach, K., & Grabe, S. (2003). Health-related disorders. In E. J. Mash & R. A. Barkley (Eds.), *Child psychopathology* (2nd ed., pp. 716–749). New York: Guilford Press.

Phipps, S., & Srivastava, D. K. (1997). Repressive adaptation in children with cancer. *Health Psychology, 16*, 521–528.

Pianta, R. C., & Kraft-Sayre, M. (1999). Parents' observations about their children's transitions to kindergarten. *Young Children, 54,* 47–52.

Piaget, J. (1948). *The moral judgment of the child.* Glencoe, IL: Free Press.

Piaget, J. (1951). *Judgment and reasoning in the child.* London: Routledge & Kegan Paul.

Piaget, J. (1952a). *The language and thought of the child.* London: Routledge & Kegan Paul.

Piaget, J. (1952b). *The origins of intelligence in children.* New York: International Universities Press.

Piaget, J. (1962). *Play, dreams and imitation in childhood.* New York: Norton.

Piaget, J., & Inhelder, B. (1969). *The psychology of the child.* New York: Basic Books.

Porter, C. L., & Hsu, H.-C., (2003). First-time mothers' perceptions of efficacy during the transition to motherhood: Links to infant temperament. *Journal of Family Psychology, 17,* 54–64.

Pomerantz, E. M., & Saxon, J. L. (2001). Children's conceptions of ability as stable and self-evaluative processes: A longitudinal investigation. *Child Development, 72,* 152–173.

Posada, G., Jacobs, A., Richmond, M. K., Carbonell, O. A., Alzate, G., Bustamante, M. R., & Quiceno, J. (2002). Maternal caregiving and infant security in two cultures. *Developmental Psychology, 38,* 67–78.

Posner, M. I., & Rothbart, M. K. (1994). Constructing neuronal theories of mind. In C. Koch & J. Davis (Eds.), *High level neuronal theories of the brain* (pp. 183–199). Cambridge, MA: MIT Press.

Posner, M. I., & Rothbart, M. K. (2000). Developing mechanisms of self-regulation. *Development and Psychopathology, 12,* 427–441.

Powell, J. (1998). First person account: Paranoid schizophrenia—a daughter's story. *Schizophrenia Bulletin, 24,* 175–177.

Provence, S., Erickson, J., Vater, S., & Palmeri, S. (1995). *Infant–Toddler Developmental Assessment: IDA.* Chicago: Riverside.

Pruett, M. K., Williams, T. Y., Insabella, G., & Little, T. D. (2003). Family and legal indicators of child adjustment to divorce among families with young children. *Journal of Family Psychology, 17,* 169–180.

Putnam, F, W. (2003). Ten year research update review: Child sexual abuse. *Journal of the American Academy of Child and Adolescent Psychiatry, 42,* 269–278.

Putnam, F. W., & Trickett, P. (1997). The psychobiological effects of sexual abuse: A longitudinal study. *Annals of the New York Academy of Sciences, 821,* 150–159.

Pynoos, R. S., Steinberg, A. M., & Goenjian, A. (1996). Traumatic stress in childhood and adolescence: Recent developments and current controversies. In B. van der Kolk, A. C. McFarlane, & L. Weisaeth (Eds.), *Traumatic stress* (pp. 331–358). New York: Guilford Press.

Pynoos, R. S., Steinberg, A. M., & Piacentini, J. C. (1999). A developmental psychopathology model of childhood traumatic stress and intersection with anxiety disorders. *Biological Psychiatry, 46,* 1542–1554.

Quintana, S. M., & Vera, E. M. (1999). Mexican American children's ethnic identity, understanding of ethnic prejudice, and parental ethnic socialization. *Hispanic Journal of Behavioral Sciences, 21,* 387–404.

Radke-Yarrow, M., McCann, K., DeMulder, E., Belmont, B., Martinez, P., & Richardson, D. T. (1995). Attachment in the context of high-risk conditions. *Development and Psychopathology, 7,* 247–265.

Radke-Yarrow, M., & Sherman, T. (1990). Hard growing: Children who survive. In J. Rolf, A. S. Masten, D. Cicchetti, K. H. Neuchterlin, & S. Weintraub (Eds.), *Risk and protective factors in the development of psychopathology* (pp. 87–119). New York: Cambridge University Press.

Ramey, C. T., & Ramey, S. L. (1998). Early intervention and early experience. *American Psychologist, 53,* 109–120.

Ramey, S., Lanzi, R., Phillips, M., & Ramey, C. (1998). Perspectives of former Head Start children and their parents on the transition to school. *Elementary School Journal, 98,* 311–327.

Rao, R., & Georgieff, M. K. (2000). Early nutrition and braindevelopment. In C. A. Nelson (Ed.), *The Minnesota symposia on child psychology: The effects of early adversity on neurobehavioral development* (Vol. 24, pp. 1–30). Mahwah, NJ: Erlbaum.

Rapport, M. D., Denney, C., DuPaul, G. J., & Gardner, M. J. (1994). Attention deficit disorder and methylphenidate normalization rates, clinical effectiveness, and response prediction in 76 children. *Journal of the American Academy of Child and Adolescent Psychiatry, 33,* 882–893.

Reed, E. S. (1995). Becoming a self. In P. Rochat (Ed.), *The self in infancy: Theory and research* (pp. 431–448). Amsterdam: Elsevier Science.

Reese, E., & Cox, A. (1999). Quality of adult book reading affects children's emergent literacy. *Developmental Psychology, 35,* 20–28.

Reiss, D. (1989). The represented and practicing family: Contrasting visions of family continuity. In A. J. Sameroff & R. N. Emde (Eds.), *Relationship disturbances in early childhood* (pp. 191–220). New York: Basic Books.

Reiss, D., & Neiderhiser, J. M. (2000). The interplay of genetic influences and social processes in developmental theory: Specific mechanisms coming into view. *Development and Psychopathology, 12,* 357–374.

Rende, R., & Plomin, R. (1993). Families at risk for psychopathology: Who becomes affected and why? *Developmental Psychopathology, 5,* 529–540.

Renken, B., Egeland, B., Marvinney, D., Mangelsdorf, S., & Sroufe, L. A. (1989). Early childhood antecedrents of aggression and passive-withdrawal in early elementary school. *Journal of Personality, 57,* 257–281.

Repacholi, B. (1998). Infants' use of attentional cues to identify the referent of another person's emotional expression. *Developmental Psychology, 34,* 1017–1025.

Reschovsky, J. D., & Cunningham, P. J. (1998). CHIPing away at the problem of uninsured childen. *HSC Issue Briefs* (No. 14). Washington, DC: Center for Studying Health System Change.

Reyna, V. F., & Brainerd, C. J. (1995). Fuzzy-trace theory: An interim synthesis. *Learning and Individual Differences, 7,* 1–75.

Ribaudo, J., & Glovak, S. (2002). Becoming whole: Combining infant mental health and occupational therapy on behalf of a toddler with sensory integration difficulties and his family. In J. J. Shirilla & D. J. Weatherston (Eds.), *Case studies in infant mental health: Risk, resiliency, and relationships* (pp. 85–104). Washington, DC: Zero to Three.

Rice, M. L. (1989). Children's language acquistion. *American Psychologist, 42,* 149–156.

Richards, J. E. (1997). Effects of attention on infant's preference for briefly exposed visual stimuli in the paired-comparison recognition-memory paradigm. *Developmental Psychology, 32,* 22–31.

Richters, J. E., & Martinez, P. E. (1993). The NIMH community violence project: I. Children as victims of and witnesses to violence. *Psychiatry, 56,* 7–21.

Ridgeway, D., Waters, E., & Kuczaj, S. A. (1985). Acquisition of emotion-descriptive language: Receptive and productive vocabulary norms for ages 18 months to 6 years. *Developmental Psychology, 21,* 901–908.

Riggs, S. A., & Jacobvitz, D. (2002). Expectant parents representations of early attachment relationships: Associations with mental health and family history. *Journal of Consulting and Clinical Psychology, 70,* 195–204.

Rimm-Kaufman, S. E., & Pianta, R. C. (2000). An ecological perspective on the transition to kindergarten: A theoretical framework to guide empirical research. *Journal of Applied Developmental Psychology, 21,* 491–511.

Rimm-Kaufman, S. E., Pianta, R. C., & Cox, M. J. (2000). Teachers' judgments of problems in the transition to kindergarten. *Early Childhood Research Quarterly, 15,* 147–166.

Rogoff, B. (1998). Cognition as a collaborative process. In W. Damon, D. Kuhn, & R. S. Siegler (Eds.), *Handbook of child psychology* (5th ed.): *Vol. 2. Cognition, perception, and language* (pp. 745–800). New York: Wiley.

Rosser, R. (1994). *Cognitive development: Psychological and biological perspectives.* Needham Heights, MA: Allyn & Bacon.

Rothbart, M. K., & Bates, J. E. (1998). Temperament. In W. Damon & N. Eisenberg (Eds.), *Handbook of child psychology* (5th ed.). *Vol. 3: Social, emotional, and personality development* (pp. 105–176). New York: Wiley.

Rothbart, M. K., Posner, M. I., & Hershey, K. L. (1995). Temperament, attention, and developmental psychopathology. In D. Cicchetti & D. J. Cohen (Eds.), *Manual of developmental psychopathology* (Vol. 1, pp. 315–340). New York: Wiley.

Rovee-Collier, C., Hartshorn, K., & DiRubbo, M. (1999). Long-term maintenance of infant memory. *Developmental Psychobiology, 35,* 91–102.

Rovee-Collier, C., & Hayne, H. (2000). Memory in infancy and early childhood. In E. Tulving (Ed.), *The Oxford handbook of memory* (pp. 267–282). New York: Oxford University Press.

Rowland, J. H. (1989). Developmental stage and adaptation: Child and adolescent model. In J. C. Holland & J. H. Rowland (Eds.), *Handbook of psychooncology* (pp. 519–543). New York: Oxford University Press.

Rubin, K. H., Bukowski, W., & Parker, J. G. (1998). Peer interactions, relationships, and groups. In W. Damon & N. Eisenberg (Eds.), *Handbook of child psychology* (5th ed.). *Vol. 3: Social, emotional and personality development* (pp. 619–700). New York: Wiley.

Rubin, K. H., Burgess, K, B., Kennedy, A. E., & Stewart, S. L. (2003). Social withdrawal. In E. J. Mash & R. J. Barkley (Eds.), *Child psychopathology* (2nd ed., pp. 330–371). New York: Guilford Press.

Rubin, K. H., Coplan, R. J., Fox, N. A., & Calkins, S. D. (1995). Emotionality, emotion regulation, and preschoolers' social adaptation. *Development and Psychopathology, 7,* 49–62.

Ruble, D. N., & Martin, C. L. (1998). Gender development. In W. Damon & N. Eisenberg (Eds.), *Handbook of child psychology* (5th ed.). *Vol. 3: Social, emotional and personality development* (pp. 553–618). New York: Wiley.

Rudolph, K. D., Lambert, S. F., Clark, A. G., & Kurlakowsky, K. D. (2001). Negotiating the transition to middle school: The role of self-regulatory processes. *Child Development, 72,* 929–946.

Rumm, P. D., Cummings, P., Krauss, M. R., Bell, M. A., & Rivara, F. P. (2000). Indentified spouse abuse as a risk factor for child abuse. *Child Abuse and Neglect, 24,* 1375–1381.

Russ, S. W., Robins, A. L., & Christiano, B. A. (1999). Pretend play: Longitudinal Prediction of creativity and affect in fantasy in children. *Creativity Research Journal, 12,* 129–139.

Russell, J., & Hill, E. (2001). Action monitoring and intention reporting in children with autism. *Journal of Child Psychiatry and Psychology, 42,* 317–328.

Rutter, M. (1981). Stress, coping and development: Some issues and some questions. *Journal of Child Psychology and Psychiatry, 22,* 326–356.

Rutter, M. (1985). Resilience in the face of adversity: Protective factors and resistance to psychiatric disorder. *British Journal of Psychiatry, 147,* 598–611.

Rutter, M. (1989). Psychological sequelae of brain damage in children. *American Journal of Psychiatry, 138,* 1533–1544.

Rutter, M., Kreppner, J. M., & O'Connor, T. G. (2001). Specificity and heterogeneity in children's responses to profound institutional privation. *British Journal of Psychiatry, 179,* 97–103.

Ryan, G. (2000). Childhood sexuality: A decade of study. Part II. Dissemination and future directions. *Child Abuse and Neglect, 24,* 49–61.

Saarni, C. (1997). Coping with aversive feelings. *Motivation and Emotion, 21,* 45–63.

Saarni, C. (1999). *The development of emotional competence.* New York: Guilford Press.

Saarni, C., Mumme, D. L., & Campos, J. J. (1998). Emotional development: Action, communication, and understanding. In W. Damon & N. Eisenberg (Eds.), *Handbook of child psychology* (5th ed.). *Vol. 3. Social, emotional and personality development* (pp. 237–310). New York: Wiley.

Sadeh, A., Dark, I., & Vohr, B. (1996). Newborns' sleep–wake patterns: The role of maternal, delivery, and infant factors. *Early Human Development, 44,* 311–322.

Sagi, A., Lamb, M. E., Lewkowicz, K. S., Shoham, R., Dvir, R., & Estes, D. (1985). Security of infant–mother, –father, and –*metaplet* attachments among kibbutz-reared Israeli children. In I. Bretherton and E. Waters (Eds.), Growing points of attachment theory and research. *Monographs of the Society for Research in Child Development. 50*(1–2, Serial No. 209), 257–255.

Sagi, A., van IJzendoorn, M. H., Aviezer, O., Donnell, F., & Mayseless, O. (1994). Sleeping out of home in a kibbutz communal arrangement: It makes a difference for infant–mother attachment. *Child Development, 65,* 992–1004.

Saldinger, A., Cain, A., Kalter, N., Lohnes, K. (1999). Anticipating parental death in families with young children. *American Journal of Orthopsychiatry, 69,* 39–48.

Salmon, K., & Bryant, R. (2001). Posttraumatic stress disorder in children: The influence of developmental factors. *Clinical Psychology Review, 22,* 163–188.

Sameroff, A. J. (1993). Models of development and developmental risk. In C. H. Zeanah, Jr. (Ed.), *Handbook of infant mental health* (pp. 3–13). New York: Guilford Press.

Sameroff, A. J., Bartko, W. T., Baldwin, A., Baldwin, C., & Seifer, R. (1998). Family and social influences on the development of child competence. In M. Lewis & C. Feiring (Eds.), *Families, risk, and competence* (pp. 161–186). Hillsdale, NJ: Erlbaum.

Sameroff, A. J., & Chandler, M. J. (1975). Reproductive risk and the continuum of caretaking casualty. In F. D. Horowitz, E. M. Hetherington, S. Scarr-

Salapatek & G. Siegel (Eds.), *Review of child development research* (Vol. 4, pp. 187–244). Chicago: University of Chicago Press.

Sameroff, A. J., & Fiese, B. H. (2000). Transactional regulation: The developmental ecology of early intervention. In J. P. Shonkoff & S. J. Meisels (Eds.), *Handbook of early childhood intervention* (2nd ed., pp. 135–159). Cambridge, UK: Cambridge University Press.

Sameroff, A. J., Seifer, R., Barocas, R., Zax, M., & Greenspan, S. (1987). Intelligence quotient scores of 4–year-old children: Social environmental risk factors. *Pediatrics, 79*, 343–350.

Samuels, A., & Taylor, M. (1994). Children's ability to distinguish fantasy events from real life events. *British Journal of DevelopmentalPsychology, 12*, 417–427.

Sander, L. (1975). Infant and caretaking environment: Investigation and conceptualization of adaptive behavior in a system of increasing complexity. In E. J. Anthony (Ed.), *Explorations in child psychiatry* (pp. 129–166). New York: Plenum Press.

Sanson, A. V., & Rothbart, M. K. (1995). Child temperament and parenting. In M. Bornstein (Ed.), *Parenting* (Vol. 4, pp. 299–321). Hillsdale, NJ: Erlbaum.

Sarnoff, C. A. (1976). *Latency.* Northvale, NJ: Jason Aronson.

Sarnoff, C. A. (1987). *Psychotherapeutic strategies in the latency years.* Northvale, NJ: Jason Aronson.

Savin-Williams, R. C. (2001). *Mom, Dad. I"m gay: How families negotiate coming out.* Washington, DC: American Psychological Association.

Sawyer, R. K. (1997). *Pretend play as improvisation: Conversation in the preschool classroom.* Mahwah, NJ: Erlbaum.

Schaefer, C. E., & Reid, S. E. (Eds.). (1986). *Game play.* New York: Wiley.

Scaife, M., & Bruner, J. (1975). The capacity for joint visual attention in the infant. *Nature, 253*, 265–266.

Scarr, S. (1998). American child care today. *American Psychologist, 53*, 95–108.

Scheeringa, M. S. (1999). Treatment for posttraumatic stress disorder in infants and toddlers. *Journal of Systemic Therapies, 18*, 20–31.

Scheeringa, M. S., & Gaensbauer, T. J. (2000). Posttraumatic stress disorder. In C. H. Zeanah (Ed.), *Handbook of infant mental health* (2nd ed., pp. 369–381). New York: Guilford Press.

Scheeringa, M. S., & Zeanah, C. H. (2001). A relational perspective on PTSD in early childhood. *Journal of Traumatic Stress, 14*, 799–815.

Schneider, W. (2002). Memory development in childhood. In U. Goswami (Ed.), *Blackwell handbook of childhood cognitive development* (pp. 236–256). Malden, MA: Blackwell.

Schneider, W., & Bjorklund, D. F. (1998). Memory. In W. Damon, D. Kuhn, & R. S. Siegler (Eds.), *Handbook of child psychology* (5th ed.): *Vol. 2. Cognition, perception, and language* (pp. 467–521). New York: Wiley.

Schneider, W., Gruber, H., Gold, A., & Opwis, K. (1993). Chess expertise and memory for chess positions in children and adults. *Journal of Experimental Child Psychology, 56*, 328–349.

Schneider-Rosen, K. (1990). The developmental reorganization of attachment relationships: Guidelines for classification beyond infancy. In M. T. Greenberg, D. Cicchetti, & E. M. Cummings (Eds.), *Attachment in the preschool years: Theory, research and intervention* (pp. 185–220). Chicago: University of Chicago Press.

Schore, A. N. (2001). Effects of a secure attachment relationship on right brain development, affect regulation, and infant mental health. *Infant Mental Health Journal, 22,* 7–66.

Sears, W., & Sears, M. (1995). *The discipline book: How to have a better-behaved child from birth to age 10.* Boston: Little, Brown.

Sebanc, A. M., Pierce, S. L., Cheatham, C. L., & Gunnar, M. R. (2003). Gendered social worlds in preschool: Dominance, peer acceptance and assertive social skills in boys' and girls' peer groups. *Social Development, 12,* 91–106.

Seja, A. L., & Russ, S. W. (1999). Children's fantasy play and emotional Understanding. *Journal of Clinical Child Psychology, 28,* 269–277.

Seligman, M. E. (1975). *Helplessness: On depression, development and death.* San Francisco: Freeman.

Seligman, S. (2000). Clinical interviews wiht families of infants. In C. H. Zeanah, Jr. (Ed.), *Handbook of infant mental health* (2nd ed., pp. 211–221). New York: Guilford Press.

Selner-O'Hagan, M. B., Kindlon, D. J., Buka, S. L., Raudenbush, S. W., & Earls, F. J. (1998). Assessing exposure to violence in urban youth. *Journal of Child Psychology and Psychiatry, 39,* 215–224.

Semidei, J., Radel, L. F., & Nolan, C. (2001). Substance abuse and child welfare: Clear linkages and promising responses. *Child Welfare, 80,* 109–128.

Sénéchal, M., & LeFevre, J. (2002). Parental involvement in the development of children's reading skill: A five-year longitudinal study. *Child Development, 73,* 445–460.

Sexson, S. B., & Madan-Swain, A. (1993). School reentry for the child with chronic illness. *Journal of Learning Disabilities, 26,* 115–125.

Shapiro, E. R. (1994). *Grief as a family process.* New York: Guilford Press.

Shapiro, J., & Applegate, J. S. (2002). Child care as a relational context for early development: Research in neurobiology and emerging roles for social work. *Child and Adolescent Social Work Journal, 19,* 97–114.

Share, D., Givens, C., Davies, D., Eley, E., & Chesler, J. (1992). "A Star is Born" in Ypsilanti. *American Journal of Public Health, 82,* 611–612.

Shaw, D. S., Gilliom, M., Ingoldsby, E. M., & Nagin, D. S. (2003). Trajectories leading to school-age conduct problems. *Developmental Psychology, 39,* 189–200.

Sher, K. J., Walitzer, K. S., Wood, P. K., & Brent, E. E. (1991). Characteristics of children of alcoholics: Putative risk factors, substance use and abuse, and psychopathology. *Journal of Abnormal Psychology, 100,* 427–448.

Shibusawa, T. (2001). Parenting in Japanese American families. In N. B. Webb (Ed.), *Culturally diverse parent–child and family relationships: A guide for social workers and other practitioners* (pp. 235–260). New York: Columbia University Press.

Shonkoff, J. P., & Marshall, P. C. (2000). The biology of developmental vulnerability. In J. P. Shonkoff & S. J. Meisels (Eds.), *Handbook of early childhood intervention* (2nd ed., pp. 35–53). Cambridge, UK: Cambridge University Press.

Shonkoff, J., & Phillips, D. (Eds.). (2000). *From neurons to neighborhoods: The science of early childhood development.* Washington, DC: National Academy Press.

Siegel, D. J. (1999). *The developing mind: Toward a neurobiologyof interpersonal experience.* New York: Guilford Press.

Siegel, D. J. (2001). Toward an interpersonal neurobiology of the developing mind: Attachment relationships, "mindsight," and neural integration. *Infant Mental Health Journal, 22,* 67–94.

Siegler, R. S. (1996). *Emerging minds: The process of change in children's thinking.* New York: Oxford University Press.

Silverman, P. R., Nickman, S., & Worden, J. W. (1992). Detachment revisited: The child's reconstruction of a dead parent. *American Journal of Orthopsychiatry, 62,* 494–503.

Simcock, G., & Hayne, H. (2003). Age-related changes in verbal and nonverbal memory during early childhood. *Developmental Psychology, 39,* 805–814.

Simons, R. L., Murry, V., McLoyd, V., Lin, K., Cutrona, C., & Conger, R. D. (2002). Discrimination, crime, ethnic identity, and parenting as correlates of depressive symptoms among African American children. *Development and Psychopathology, 14,* 371–393.

Simpson, J. A. (1999). Attachment theory in modern evolutionary perspective. In J. Cassidy & P. R. Shaver (Eds.), *Handbook of attachment: Theory, research, and clinical applications* (pp. 115–140). New York: Guilford Press.

Singer, D. G., & Singer, J. L. (1990). *The house of make-believe: Play and the developing imagination.* Cambridge, MA: Harvard University Press.

Singer, J. L. (1993). Imaginative play and adaptive development. In J. H. Goldstein (Ed.), *Toys, play and child development* (pp. 6–26). Cambridge, UK: Cambridge University Press.

Slade, A. (1994). Making meaning and making believe: Their role in the clinical process. In A. Slade & D. P. Wolf (Eds.), *Children at play* (pp. 81–107). New York: Oxford University Press.

Small, M. (1998). *Our babies, ourselves: How biology and culture shape the way we parent.* New York: Anchor Books.

Smetana, J. G. (1995). Morality in context: Abstractions, ambiguities, and applications. *Annals of Child Development, 10,* 83–130.

Smith, J., Brooks-Gunn, J., & Klebanov, P. (1997). Consequences of living in poverty for young children's cognitive and verbal ability and early school achievement. In G. Duncan & J. Brooks-Gunn (Eds.), *Consequences of growing up poor* (pp. 132–189). New York: Russell Sage Foundation.

Smith, P. K., & Brain, P. (2000). Bullying in schools: Lessons from two decades of research. *Aggressive Behavior, 26,* 1–9.

Smith, P. K., & Cowie, H. (1991). *Understanding children's development.* (2nd ed.). Cambridge, MA: Blackwell.

Smyth, M. M., & Anderson, H. I. (2000). Coping with clumsiness in the school playground: Social and physical play in children with coordination impairments. *British Journal of Developmental Psychology, 18,* 389–413.

Snow, C. W., & McGaha, C. G. (2003). *Infant development* (3rd ed.). Upper Saddle River, NJ: Prentice Hall.

Snyder, J. J., & Patterson, G. R. (1995). Individual differences in social aggression: A test of a reinforcement model of socialization in the natural environment. *Behavior Therapy, 26,* 371–391.

Solomon, J., George, C., & de Jong, A. (1995). Children classified as controlling at age six: Evidence of disorganized representational strategies and aggression at home and at school. *Development and Psychopathology, 7,* 447–463.

Sonnenschein, S. (1988). The development of referential communication: Speaking to different listeners. *Child Development, 59,* 694–702.

Sorce, J. F., Emde, R. N., Campos, J. J., & Klinnert, M. D. (1985). Maternal emotional signaling: Its effect on visual cliff behavior of one-year-olds. *Developmental Psychology, 21,* 195–200.

Spangler, G., & Grossman, K. E. (1993). Biobehavioral organization in securely and insecurely attached infants. *Child Development, 64,* 1439–1450.

Spencer, M. B. (1985). Cultural cognition and social cognition as identity factors in black children's personal-social growth. In M. B. Spencer, G. K. Brookins, & W. R. Allen (Eds.), *Beginnings: The social and affective development of black children* (pp. 215–230). Hillsdale, NJ: Erlbaum.

Spencer, M. B. (1987). Black children's identity formation: Risk and resilience of castelike minorities. In J. S. Phinney & M. J. Rotherham (Eds.), *Children's ethnic socialization: Pluralism and Development* (pp. 103–116). Newbury Park, CA: Sage.

Spencer, M. B. (1990). Development of minority children: An Introduction. *Child Development, 61,* 267–269.

Spencer, M. B., & Horowitz, F. D. (1973). Racial attitudes and color concept–attitude modification in black and caucasian preschool children. *Developmental Psychology, 9,* 246–254.

Spencer, M. B., & Markstrom-Adams, C. (1990). Identity processes among racial and ethnic minority children in America. *Child Development, 61,* 290–310.

Spitz, R. (1945). Hospitalism: An inquiry into the genesis of psychiatric conditions in early childhood. *Psychoanalytic Study of the Child, 1,* 53–74.

Squires, J., Bricker, D., Yockelson, S., Davis, M. S., & Kim, Y. (2002). *Ages and stages questionnaires: Social-emotional. A parent-completed, child-monitoring system for social-emotional behaviors.* Baltimore: Brookes.

Sroufe, L. A. (1983). Infant–caregiver attachment and patterns of adaptation in preschool: The roots of adaptation and competence. In M. Pelmutter (Ed.), *Minnesota Symposium on Child Psychology* (Vol.16, pp. 41–83). Hillsdale, NJ: Erlbaum.

Sroufe, L. A. (1989). Relationships, self and individual adaptation. In A. J. Sameroff & R. N. Emde (Eds.), *Relationship disturbances in early childhood* (pp. 70–94). New York: Basic Books.

Sroufe, L. A. (1990). Considering normal and abnormal together: The essence of developmental psychopathology. *Development and Psychopathology, 2,* 335–347.

Sroufe, L. A. (1997). Psychopathology as an outcome of development. *Development and Psychopathology, 9,* 251–268.

Sroufe, L. A., Carlson, E. A., Levy, A. K., & Egeland, B. (1999). Implications of attachment theory for developmental psychopathology. *Development and Psychopathology, 11,* 1–13.

Sroufe, L. A., Egeland, B., & Kreutzer, T. (1990). The fate of early experience following developmental change: Longitudinal approaches to individual adaptation. *Child Development, 61,* 1363–1373.

Sroufe, L. A., & Jacovitz, D. (1989). Diverging pathways, developmental transformations, multiple etiologies and the problem of continuity in development. *Human Development, 32,* 196–203.

St. James-Roberts, I., & Plewis, I. (1996). Individual differences, daily fluctuations, and developmental changes in amounts of infant waking, fussing, crying, feeding and sleeping. *Child Development, 67,* 2527–2540.

Steele, C. M. (1997). A threat in the air: How stereotypes shape intellectual identity and performance. *American Psychologist, 52,* 613–629.

Steinglass, P. (1987). *The alcoholic family.* New York: Basic Books.

Steir, A. J., & Lehman, E. B. (2000). Attachment to transitional objects: Role of maternal personality and mother–toddler interaction. *American Journal of Orthopsychiatry, 70,* 340–350.

Stern, D. N. (1974). The goal and structure of mother–infant play. *Journal of the American Academy of Child Psychiatry, 13,* 402–421.

Stern, D. N. (1977). *The first relationship: Mother and infant.* Cambridge, MA: Harvard University Press.

Stern, D. N. (1983). The early development of schemas of self, other and "self with other." In J. D. Lichtenberg & S. Kaplan (Eds.), *Reflections on self psychology.* Hillsdale, NJ: Erlbaum.

Stern, D. N. (1985). *The interpersonal world of the infant.* New York: Basic Books.

Stern, D. N. (1995a). Self/other differentiation in the domain of intimate socio-affective interactions: Some considerations. In P. Rochat (Ed.), *The self in infancy: Theory and research* (pp. 419–430). Amsterdam: Elsevier.

Stern, D. N. (1995b). *The motherhood constellation: A unified view of parent–infant psychotherapy.* New York: Basic Books.

Strunk, B. J., & Reschovsky, J. D. (2002). Working families' health insurance coverage, 1997–2001. *Health System Change Tracking Report, 4,* 1–4.

Sullivan, P. M., & Knutson, J. F. (2000). Maltreatment and disabilities: A population-based epidemiological study. *Child Abuse and Neglect, 24,* 1257–1273.

Szkrybalo, J., & Ruble, D. N. (1999). "God made me a girl": Sex category constancy judgments and explanations revisited. *Developmental Psychology, 35,* 393–402.

Takahashi, K. (1990). Are the key assumptions of the "Strange Situation" procedure universal? *Human Development, 33,* 23–30.

Tallal, P., & Benasich, A. A. (2002). Developmental language learning impairments. *Development and Psychopathology, 14,* 559–579.

Tamis-LeMonda, C. S., Bornstein, M. H., & Baumwell, L. (2001). Maternal responsiveness and children's achievement of language milestones. *Child Development, 72,* 748–767.

Tanner, E. M., & Finn-Stevenson, M. (2002). Nutrition and brain development: Social policy implications. *American Journal of Orthopsychiatry, 72,* 182–193.

Taylor, R. D., & Roberts, D. (1995). Kinship support and maternal and adolescent well-being in economically disadvantaged African-American families. *Child Development, 66,* 1585–1597.

Telingator, C. J. (2000). Children, adolescents, and families infected and affected by HIV and AIDS. *Child and Adolescent Psychiatric Clinics of North America, 9,* 295–312.

Terr, L. (1991). Childhood traumas: An outline and an overview. *American Journal of Psychiatry, 148,* 10–20.

Teti, D. M., Gelfand, D. M., Messinger, D. S., & Isabella, R. (1995). Maternal depression and the quality of early attachment: An examination of infants, preschoolers and their mothers. *Developmental Psychology, 31,* 364–376.

Teti, D. M., Sakin, J., Kucera, E., Corns, K. M., & Das Eisen, R. (1996). And baby makes four: Predictors of attachment security among preschool-aged firstborns during the transition to siblinghood. *Child Development, 67,* 579–596.

Thelen, E. (1995). Motor development: A new synthesis. *American Psychologist, 50,* 79–95.

Thoman, E. B. (1990). Sleeping and waking states in infants: A functional perspective. *Neuroscience and Behavioral Review, 14,* 93–107.

Thomas, A., & Chess, S. (1977). *Temperament and development*. New York: Brunner-Mazel.

Thomas, A., Chess, S., & Birch, H. G. (1968). *Temperament and behavior diosrders in children*. New York: New York University Press.

Thomas, D. G., Whitaker, E., Crow, C. D., Little, V., Love, L., Lykins, M. S., & Letterman, M. (1997). Event-related potential variability as a measure of information storage in infant development. *Developmental Neuropsychology, 13,* 205–232.

Thomas, J. M., & Guskin, K. A. (2001). Disruptive behavior in young children: What does it mean? *Journal of the American Academy of Child and Adolescent Psychiatry, 40,* 44–51.

Thomasgard, M., & Metz, W. P. (1996). The 2–year stability of parental perceptions of child vulnerability and parental overprotection. *Journal of Developmental and Behavioral Pediatrics, 17,* 222–228.

Thompson, L. A., & Kelly-Vance, L. (2001). The impact of mentoring on academic achievement of at-risk youth. *Children and Youth Services Review, 23,* 227–242.

Thompson, R. A. (1998). Early sociopersonality development. In W. Damon & N. Eisenberg (Eds.), *Handbook of child psychology* (5th ed.). *Vol. 3: Social, emotional and personality development* (pp. 25–104). New York: Wiley.

Thompson, R. A. (2000). The legacy of early attachments. *Child Development, 71,* 145–152.

Tomasello, M. (1995). Understanding the self as social agent. In P. Rochat (Ed.), *The self in infancy: Theory and research* (pp. 449–460). Amsterdam: Elsevier Science.

Toth, S. L., Maughan, A., Manly, J. T., Spagnola, M., & Cicchetti, D. (2002). The relative efficacy of two interventions in altering maltreated preschool children's representational models: Implications for attachment theory. *Development and Psychopathology, 14,* 877–908.

Trevarthen, C., Murray, L., & Hubley, P. (1981). Psychology of infants. In J. A. Davis & J. Dobbing (Eds.), *Scientific foundations of pediatrics* (2nd ed., pp. 211–274). London: Heinemann.

Tronick, E. Z., Als, H., Adamson, L., Wise, S., & Brazelton, T. B. (1978). The infant's response to intrapment between contradictory messages in face-to-face interaction. *Journal of Child Psychiatry, 17,* 1–13.

Tronick, E. Z., & Gianino, Jr., A. F. (1986a). The transmission of maternal disturbance to the infant. In E. Z. Tronick and T. Field (Eds.), *Maternal depression and infant disturbance* (pp. 5–13). San Franciso: Jossey-Bass.

Tronick, E. Z., & Gianino, Jr., A. F. (1986b). Interactive mismatch and repair: Challenges to the coping infant. *Zero to Three, 6,* 1–6.

Troy, M., & Sroufe, L. A. (1987). Victimization among preschoolers: The role of attachment relationship history. *Journal of the American Academy of Child and Adolescent Psychiatry, 26,* 166–172.

True, M. M., Pisani, L., & Oumar, F. (2001). Infant–mother attachment among the Dogon of Mali. *Child Development, 72,* 1451–1466.

Turiel, E. (1998). The development of morality. In W. Damon & N. Eisenberg (Eds.), *Handbook of child psychology* (5th ed.). *Vol. 3: Social, emotional and personality development* (pp. 863–932). New York: Wiley.

Tyson, P., & Tyson, R. (1991). *Psychoanalytic theories of development*. New Haven: Yale University Press.

Ullman, R., Sleator, E., & Sprague, R. (1984). A new rating scale for diagnosis and monitoring of ADD children. *Psychopharmacology Bulletin, 20,* 160–164.

UNICEF Innocenti Research Centre (2000). A league table of child poverty in rich nations. *Innocenti Report Cards* (No. 1, pp. 1–32). Florence, Italy: Author.

U.S. Department of Health and Human Services. (1999). *Blending perspectives and building common ground.* Washington, DC: Author.

Uzgiris, I., & Raeff, C. (1995). Play in parent–child interactions. In M. Bornstein, (Ed.), *Handbook of parenting* (Vol. 4, pp. 353–376). Mahwah, NJ: Erlbaum.

Valeski, T. N., & Stipek, D. J. (2001). Young children's feelings about school. *Child Development, 72,* 1198–1213.

van den Boom, D. C. (1994). The influence of temperament and mothering on attachment and exploration: An experimental manipulation of sensitive responsiveness among lower-class mothers with irritable infants. *Child Development, 65,* 1457–1477.

van den Boom, D. C., & Hoeksma, J. B. (1994). The effect of infant irritability on mother–infant interaction: A growth-curve analysis. *Developmental Psychology, 30,* 581–590.

van der Kolk, B. (1987). *Psychological trauma.* Washington, DC: American Psychiatric Press.

van der Kolk, B., & Fisher, R. (1994). Childhood abuse and neglect and loss of self-regulation. *Bulletin of the Menninger Clinic, 58*(2), 145–168.

van IJzendoorn, M. H., & Sagi, A. (1999). Cross-cultural patterns of attachment: Universal and contextual dimensions. In J. Cassidy & P. R. Shaver (Eds.), *Handbook of attachment: Theory, research, and clinical applications* (pp. 198–225). New York: Guilford Press.

van IJzendoorn, M. H., Schuengel, C., & Bakermans-Kranenberg, M. J. (1999). Disorganized attachment in early childhood: Meta-analysis of precursors, concomitants, and sequelae. *Development and Psychopathology, 11,* 225–249.

Vaughn, B. E., & Bost, K. K. (1999). Attachment and temperament: Redundant, independent, or interacting influences on interpersonal adaptation and personality development? In J. Cassidy & P. R. Shaver (Eds.), *Handbook of attachment: Theory, research, and clinical applications* (pp. 198–225). New York: Guilford Press.

Verkuyten, M., & Thijs, J. (2001). Ethnic and gender bias among Dutch and Turkish children in late childhood: The role of social context. *Infant and Child Development, 10,* 203–217.

Volterra, V. (1984). Waiting for the birth of a sibling: The verbal fantasies of a 2–year-old boy. In I. Bretherton (Ed.), *Symbolic Play: The development of social understanding* (pp. 219–248). Orlando, FL: Academic Press. Vondra, J. I., Hommerding, K. D., & Shaw, D. S. (1999). Stability and change in infant attachment for a low-income sample. *Monographs of the Society for Research in Child Development, 64,* 119–144.

Vondra, J. I., Shaw, D. S., Swearingen, L., Cohen, M., & Owens, E. B. (2001). Attachment stability and emotional and behavioral regulation from infancy to preschool age. *Development and Psychopathology, 13,* 13–33.

Von Hofsten, C. (1992). Studying the development of goal-directed behavior. In A. Kalverboer, B. Hopkins, & R. Gueze (Eds.), *Motor development in early and later childhood: Longitudinal approaches* (pp. 89–108). Cambridge, UK: Cambridge University Press.

Vygotsky, L. S. (1978). *Mind in society.* Cambridge, MA: Harvard University Press.

Wachs, T. D., & Kohnstamm, G. A. (2001). *Temperament in context.* Mahway, NJ: Erlbaum.

Wakschlag, L. S., & Hans, S. L. (2000). Early parenthood in context: Implications for development and intervention. In C. H. Zeanah, Jr. (Ed.), *Handbook of infant mental health* (2nd ed., pp. 129–144). New York: Guilford Press.

Waldfogel, J. (2001). What other nations do: International policies toward parental leave and child care. *The Future of Children, 11,* 99–111.

Waldinger, R. J., Toth, S. L., & Gerber, A. (2001). Maltreatment and internal representations of relationships: Core relationship themes in the narratives of abused and neglected preschoolers. *Social Development, 10,* 41–58.

Walker, L. J., Hennig, K. H., & Krettenauer, T. (2000). Parent and peer contexts for children's moral reasoning development. *Child Development, 71,* 1033–1048.

Walker-Andrews, A. S., & Kahana-Kalman, R. (1999). The understanding of pretence across the second year of life. *British Journal of Developmental Psychology, 17,* 523–536. Wang, Q., & Leichtman, M. D. (2000). Same beginnings, different stories: A comparison of American and Chinese children's narratives. *Child Development, 71,* 1329–1346.

Ward, M. J., & Carlson, E. A. (1995). Associations among adult attachment representations, maternal sensitivity and infant–mother attachment in a sample of adolescent mothers.*Child Development, 66,* 69–79.

Waters, E., & Cummings, E. M. (2000). A secure base from which to explore close relationships. *Child Development, 71,* 164–172.

Waters, E., Merrick, S., Treboux, D., Crowell, J., & Albersheim, L. (2000). Attachment security in infancy and early adulthood: A twenty-year longitudinal study. *Child Development,71,* 684–689.

Weatherston, D. J. (2002). Introduction to the infant mental health program. In J. J. Shirilla & D. J. Weatherston (Eds.), *Case studies in infant mental health: Risk, resiliency, and relationships* (pp. 1–14). Washington, DC: Zero to Three.

Webb, N. B. (2001). Working with culturally diverse children. In N. B. Webb (Ed.), *Culturally diverse parent–child and family relationships: A guide for social workers and other practitioners* (pp. 3–28). New York: Columbia University Press.

Webb, N. B. (2002). Assessment of the bereaved child. In N. B. Webb (Ed.), *Helping bereaved children* (2nd ed., pp. 19–42). New York: Guilford Press.

Webb, N. B. (2003). *Social work practice with children* (2nd ed.). New York: Guilford Press.

Weikart, D. P., & Schweinhart, L. J. (1992). High/Scope preschool program outcomes. In J. McCord & R. E. Tremblay (Eds.), *Preventing antisocial behavior: Interventions from birth to adolescence* (pp. 67–86). New York: Guilford Press.

Weinfield, N. S., Ogawa, J. R., & Egeland, B. (2002). Predictability of observed mother–child interaction from preschool to middle childhood in a high-risk sample. *Child Development, 73,* 528–543.

Weinfield, N. S., Sroufe, L. A., & Egeland, B. (2000). Attachment from infancy to early adulthood in a high-risk sample: Continuity, discontinuity, and their correlates. *Child Development, 71,* 695–702.

Weiss, B., Dodge, K. A., Bates, J. E., & Pettit, G. S. (1992). Some consequences of early harsh discipline: Child aggression and a maladaptive social information processing style. *Child Development, 63,* 1321–1335.

Wellman, H. M. (1990). *The child's theory of mind.* Cambridge, MA: MIT Press.

Wellman, H. M., & Gelman, S. A. (1998). Knowledge acquisition in foundational domains. In W. Damon, D. Kuhn, & R. S. Siegler (Eds.), *Handbook of child psychology* (5th ed.). *Vol. 2: Cognition, perception, and language* (pp. 523–573). New York: Wiley.

Wentzel, K. R. (1999). Social-motivational processes and interpersonal relationships: Implications for understanding motivation at school. *Journal of Educational Psychology, 91,* 76–97.

Werner, E. E. (1993). Risk, reslience and recovery: Perspectives from the Kauai longitudinal study. *Development and Psychopathology, 5,* 503–515.

Werner, E. E. (2000). Protective factors and individual resilience. In J. P. Shonkoff & S. J. Meisels (Eds.), *Handbook of early childhood intervention* (2nd ed., pp. 115–132). Cambridge, UK: Cambridge University Press.

Werner, L., & VandenBos, G. (1993). Developmental psychoacoustics: What infants and children hear. *Hospital and Community Psychiatry, 44,* 624–626.

White, B. P., Gunnar, M. R., Larson, M. C., Donzella, B., & Barr, R. G. (2000). Behavioral and physiological responsivity, sleep, and patterns of daily cortisol production in infants with and without colic. *Child Development, 71,* 862–877.

White, S. H. (1996). The child's entry into the "age of reason." In A. J. Sameroff & M. M. Haith (Eds.), *The five to seven year shift: The age of reason and responsibility* (pp. 17–32). Chicago: University of Chicago Press.

Whiteside, M. F., & Becker, B. J. (2000). Parental factors and the young child's postdivorce adjustment: A meta-analysis with implications for parenting arrangements. *Journal of Family Psychology, 14,* 5–26.

Williams, J. S., Singh, B. K., & Singh, B. B. (1994). Urban youth, fear of crime, and resulting defensive actions. *Adolescence, 29,* 323–330.

Williams-Gray, B. (2001). A framework for culturally responsive practice. In N. B. Webb (Ed.), *Culturally diverse parent–child and family relationships: A guide for social workers and other practitioners* (pp. 157–180). New York: Columbia University Press.

Williamson, G. G. (1996). Assessment of adaptive competence. In S. J. Meisels & E. Fenichel (Eds.), *New visions for the developmental assessment of infants and young children* (pp. 193–206). Washington, DC: Zero to Three.

Wilson, G. T., Becker, C. B., & Heffernan, K. (2003). Eating disorders. In E. J. Mash & R. J. Barkley (Eds.), *Child psychopathology* (2nd ed., pp. 687–715). New York: Guilford Press.

Winicki, J. (2003). Children in homes below poverty: Changes in program participation since welfare reform. *Children and Youth Services Review, 25,* 651–668.

Winnicott, D. W. (1958). *Collected papers: Through paediatrics to psychoanalysis.* London: Tavistock Publications.

Winnicott, D. W. (1965). *The maturational processes and the facilitating environment.* London: Hogarth Press & The Institute for Psychoanalysis.

Winnicott, D. W. (1971). *Playing and reality.* London: Routledge.

Wooley, J. D. (1995). The fictional mind: Young children's understanding of imagination, pretense and dreams. *Developmental Review, 15,* 172–211. Woolley, J. (1997). Thinking about fantasy: Are children fundamentally different thinkers and believers from adults? *Child Development, 68,* 991–1001.

Wooley, J. D., Phelps, K. E., Davis, D. L., & Mandell, D. J. (1999). Where theories of mind meet magic: The development of children's beliefs about wishing. *Child Development, 70,* 571–587.

Worden, J. W. (1996). *Children and grief: When a parent dies.* New York: Guilford Press.

Zahn-Waxler, C., & Kochanska, G. (1990). The development of guilt. In R. Thompson (Ed.), *Nebraska Symposium on Motivation, 1988: Socioemotional development* (pp. 109–137). Lincoln: University of Nebraska Press.

Zahn-Waxler, C., & Smith, K. D. (1992). The development of prosocial behavior. In V. B. Van Hasselt & M. Hersen (Eds.), *Handbook of social development: A lifespan perspective* (pp. 229–256). New York: Plenum Press.

Zeanah, C. H., Danis, B., Hirshberg, L., Benoit, D., Miller, D., & Miller, S. S. (1999). Disorganized attachment associated with partner violence: A research note. *Infant Mental Health Journal, 20,* 77–86.

Zeanah, C. H., Jr., Larrieu, J. A., Heller, S. S., & Valliere, J. (2000). Infant–parent relationship assessment. In C. H. Zeanah, Jr. (Ed.), *Handbook of infant mental health* (2nd ed., pp. 485–493). New York: Guilford Press.

Zero to Three. (1994). *Diagnostic classification 0–3: Diagnostic classification of mental health and developmental disorders of infancy and early childhood.* Washington, DC: Author.

Zhou, M. (1997). Growing up American: The challenge confronting immigrant children and children of immigrants. *Annual Review of Sociology, 23,* 63–96.

Zigler, E., & Hall, N. W. (2000). *Child development and social policy: Theory and applications.* New York: McGraw-Hill.

Zito, J. M., Safer, D. J., dosReis, S., Gardner, J. F., Boles, M., & Lynch, F. (2000). Trends in the prescribing of psychotropic medications to preschoolers. *Journal of the American Medical Association, 283,* 1025–1030.

Zuckerman, B., & Bresnahan, K. (1991). Developmental and behavioral consequences of prenatal drug and alcohol exposure. *Pediatric Clinics of North America, 83,* 1387–1407.

Zuckerman, B., & Brown, E. R. (1993). Maternal substance abuse and infant development. In C. H. Zeanah, Jr. (Ed.), *Handbook of infant mental health* (pp. 143–158). New York: Guilford Press.

Index

"A-B-C analysis," 237, 245, 246
  case example, 245, 246
  in functional assessment, 237, 245, 246
Abuse (*see* Child maltreatment)
Accident proneness, 235, 236
Accumulating risk factors, 119, 120
Achievement motivation, 377, 378
Acting-out, psychodynamics, 402, 403
Adaptation
  caregiver, in infant development, 141, 142
  as protective factor, 62
  to risk, assessment of, 121, 122
  in transactional model of development, 4-6
Adolescence, 385
Adult Attachment Interview, 25, 30
Affective functioning
  beginnings of infant interaction, 149, 150
  cultural regulation, 373
  middle childhood development, 367-373,
    387, 388
  preschool development, 287-294
  preschooler reality testing, 284-287
  regulation of, 211-217
  toddler development, 198, 211-217
  toddler moral development, 216, 217
African Americans
  racial identity, preschoolers, 306, 307
  racism, 98-100, 383, 384
  risk and protective factors, 99, 100
Ages 1-3 (*see* Toddler development)
Ages 3-6 (*see* Preschool development)
Ages 6 to puberty (*see* School-aged children)
Aggressive behavior
  displacement of, 291
  intervention, 419-421
  and language delays, 206
  in middle childhood, 352, 353
  in preschoolers, 267, 268, 288
  in pretend play, 267, 296

retrospective assessment, case example,
    123-129
  in toddlers, 213, 214, 216, 217
Ainsworth, Mary, 11, 12
Alcohol abuse, 90-92
Altruistic behavior, 347 (*see also* Prosocial
    behavior)
Ambivalent/resistant attachment, 16, 17
  in adults, 26, 27
  case examples, 16, 17, 30-38
  classification, 12, 16
  maternal depression link, 36, 37
  parental inconsistency role in, 150
  in "pursuer-distancer" interactions, 29
Animism, 281
Antisocial behavior
  family processes in development of, 76, 77
  risk factors, 76, 77
  school-age peer relationships, 351
  school-age social development, 352, 353
Anxiety
  coping strategies, preschoolers, 291-294
  middle childhood, 367, 368
  psychodynamic perspective, 402, 403
  sources of, 212, 288-290
Approach/avoidance conflict, 18
Arousal
  child maltreatment effects, 80
  infant regulation of, 154, 155
  middle childhood regulation of, 369, 370
  neonate development, 145
  regulation of, 8, 9
  toddler regulation of, 216, 217
Assessment
  attachment, 29-38
  developmental perspective, 136
  infant-caregiver interaction, 173-183, 191,
    192
    case example, 175-183

infant instruments, 174
infant observation exercises, 191, 192
during intervention, 250
middle childhood development, 389-396
preschooler, 301, 302
retrospective analysis, 121-129
risk/protective factors, 111-137
toddler development, 234-238, 257, 258
case example, 238-249
Attachment processes
ambivalent/resistant (*see* Ambivalent/
resistant attachment)
assessment, 29-38
avoidant (*see* Avoidant attachment)
biological factors, 43-45, 68
changes in patterns of, 24
child maltreatment effects, 18, 27
classification, 12-19
development of, 8
disorganized (*see* Disorganized/disoriented
attachment)
family systems theory, 28, 29
foster care experience, 23, 83
functions, 8-11
future development implications, 21-24
implications for practice, 38, 253, 254, 421
infant development, 151, 152
intergenerational transmission, 25, 28, 29,
301
internalization, 22, 23
in middle childhood, 343-345
parent-child therapy basis, 253-259
parental depression and, 36, 37
patterns, 11, 12
preschool development, 261-264, 290, 307
secure (*see* Secure attachment)
separation-individuation, 224, 225
sociocultural context, 19-21
toddler assessment, 234-236
toddler development, 194-200
universality, 21
Attention-deficit/hyperactivity disorder
assessment, 394-396
cultural context, 396
executive processing deficits, 367
and learning disabilities, 395, 396
Romanian orphanage children, 58-60
stigma, 375
Attentional processes
infants, 163
middle childhood development, 363, 364
preschooler assessment, 311
Auditory processing, 363
Authority, acceptance of, 375
Autism
communication deficits distinction, 246
executive processing deficits, 367
theory of mind relative absence, 227
Autonomy orientation, gender roles, 381

Avoidant attachment, 13-16
in adults, 26
case example, 15, 16
as defensive strategy, 14
preschooler behavior, 290
in "pursuer-distancer" interactions, 29

Babbling, in language development, 165, 166
Baby games, 154-156
Bayley Scales of Infant Development-II, 74
Behavioral inhibition
parenting interaction, 71
and peer relations, 349, 350
transactional processes, 71-73
as vulnerability factor, 70-72
Behavioral interventions, 398, 399
Betrayal trauma, sexual abuse, 79
Bilingualism, immigrant children, 355, 356
Body rhythms, neonates, 146, 147
Bonding, and brain development, 43-45
Brain development, 39-60
attachment effects, 43-45
infants, 140
institutionally-deprived children, 49, 50, 55-
60
intensive stimulation effects, 45
and language, 201, 202
plasticity and experience, 43, 58-60
premature infants, 148
preschoolers, 260
school-age children, 338
sequence of, 40
stress and trauma effects, 48-60
toddlers, 194, 201, 202
Brain tumors, 320, 322-333
Breast feeding, nutritional benefits, 47
Brief reactive psychosis, 116-118
Bullying, 267, 352, 353

Cancer
case study, preschooler, 322-333
developmental interference, 320-322
Cause-and-effect thinking, 360
and cognitive-behavioral interventions, 397,
398
and egocentrism, 280
and narrative construction, 318
play function, 276
Chess playing, 361
Child care, 96-98, 341
Child care centers, assessment in, 311-313
Child-caregiver interaction
assessment, case examples, 112-114
attachment theory, 9-19, 28, 29
depressed parent, 36-37, 89, 90, 179, 182
development of internal representations,
163-165
development of self-efficacy beliefs, 167, 168
development of self-esteem, 167, 168, 300-302

difficult temperament infant, 149, 150
goodness of fit, 70-72, 149
infant development, 139-141, 149-151, 156-159, 173-175
infant play behaviors, 153-156
in mastery motivation, 168, 169
metaphors of development, 140, 141
mutual adaptation, 146-148
normal parent-infant, 156-159
regulation of arousal, 8, 9
risk factors, 73-92
synchrony degrees, 10
toddler development, 197, 198
in transactional model of development, 4-6
Child maltreatment
attachment effects, 18, 27, 81
brain development, 50-53
developmental effects, 79-81
as risk factor, 78-81, 125-129
case example, 125-129
and self-regulation difficulties, toddlers, 217
substance abusing parents, 91
toddler intervention, 255-257
Children's Protective Services, 86, 87
Circadian rhythms, neonates, 146, 147
Classroom environment, as protective factor 65, 66
Coercive family processes
and choice of antisocial friends, 349
and internalization of values, 221
as risk factor, 76-78
and self-regulation difficulties, 217
Cognitive-behavioral interventions, 397, 398
Cognitive development
bilingualism and, 355, 356
concrete operations, 357-360
egocentric thinking, 222, 223, 279-282, 336
executive processes, 365-367
infant, 161-169
language development and, 353, 354
logical thinking, 360
magical thinking, 282-284
maturation role, 360, 361
in middle childhood, 336, 353-356, 359-367, 386
moral development, in toddlers, 217-223
perspective-taking skills, 276, 279, 346, 347, 354
in play, 209, 276, 277
preschool, 277-287, 308, 309
toddler, 200, 201, 231
transductive reasoning, 280
understanding of causality, 280
Colic, 148, 182
Communication (see also Language development)
attachment processes link, 9, 10
functional assessment, toddler, 245, 246

infant development, 165, 166
intervention, 249-254
preschool development, 270-274, 308
school-age children, 353-356
toddler development, 198, 201-207
in toddler play behaviors, 207-211
Community risk factors, 92-103
Compadres, 100
"Compulsive caregiving," 28
Concrete operations, 359, 360
Conduct disorder, risk factors, 76, 77
Conflict resolution, 266, 267
preschoolers, 266, 267
school-age development, 348, 349
Conformist moral orientation, 375
Conscience development
parents' contribution, 220, 221
preschoolers, 294, 300
school-age children, 336, 343
Conservation abilities
preschoolers, 281, 282
school-age children, 360
Cooperative play, 269, 270, 303
Coping strategies
and medical treatment, 320-322
preschoolers, 291-294
school-age children, 368-372
toddlers, 214-216
transactional model of failures in, 103, 104
Corporal punishment, 76-78, 217, 298
moral development effect, 298
as risk factor, 76-78
Corpus callosum, myelination, 260
Cortisol levels, 48-50
Counterphobic reckless behavior, 235, 236
Crib talk, 204-206
Critical periods, brain development, 42
Cross-modal perception, infants, 143, 144
Cross-sex play, 304
Crying
assessment, case example, 176-192
neonatal differences, 145
transactional aspects, 182, 183
Cultural context
attachment patterns, 19-21
learning disabilities, 393
self-regulation, 373
social development, 270
Custody arrangements, 75, 76

Death of parent, 87, 88
Defenses
avoidant behaviors, 13, 14
insecure attachment, 14-16, 27, 28
middle childhood development, 371, 372, 400, 401
preschool development, 293, 294
retrospective assessment, 122-129
rigidity in, 104

Delayed gratification, 370
Denial, preschooler coping, 293, 294
Depressed parent (see Maternal depression)
Development, generally
    dynamics, 135
    and intervention, 5, 6
    maturational perspective, 3, 4, 135, 136
    mutual adaptation in, 4
    transactional model, 4-6
Developmental delay, 245-254
Developmental pathways, 5, 6
"Difficult" temperament, 70-73, 148, 149
Disabilities
    peer relationships, 350
    transactional model, 68, 69
Discipline (see Harsh parenting)
Disorganized/disoriented attachment, 17-19
    in adults, 27
    classification, 12, 17, 18
    developmental patterns, 17-19
    maltreatment outcome, 18, 27, 81
Displacement
    preschooler coping strategy, 288, 291, 293
    in school-age children, 400, 401, 406-408,
        412, 413
Dissociation, 52, 53, 391
Divorce
    middle childhood intervention, 409-411,
        413, 414
    as risk factor, 74-76
Dramatic play
    function, 275, 276, 292
    gender roles, 303
Drawing, traumatized child, 405-407, 413, 414
Dreams, and magical thinking, 282, 283
Dyslexia, 392, 393

Early intervention (see Intervention)
Ecological approach, immigrant children, 317
"Effortful control," 215, 216, 288
Egocentrism
    and moral development, 222, 223
    preschooler development, 265, 278-282
    school-age children, 336
    toddlers, 211
Emotions (see Self-regulation)
Empathy
    in moral development, 299
    preschooler development, 299
    and theory of mind, 227, 228
    toddler development, 221-223
Environmental/social factors
    community violence, 100-102
    maturational interactions, 135, 136
    policy issues, 92-98
    poverty, 93-99
    protective factors, 65, 66
    risk factors, 92-103
    transactional model of development, 4

Ethnicity (see Race/ethnicity)
Executive function, 365-367
Exploratory behaviors
    attachment relationship basis for, 10, 11
    infant play, 153
    toddler assessment, 236
    toddler development, 196, 197
Exposure to violence, 100-103
Externalized adaptations, 121, 122

Facial expressions, infant reactions, 149, 150
Family functioning
    assessment, 116-118
        case example, 175-192
    child exposure to violence, 84-87
    and parental conflict, 74-76
Family-leave policies, 96
Family systems theory, 28, 29
Fantasy play, 288, 296, 357, 358
Fantasy/reality
    assessment, 123, 126, 127
    magical thinking, 282-284
    middle childhood development, 336, 358,
        359, 386
    in play behavior, 209
    preschool development, 266-270, 273-
        276
    reality testing, 266-270, 273-276, 282-287,
        317, 318
Fathers
    absence of, 76
    and attachment, 19
    as protective factor, 177
Feeding patterns, neonates, 146, 147
Fetal health, 46, 90-92
Food Stamps and School Lunch programs,
    94
Foster care, 23, 82-84
Freud, A., 136, 358, 372
Friendships
    preschool development, 268, 269
    school-age children, 348, 349
    and school transition, 339
Functional assessment, 236-238, 245, 246
"Fuzzy trace theory," 365

Games
    infants, 154-156
    school-age children, 356, 357
Gay/lesbian orientation, 381, 382
Gender constancy, 304, 380
Gender differences
    aggression, 351
    prosocial behavior, 347, 348
    social roles, 381
Gender identity
    preschool development, 302-304
    school-age children, 380, 381
    toddlers, 230, 233

Generational transmission, 25, 28, 29, 301
Genetic risk, 67, 68
Gestural communication, toddlers, 202
Goal-directed behavior
    school-age children, 370
    toddlers, 201
"Good enough" parents, 73
Goodness of fit, 70-72, 149, 190
Grandparent support, 65
Grief, death of parent, 88
Group therapy, 399
Guilt, preschool development, 295

Habituation, in neonates, 144, 145
Harsh parenting
    moral development effect, 221, 298
    as risk factor, 76-78
    and self-regulation difficulties, 217
Head Start, 339-341
Heart rate, and attachment patterns, 14
Heterosexuality, 381, 382
Hobbies, 358
Home visits, natural setting advantages, 172, 177
Homosexual orientation, 381, 382
Hospitalization, coping, 321
Hyperarousal, 9, 50, 51

Identification with the aggressor, 86, 128, 129, 267
Imitative behaviors
    infants, 164
    preschool development, 312-317
    toddler development, 201
Immigrant children, 312-317, 355, 356
Implicit memory, and trauma, 51, 52
Individual differences
    developmental lag, 343
    protective factors, 63, 64
    risk factors, 70-73
Individuals with Disabilities Education Act, 173, 174
Infant development
    age 1-2 months, 145-151
    age 3-6 months, 151-159
    age 6-12 months, 151-153
    attachment categories, 12-19
    attachment processes, 151, 152
    beginnings of interaction, 149-151
    brain development, 140
    caregiver adaptation, 141, 142
    caregiver role, 139-141
    cognitive, 161-169
    difficult temperament, 148, 149
    language and communication skills, 165, 166
    mastery motivation, 168, 169
    motor skills, 161
    neonatal period, 142-145

parent interaction, assessment, 149-151, 155-159
    case example, 156-159
    physical, 160, 161
    play behaviors, 152-156
    scaffolding, 141
    self regulation in, 144-148
    sense of self, 166-168
Inner speech, and self-control, 287, 288
Insecure attachment
    change to secure attachment, 24
    classification, 12-19
    defensive processes, 27, 28
    family systems theory, 28, 29
    maternal unresponsiveness link, 182
    preschool development, 262-264, 266
Institutionally-deprived children, 49, 50, 55-60
Intentionality
    infant development, 164
    preschooler moral development, 295
    and theory of mind, 226-228
    toddlers, 228, 229
Intergenerational transmission, attachment patterns, 25, 28, 29, 301
Internal locus of control, 64
Intervention
    assessment during, 250
    attachment perspective, 38, 253, 254, 421
    attention deficit/hyperactivity disorder, 396
    developmental outcomes, 423
    developmental perspective, 136, 417, 419-423
    early, 105, 106
    ecological perspective, 421
    following death of parent, 88
    implications of attachment theory, 38
    infant-parent interaction, 173
    intermittent therapy, 417
    language development implications, 272
    maturational perspective, 421
    in middle childhood, 396-401
        case examples, 401-417
    minority groups, 384, 385
    parent-child therapy, 251-254
    play therapy exploration of abuse trauma, 126-128, 399-401
    with preschoolers, 311, 312, 317-320
        case examples, 312-333
    problems of middle childhood, 391-396
    theoretical basis, 5, 6
    with toddlers, 249-257
        case example, 255-257
    understanding child perspective, 133, 134
    videotaped, 186-189
IQ
    chronic trauma effect, 51
    risk factor effects on, 66, 67
Iron deficiency, brain development, 47

Joint attention
   infants, 163
   in language learning, 248
   toddlers, 226
Joint custody, 75, 76

Kibbutz infants, attachment patterns, 20, 21
Kindergarten, transition to, 339, 340

Language delays, 245-254, 273
Language development
   brain development link, 39
   child maltreatment effects, 80
   cognitive development and, 353, 354
   construction of meaning, 204-206
   immigrant children, 355, 356
   infant, 165, 166
   middle childhood, 353-356, 386, 391, 392
   preschool, 270-272, 308
   scaffolding, 198, 271, 272
   self-regulation and, 206, 354, 355
   toddler, 198, 201-207, 215
   word play, 353
Latency period, 336
Learned helplessness, 104
Learning disorders, 392, 393
   assessment, 392, 393, 395, 396
   secondary effects, 378, 379, 393
Limit setting, toddlers, 198
Logical thinking, 360
Lying, preschool children, 297

Magical thinking, 282-284, 290
Malnutrition, and brain development, 46, 47
Marital conflict, as risk factor, 74-76
Mastery motivation, 168, 169
Maternal depression
   and attachment, 36, 37
   child cortisol levels, 49, 50
   effect on infant, 179, 182
   risk and protective factors, 89, 90
Maternal deprivation, 49, 50
Maturation, 3, 4
   and cognitive development, 360, 361
   environmental interactions, 135, 136
   implications for treatment, 421
   infant development, 139, 140
Media influences, 99, 102, 103
Medical treatment, coping, 320-333
Medication use, toddlers, 250, 251
Memory
   infant development, 161-163
   middle childhood development, 364, 365
   preschool development, 262, 277
   stress/trauma effects on, 284-287
   toddler development, 202, 203
Mentoring programs, protective factor, 66
Metacognition, 365-367
Middle childhood (see School-age children)

Minority populations, 98-100, 382-385
Moral development
   empathy link, 222
   internalization of moral controls, 219-223,
      297-300
   middle childhood, 336, 374, 375, 388
   parental contribution, 220, 221, 298, 299
   preschool age, 294-300
   toddler, 217-223, 232, 233
Mother-child interactions (see Child-caregiver
      interaction)
Motivation
   in strengths assessment, 248
   toddlers, 193, 194
Motor skills development
   infant, 161
   preschool age, 260, 261
   school-age, 337, 338
   toddler, 194
Multiple attachments, 19
Mutual regulation
   baby games, 155
   caregiver-neonates, 145, 146
   and internalization, 291, 292
   toddlers, 214
Myelination, 41, 260, 338

Narratives
   in toddlers, 203-206
   in understanding of experience, 318, 319
Neglect, developmental effects, 81
Neonatal development, 142-145
Nutrition, brain development, 46, 47

Obesity, school-age children, 337
Object constancy, 225, 226
Object permanence, 162
Observational assessment
   in child care centers, 311-313
   functional, 236-238
   infants, 175, 191, 192
   preschoolers, 311-313, 333, 334
   structured testing comparison, 234
   toddlers, 234, 236-238, 257, 258
Oedipus complex, 229, 305, 306
Orphanage studies, 49, 50, 55-60
Oxytocin, 43

Parallel play, toddlers, 199
Parent-child therapy, 251-254
"Parental child," 28
Parental conflict, 74-76
"Parentese," 150, 151
Parenting (see also Child-caregiver
      interaction)
   and attachment, 17, 18, 24-28
      case example, 30-38
   child temperament interactions, 70-73
   effects on preschooler self-image, 300, 301

harsh/coercive, 76-78
and moral development, 298, 299, 374
parental conflict, 74-76
protective factors, 64, 65
risk factors, 73-92, 103, 104
and school transition, 341
in transactional model of development, 4
Peer rejection, 289, 349, 350
Peer relationships
  antisocial school-age children, 350
  aggressive behavior in middle childhood,
    352, 353
  in moral development, 299
  preschooler development, 265-268
  school-age development, 336, 349-353
  sense of self in middle childhood, 376
  status hierarchies in middle childhood, 350,
    351
Perceptual abilities, neonates, 142-144
Personalism, 280, 281
Personality characteristics (see Temperament)
Perspective taking
  egocentrism effect, 279
  and play, 276
  school-age children, 346, 347, 354
Pharmacotherapy, toddlers, 250, 251
Physical development
  infant, 160, 161
  preschooler, 260, 261
  school-age children, 337, 338
  toddler, 194
Plasticity, brain development, 43, 58-60
Physical development
  infant, 160, 161
  preschooler, 260, 261
  school-age children, 337, 338
  toddler, 194
Play behaviors
  and cognitive development, 276, 277
  in conflict resolution, 266, 267
  as coping strategy, 209, 210
  cultural differences, 270
  displacement of negative affect, 291
  gender development, 303
  hobbies as, 358
  infant development, 152-156
  in middle childhood, 356-359, 386
  mutually regulating dyadic systems, 155
  preschool development, 260, 266-270, 273,
    274, 291, 303, 308
  preschooler assessment/treatment, 319,
    320, 322-333
  preschooler moral development, 296, 297
  as representation of experience, 210, 211
  social development and, 269, 270
  symbolic communication and, 207-211
  toddler assessment, 241, 242
  toddler development, 195, 198-200, 204,
    215, 251-253

traumatized children, 126-128, 403, 404
  types of, in infants, 153, 154
Play therapy
  cancer survivors, 320, 322-333
  preschoolers, 317-320
  school-age children, 399-401
  toddlers, 251-253
  trauma intervention, 126-128
Policy issues, 92-98
Possessive behavior, 200
Posttraumatic stress disorder
  death of parent, 87, 88
  diagnosis, 125, 126
  and exposure to violence, 101, 125
  maltreatment outcome, 79
    case example, 125-129
  psychodynamics, 125-129
Poverty, 93-99
Precocious competence, 236, 321
Premature birth
  attachment patterns, case example, 32-38
  and brain development, 47, 148
  self-regulation consequences, 148
Prenatal period
  developmental influences, 144
  drug/alcohol exposure, 46, 90, 91
Preoperational period, 278
Preschool development
  ages, 259
  aggressive feelings/behavior, 267, 291, 296
  assessment, 311, 312
  attachment, 261-264
  cognitive, 277-287, 308, 309
  defense mechanisms, 293, 294
  friendships, 268
  gender identity, 302-304
  language and communication, 270-274, 308
  main features, 259, 260
  medical treatment, 320-333
  moral, 294-300
  new sibling, 289
  physical, 260, 261
  play behaviors, 260, 274-276, 302, 303
  play therapy, 317-320
  peer relationships, 265-268, 289
  prosocial behavior, 263, 265
  rule recognition, 296, 297
  self-regulation, 287-294
  sense of self, 300-307, 310
  social, 263-270
  sources of anxiety for preschoolers, 288-290
Pretend play
  preschool development, 267, 319, 320
  toddlers, 195, 199, 208, 209
Prevention programs, effectiveness elements,
    105, 106
Private speech, 287, 288
Problem solving, executive processes, 365, 366
Projection (defense mechanism), 293

Projective identification, parents, 301
Prosocial behavior
  gender differences, 347, 348
  preschool development, 263, 265
  as protective factor, 64
  school-age development, 347, 348
  and theory of mind, 227, 228
  toddler development, 221, 222
Protective factors
  assessment, 111-137
  attachment theory, 13, 69
  in case management decisions, 120, 121
  child-based, 63, 64
  and early intervention programs, 105, 106
  orphanage-reared children, 57
  parent characteristics, 64, 65
  in parental psychopathology, 90
  retrospective analysis, 121-129
  risk factor interaction, 105, 106, 130
  transactional model, 62
Psychopathology, parental, 89, 90
  assessment, 115-120
  protective factors, 90
  and risk factors, 89, 90
Puberty, 385
Public assistance programs, 94, 96
"Pursuer-distancer" interactions, 29

Race/ethnicity, 98-100
  media influences, 99
  middle childhood sense of self, 382-385
  preschooler sense of self, 306, 307
Rapprochement crisis, 225
Reading/writing disorders, 392, 393
Reality testing, 273-276, 282-284, 290, 336
Regression
  and birth of sibling, 289
  preschooler coping strategy, 294
"Relational aggression," 351
"Relational self," 381
"Representational competence," 276, 277, 369
Research, and practice, 38
Resilience
  child characteristics, 63-69
  definition, 61, 62
  parenting factor, 64, 65
  and risk factors, 61-63
  Romanian orphanage children, 58-60
  transactional model, 62
Reversible thinking, 360, 397
Risk factors, 61-108
  accumulation of, 66, 67, 104, 105
  assessment, 111-137
  biological vulnerabilities, 67-69
  in case management decisions, 120, 121
  child-based, 67-73, 106
  child maltreatment, 78-81
  divorce as, 74-76
  exposure to violence, 84-87, 100-103

  foster care, 82-84
  parental, 73-92, 106, 107
  parental psychopathology, 89, 90
  protective factor interaction, 105, 106, 130
  retrospective analysis, 121-129
  social/environmental, 92-103
  temperament as, 70-73
  transactional model, 62, 105
Role models, school-age children, 376, 377
Romanian orphans, 49, 50, 55-60
Rule learning/acceptance
  preschoolers, 296, 297
  school-age children, 375
  toddler internalization process, 219-221

Same-sex attractions, 381, 382
Scaffolding
  executive processes development, 367
  infant development, 141
  and mastery motivation, 168
  and play behavior, 154, 158, 159
  toddler development, 271, 272
School-age children, 335-418
  anxiety, 367, 368
  assessment, 389-396
  attachment history effects, 345
  attachment processes, 343-345
  bullying, 352, 353
  cognitive development, 336, 353, 354, 359-
    367, 386
  communication skills deficits, 353, 354
  coping in dangerous environments, 373
  defense mechanisms, 371, 372
  displacement therapy, 400, 401, 406-408,
    412-415
  executive processes, 365-367
  fantasizing, 356-359
  friendships, 348, 349
  intervention, 396-401
    case examples, 401-417
  language and communication, 353-356,
    386
  as latency period, 336
  main features of development, 335, 336,
    386-388
  memory processes, 364, 365
  moral development, 336, 374, 375, 388
  peer relationships, 336, 349-353
  physical development, 337, 338
  play behaviors, 356-359, 387
  presenting problems, 389
  prosocial behavior, 347, 348
  racial identity, 382-385
  role model selection, 376, 377
  self-regulation, 336, 367-373, 387, 388
  sense of self, 349, 376-385, 388
  signs of developmental lag, 342, 343
  skill-building activities, 335, 336
  social development, 345-353, 386

stresses for beginning student, 338-343
superego development, 336, 343
transitional tasks/stresses, 338-343
School transition, 338-343
Secure attachment
change to insecure attachment, 24
classification, 12
developmental outcomes, 12, 23, 24
and exploratory behavior, 10
family systems, 29, 30
and preschool development, 261-264
as protective factor, 69
in toddler development, 193, 194
Secure base behavior
and exploratory behavior, 196, 197
toddler development, 194-200, 234-236, 257
universality, 21
Security, as goal of attachment, 8
Self-consciousness, in toddlers, 228
Self-control
preschooler development, 287, 288
school-age children, 369, 370
self-concept link, 378, 379
Self-efficacy
infant development, 167, 168
toddler development of persistence, 229
toddler development of self-evaluation,
218, 219
Self-esteem
gender identity, 302, 303, 380, 381
identification with parents, 301, 302
infant development of self-efficacy, 167,
168
infant development of self-esteem, 167, 168
infant development of self-sense, 166, 167
maternal depression effects, 89
middle childhood self-sense, 349, 376-385
preschooler self-sense, 300-307
racial identity, 306, 307
role of friendships in school, 348, 349
self-control and, 369, 370
social comparison in middle childhood,
371
social reputation in middle childhood, 349,
350
status hierarchies in middle childhood, 350,
351
toddler development of self-sense, 193, 194,
223-230
working models of attachment, 22, 23, 37,
38
Self-regulation
infants, 145-148
neonates, 144, 145
preschooler strategies, 290-294, 309
school-age children, 367-373, 387, 388
toddlers, 211-217
Self-stimulation, 214, 215
Sensitive periods, 42, 49, 50, 58-60

Sensory functioning, neonates, 142-144
Separation anxiety (see also Strange Situation)
infant development, 162, 163, 182, 183
mastery, 225, 226
transactional aspects, 182, 183
Separation-individuation, 224, 225
Seriation, 362
Sex differences (see Gender differences)
Sex roles (see Gender identity)
Sexual abuse
betrayal trauma, 79
middle childhood trauma intervention, 401-
409
Sexual orientation, precursors, 381, 382
Sexuality/sexual behavior
latency concept, 336
preschooler development, 304-306
school-age development, 381, 382
Shame, 371
Sharing behavior, toddlers, 199, 200
Shyness, and peer relations, 349, 350
Sibling rivalry, 178, 179
Sleep patterns, neonates, 146, 147
Social comparison, school-age children, 371
Social development
preschooler, 263-270
school-age children, 345-353
toddlers, 199, 200, 231
Social play, 92-98
Social referencing
in infant development, 163, 164
in toddler development, 197, 243, 244
Social withdrawal, 349, 350
Sole custody, 75, 76
Speech therapy, 250
Storytelling
cultural differences, 270
preschoolers, 272
in therapy, 281
toddlers, 204
Strange Situation, 11-19, 30
Stranger anxiety, 162
Strengths orientation, 6
assessment, 420
middle childhood interventions, 409-417
Stress response system, 48-55
Structured testing, limitations, 241
Substance abuse, 90-92
Superego (see Conscience)
Symbolic play, 204, 206-211
Synaptic pruning, 42, 338
Synchrony, in attachment processes, 10

Tantrums, 245, 246, 248
Television, violence exposure, 102, 103
Temperament, 70-73
"difficult," 148, 149
and goodness of fit, 70-72, 149
and peer relations, case example, 349, 350

Temperament (cont.)
   transactional model, 71-73
   as vulnerability factor, 70-73
Terrible 2's, 213, 229
Theory of mind
   in autism, 227
   and egocentrism, 278, 279
   empathy basis, 227, 228
   preschooler development, 271, 272, 276,
      278, 279
   toddler development, 226-228
Therapeutic relationship
   and attachment relationship, 127
   middle childhood trauma intervention, 404,
      405
   transference, 412-415
Time orientation, school-age children, 361,
      362
Toddler development, 193-258
   aggressive behavior, 213, 214
   assessment, 234-238
      case example, 238-249
   attachment assessment, 234-236
   attachment processes, 193-200, 230, 231,
      254, 255
   cognitive, 200, 201, 231
   exploratory behaviors, 196, 197
   intervention, 249-257
   language and communication skills, 198,
      201-207, 215
   medication question, 250, 251
   main features, 193, 194
   mastery of autonomy, 225, 226
   moral sense and behavior, 217-223, 232,
      233
   physical, 194
   play behaviors, 198-200, 251-254
   prosocial behavior, 221, 222
   self-regulation, 206, 211-217
   self-stimulation, 214, 215
   sense of self, 193, 194, 223-230
   social, 199, 200
   sources of anxiety for toddler, 212, 213
   terrible 2's, 213
   transitional objects, 195, 196
Toilet training, 289
Token economies, 398, 399

Transactional model of development, 4-6
   and assessment, 122, 123
   and disabilities, 68, 69
   and infant crying, case example, 182-186
   risk and protective factors, 62, 103, 104
   temperament, 71-73
Transductive reasoning, 280
Transference, 412-415
Transgenerational transmission, attachment
      patterns, 25, 28, 29, 301
Transitional objects, 195, 196
Trauma (see also Posttraumatic stress
      disorder)
   assessment, 122-129
   and brain development, 48-60
   child maltreatment, 255-257
   displacement, 401, 402, 406-408
   implicit memory of, 51, 52, 284-287
   internal representation, 253, 254
   medical treatment survivors, 325-333
   middle childhood intervention, 401-409
   play behavior, 403, 404
   reality testing effects of, 284-287
   toddler intervention, 255-257
   witnessing violence, 84-86, 100-102
Trauma story, 403, 404, 408, 409
Triangulated families, 29

Videotaped sessions, 186-189
Violence
   child exposure to, 84-86, 100-102
   representations in play, 210, 211
Visual processing, 362
Vocabulary
   preschool development, 270, 271
   school-age children, 353
   toddler development, 202, 203
Vulnerability (see Risk factors)

Weaning practices, and attachment, 20
Welfare reform, 94, 96
Witnessing violence
   in community, 100-102
   in family, 84-87, 125
   play representations, 210, 211
Working models (see Attachment processes)
Working mothers, child care, 96-98